50% OFF Online HESI A2 Prep Course!

Dear Customer,

We consider it an honor and a privilege that you chose our HESI A2 Study Guide. As a way of showing our appreciation and to help us better serve you, we have partnered with Mometrix Test Preparation to offer you **50% off their online HESI A2 Prep Course.** Many HESI A2 courses are needlessly expensive and don't deliver enough value. With their course, you get access to the best HESI A2 prep material, and you only pay half price.

Mometrix has structured their online course to perfectly complement your printed study guide. The HESI A2 Prep Course contains **in-depth lessons** that cover all the most important topics, **150 video reviews** that explain difficult concepts, **2,500 practice questions** to ensure you feel prepared, and **digital flashcards**, so you can fit some studying in while you're on the go.

Online HESI A2 Prep Course

<u>Topics Covered</u>	<u>Course Features</u>
Reading	HESI A2 Study Guide

o   Key Ideas and Details
   o   Craft and Structure
   o   Integration of Knowledge & Ideas
	o Get content that complements our best-selling study guide.

English & Language Usage	7 Full-Length Practice Tests

o   Conventions of Standard English
   o   Knowledge of Language
   o   Vocabulary Acquisition
	o With over 2,500 practice questions, you can test yourself again and again.

Science	Free App Access

o   Human Anatomy & Physiology
   o   Life & Physical Sciences
   o   Scientific Reasoning
	o Subscribers to their HESI A2 course can download the free app to study on the go!

Math	HESI A2 Flashcards
o Numbers & Algebra o Measurement & Data	o Their mobile version includes a flashcard mode consisting of over 300 content cards to help you study.
	Audio Mode
	o Every lesson in their course has an audio mode, allowing you to listen to the lessons.

To receive this discount, simply head to their website: www.mometrix.com/university and add the course to your cart. At the checkout page, enter the discount code: **EXAMHESI50**

If you have any questions or concerns, please don't hesitate to contact them at universityhelp@mometrix.com.

Sincerely,

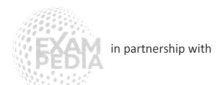 in partnership with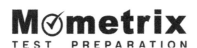

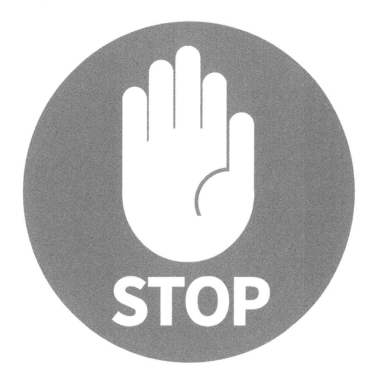

Free Exam Tips Videos/DVD

We have created a set of videos to better prepare you for your exam. We would like to give you access to these **videos** to show you our appreciation for choosing Exampedia. **They cover proven strategies that will teach you how to prepare for your exam and feel confident on test day.**

To receive your free videos, email us your thoughts, good or bad, about this book. Your feedback will help us improve our guides and better serve customers in the future.

Here are the steps:

> 1. Email **freevideos@exampedia.org**
>
> 2. Put "**Exam Tips**" in the subject line

Add the following information in the body of the email:

> 3. **Book Title:** The title of this book.
>
> 4. **Rating on a Scale of 1–5:** With 5 being the best, tell us what you would rate this book.
>
> 5. **Feedback:** Give us some details about what you liked or didn't like.

Thanks again!

HESI A2 Study Guide 2022-2023

HESI Admission Assessment Exam Prep
Book and Practice Test Questions Review
[Updated for the 5th Edition]

Andrew Smullen

Table of Contents

Preview

Congratulations! You've decided to study this guide in order to become one step closer to your educational or professional goal. This guide is designed to follow your specific test outline or educational format so that you will have the best chance at acing the test or becoming an expert in your field. Equipped with test tips, an introduction to the exam material, and content sections, we will go through each portion of the guide so that you can get a preview before you dive in.

The test tips are actionable items that assist you in preparing for the exam as well as suggestions to utilize during the exam. Studying the outline of your exam, reading thoroughly, looking for test-writing tricks, and keeping calm and collected are the basics needed in having a positive test experience. Having adequate knowledge of not just what's on a test, but *how* to take a test will set you up for success where other test takers may only be minimally prepared.

Knowing your exam content is only one of the many tools you need in order to take a test. Where will you take your test? How will it be scored? Should you still answer a question you don't know? How long will the test take? These questions and more will be answered in the Introduction portion of this guide, which goes over the exam you are studying for, who created it, what percentage of students take it and pass, and how scoring works. You will learn about your test beyond its content so that you can be fully prepared with as little distractions as possible on the day of the test.

This guide goes over the content knowledge needed to take your exam, usually in the order it will be presented on the test. Additionally, practice questions are given at the end of each guide that attempt to mimic your actual exam, along with their answer explanations. It's important that we deliver to you detailed and adequate answer explanations so that if you receive an incorrect answer, you will know why. Remember that you will make mistakes with your test questions, on subtle language or on content knowledge, but practicing taking the exam will help you read the questions more carefully and learn your content like an expert. After taking the practice exam, we hope you will be a well-prepared test taker!

In addition to the test tips below, we want to remind you of a few important things to fully prepare yourself for test-taking day.

- Avoid cramming the night before
- Get a good night's sleep and let your brain fully recover for the test ahead
- Eat a balanced breakfast in the morning
- Arrive at the test center half an hour before test time

During the test, follow these instructions to remain a calm and prepared test taker:

- Pace yourself; don't spend too much or too little time on a single question
- Use all the allotted time you have; go back and check to see that you've answered all relevant questions
- A positive mindset is key; affirmations such as "I can do this" or "I am equipped to pass this exam" will empower you to persevere throughout the day
- Remember to breathe if you find yourself holding your breath; adequate oxygen will help to clear your mind of panic and doubt

Listen—you've got this! Your decision to take time with this study guide is the first step in becoming a confident, successful test taker. Congratulations again; we wish you the best in your educational and professional journey.

If you have any questions or concerns, please feel free to contact us at:

   info@exampedia.org

Sincerely,
Exampedia Test Prep

Test Tips

1. Be Familiar with the Test

Besides being knowledgeable in your exam's content areas, the next best thing is being knowledgeable about the exam itself. Being familiar with the test means that from the time you walk into the testing center to the time you receive the test scores, you have an expectation of how things will be done. Read all about the test in our introduction section to know how much time you have to take it, what sections are in it, and what type of problems you will encounter. Be aware of how the test is scored so that you know whether to take a guess or skip a question. It's important to go into the test knowing exactly what to expect so that you can be a confident test taker.

2. Read the Directions Carefully

Before you begin the exam, read the directions carefully. These will tell you how to answer the questions. For example, are the directions asking you to choose ONE answer only, or AT LEAST TWO answers? Is the word bank showing you ANTONYMS or SYNONYMS, and which should you choose? The directions will tell you everything you need to know about answering the question correctly.

3. Read the Whole Question

It's tempting to look at the answers right away. However, if possible, cover the answers so that full focus can be given to the question first. Read every single word out loud in your head; test writers will sometime insert negatives ("which of the following is *not*..." "All of the following *except*..."), and they can be easy to miss. Reading every single word of the question with intention will help you eliminate choices that might be designed to trick you.

4. Read Every Answer Choice

There are several strategies that go into choosing a correct answer. First, read the answers without any bias; sometimes the test writers will play on test takers' bias to trip them up. A helpful tip for Reading Comprehension passages is to choose the answer choice that is true *in the world of the passage*. If the passage says the sky is purple, don't choose the answer that says the sky is blue. Remember that the passage is where you will find answers. Additionally, eliminate answers you know for a fact are incorrect. With the remaining answers, don't automatically jump to the first one you think is correct. Read all of them, and then choose. Sometimes, one answer may be *more correct* than another one. Read every word of the choices to make sure you've got the best one.

5. Look for Subtle Negatives

Sometimes test writers will insert subtle negatives into the question with words such as *not, except,* or *never*. Subtly reversing the meaning of questions examines the test taker's ability to follow directions and read thoroughly. Test takers who read each word thoroughly will not miss these subtle negatives. Look for these words in order to circle or underline them.

6. Look for Key Words

If you're taking an exam on paper, circle or underline the key words that will help you to answer the question. If you are on a computer and have scratch paper, jot down key words from the question. For Social Studies or Reading Comprehension questions, you can look for words like "main idea," "theme," "organization," or "text type" to pinpoint the exact item you should be looking for. Again, circle any subtle negatives you find, such as *not* or *except*.

7. Spot the Hedges

Words such as *almost, most, some,* and *sometimes* are words that are used in *hedging* language, which is language that denotes a claim rather than an absolute fact. Look for this type of hedging in questions and answers. Likewise, answer choices that assert something is *never* or *always* might need another look. Unless you know for sure, saying *always* or *never* may indicate an incorrect answer choice simply because of the absolutism of the term.

8. Don't Overanalyze

It's normal to be nervous while taking the test. However, be aware that with nervousness may come over-analysis. It's important not to read too much into questions and to avoid thought tangents about what the author could possibly mean behind what is actually said. If you find yourself overanalyzing or overthinking, shut your eyes, take a deep breath, and count to ten. Read the question again with a clear head so that you can answer with clarity rather than a muddled brain.

9. Don't Panic

Sometimes, you won't know the answer. In that moment, there will be nothing you can do to find the answer. To deal with this, compartmentalize each question; you may not know #27, but #28 is a new question that you are fully capable of answering. Leave the question anxiety with that question and move on to the next question. Make sure you close your eyes and take a deep breath before beginning again. This will calm your nerves. Say an affirmation, such as "I am fully competent to answer this question" or "I am calm and knowledgeable." An excellent way to understand a confusing question is to rephrase it yourself. What is the question asking you? Rewrite the question down on scratch paper and refer to the answers accordingly.

10. Retrace Your Steps

Mark any questions you know with absolute certainty right away. If you narrow the answers down to two choices, it might be worth the risk to choose one and move on. However, if you find yourself not knowing the answer at all, or having only narrowed the answers down by one (with several options left), move on. Leave the difficult questions for the end, if your exam allows you to go back and retrace your steps. One more tip; it's often prudent to go with your gut. So, don't change any answers that you've already marked as correct!

4

FREE Videos/DVD OFFER

We have created a set of Exam Tips Videos that **cover proven strategies that will teach you how to prepare for your exam and feel confident on test day.**

We want to give you access to these free videos as a token of our appreciation. All we want to know is what you thought of our product.

Here are the steps:

1. Email **freevideos@exampedia.org**

2. Put "**Exam Tips**" in the subject line

Add the following information in the body of the email:

3. **Book Title:** The title of this book.

4. **Rating on a Scale of 1–5:** With 5 being the best, tell us what you would rate our book.

5. **Feedback:** Give us some details about what you liked or didn't like.

Thanks again!

Introduction to the HESI A2 Exam

Function of the Test

The Health Education Systems, Inc. (HESI) Admission Assessment (A2) Exam is designed for high school graduates or other candidates seeking admission to nursing schools and some other post-secondary health programs in the United States. Colleges, universities, and educational institutions that use the test as part of a prospective student's application process offer the test onsite and can determine which sections they require. Test takers typically have not yet received health-specific education or training prior to sitting for the exam.

Test Administration

The individual testing site administering the HESI exam is able to determine many of the specifics for the test administration process. For this reason, candidates should inquire about the details regarding registration and the test day experience at the site where they intend to take the exam. For example, some schools offer the exam in its entirety, whereas others offer and expect scores on only certain sections. The cost and the test dates are also determined by the testing site. Test takers are typically permitted to retake the test, though again, this is often up to the discretion of the administering institution. Additionally, when retakes do occur, some schools may permit test takers to combine their top scores from each section into one total composite score, while others opt to only accept the total score from a single test administration. Candidates are encouraged to inquire about the policies for retaking the test at the school where they plan on applying and sitting for the exam.

Candidates with documented disabilities requiring accommodations for the administration of the test should contact the school where they plan to take the exam. In most cases, a variety of accommodations are permitted.

Test Format

The full HESI exam contains 340 multiple-choice questions spread over eight academic sections. Note that most schools only require that you take certain sections (rather than all eight). Accordingly, the physics section is not covered in this book since so few schools require that it be taken. The following table lists these sections and the number of questions in each:

Section	# of Questions
Mathematics	55
Reading Comprehension	55
Vocabulary	55
Grammar	55
Biology	30
Chemistry	30
Anatomy & Physiology	30
Physics	30

Five of the questions in each academic section are unscored pilot questions used to gather data on their potential effectiveness as future scored questions. Additionally, the full HESI includes a Personality

Profile and Learning Style Assessment, though not all testing sites include these sections, and in some cases, test takers can select which sections they want to take. The two non-academic sections take about 15 minutes each, and test takers do not need to study for them as there are no "right" or "wrong" answers.

Scoring

The HESI does not have a set passing score. Instead, each school or nursing program can establish their own score expectations and requirements. With that said, HESI recommends that RN and HP programs require at least a score of 75% to pass, and that LPN/LVN programs require a minimum score of 70% to pass. Candidates should inquire about score requirements at their prospective programs.

Upon completion of the exam, the test taker and their prospective educational institutions both receive detailed score reports. Individual student reports contain an explanation of the scoring procedures and the achieved scores for the different sections. The report also contains information about the incorrect answers given, such as the topics addressed in the questions. Additionally, the report may offer study tips based on the individual's Learning Style assessment and information about the test taker's dominant personality type, and strengths, weaknesses, and recommended learning strategies based on the Personality Profile.

Study Prep Plan for the HESI A2 Exam

①→ Pause

Take a breath! Don't let test anxiety keep you from doing your best.

②→ Plan

Use a study plan to help you stay organized.

③→ Prepare

Once you've taken a breath and have a plan, it's time to start studying!

1 Week Study Schedule

Day 1	Day 2	Day 3	Day 4	Day 5	Day 6	Day 7
English Language	Math	Biology	Anatomy and Physiology	Practice Test #1	Practice Test #2	Take Your Exam!

2 Week Study Schedule

Day 1	Day 2	Day 3	Day 4	Day 5	Day 6	Day 7
English Language	Usage	Math	Decimals	Biology	Cells	Chemistry

Day 8	Day 9	Day 10	Day 11	Day 12	Day 13	Day 14
Atomic Structure	Anatomy and Physiology	Skeletal System	Respiratory System	Practice Test #1	Practice Test #2	Take Your Exam!

1 Month Study Schedule

Day 1	Day 2	Day 3	Day 4	Day 5	Day 6	Day 7
Reading Comprehension	Vocabulary and General Knowledge	Grammar	Usage	Punctuation	Math	Multiplication

Day 8	Day 9	Day 10	Day 11	Day 12	Day 13	Day 14
Fractions	Ratios and Proportions	General Math Facts	Biology	Water	Metabolism	Cellular respiration

Day 15	Day 16	Day 17	Day 18	Day 19	Day 20	Day 21
Chemistry	Periodic Table	Atomic Structure	Nuclear Chemistry	Chemical Bonding	Anatomy and Physiology	Histology

Day 22	Day 23	Day 24	Day 25	Day 26	Day 27	Day 28
Integumentary System	Muscular System	Cardiovascular System	Urinary System	Practice Test #1	Answer Explanations #1	Practice Test #2

Day 29	Day 30
Answer Explanations #2	Take Your Exam!

Mathematics

Addition

The **addition** of two whole numbers means to combine the two numbers to find a total. For instance, the numbers 6 and 2 are combined to result in $6 + 2 = 8$. It is said that the **sum** of 6 and 2 is equal to 8, and 6 and 2 are known as the **addends**. To add whole numbers, the process can be done vertically. First the ones digits are added, then the tens digits, then the hundreds digits, etc. The following example outlines the sum of 877 and 946:

First, 877 is written above 946 vertically so that all the place values align. Then, the ones are added: 7 + 6 = 13. 13 ones are equivalent to 1 ten and 3 ones, so the 3 is written under the ones column and the 1 is carried over to the tens column. The 1 is placed on top of the 7 and the 4.

$$
\begin{array}{r}
1 \\
877 \\
+946 \\
\hline
3
\end{array}
$$

Next, the tens are added: $1 + 7 + 4 = 12$. 12 tens are equivalent to 10 tens and 2 tens, which is the same as 1 hundred and 2 tens. 2 is written under the tens column and the 1 is carried over to the hundreds column. Therefore, the 1 is placed on top of the 8 and 9.

$$
\begin{array}{r}
11 \\
877 \\
+946 \\
\hline
23
\end{array}
$$

Finally, the hundreds are added.

$$1 + 8 + 9 = 18$$

18 hundreds mean that 18 is written under the hundreds column, which is equivalent to 1 thousand and 8 hundreds. This final step gives us the sum. The result is 877 + 946 = 1,823. Note that the same result would be found if 946 was written above 877 vertically and the two numbers were added.

$$
\begin{array}{r}
11 \\
877 \\
+946 \\
\hline
1823
\end{array}
$$

The operation of addition adheres to two properties: the associative property of addition and the commutative property of addition. The **associative property of addition** states that grouping does not change the result of an addition problem. For example, $(1 + 5) + 6$ is equivalent to $1 + (5 + 6)$. In both expressions, the addition in the grouping symbols, in this case the parentheses, would be completed first; however, both expressions are equivalent to 12. This law is useful because numbers that have sums that are easier to compute can be grouped together. The **commutative property of addition** states that addition can be done in any order. For instance,

$$7 + 8 = 8 + 7 = 15$$

As discussed in the example above, $877 + 946$ has the same result as $946 + 877$.

The number 0 has an important property in addition. It is known as the **additive identity** because adding 0 to anything leaves it unchanged. For instance, $0 + 11 = 11$ and $198 + 0 = 198$.

These properties of addition can be helpful when adding more than two numbers together. Values can be rearranged so that easier sums are grouped together and computed first. For instance, $(11 + 14) + (19 + 33) + (7 + 4)$ can be regrouped as

$$(11 + 19) + (33 + 7) + (14 + 4) = 30 + 40 + 18 = 88$$

This second grouping allows sums that end in 0 to be completed first, which makes the final sum an easier process. In this scenario, vertical addition is unnecessary due to the ease of the sums found after regrouping. The addition can be done in one's head.

A common real-world application of addition involves finding the perimeter of a two-dimensional object. The distance around an object is defined as its **perimeter**, and it is equal to the distance one would need to travel to go around all its edges. For instance, the perimeter of a triangle is found by adding the length of its three sides, and the perimeter of a rectangle is found by adding the length of its sides. No matter how many sides an object has, its perimeter can be found by adding the lengths of all the sides. For instance, consider the following irregular shape:

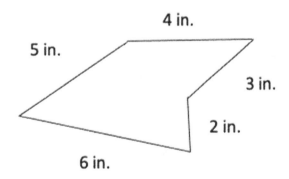

The perimeter of this shape is found by adding the length of all 5 sides, which is equal to:

$$5 + 4 + 3 + 2 + 6 = 20 \text{ inches}$$

Note that this sum can also be regrouped using the associative property of addition as $(5 + 3 + 2) + (4 + 6) = 10 + 10 = 20$ inches to make the addition process easier.

An **estimate** can help in the process of addition done in one's head. Estimation is based on the idea of rounding. In order to round a whole number to a certain place, locate the value in the specified digit. If the value to its right is 5 or higher, round up, and if the value to its right is 4 or less, round down. Then, all other values to the right of the specified digit are turned to zeros. The addition problem $92 + 106 + 56 + 45$ can be estimated by rounding each number to the nearest ten. In this case, the problem would turn into:

$$90 + 110 + 60 + 50 = 310$$

This result gives a quick answer that is close to the exact answer of 299. This process is even more convenient for larger numbers. For instance, consider the addition problem $1492 + 3455 + 6552 + 1789$.

A quick estimate from rounding to the nearest thousand results in:
$$1000 + 3000 + 7000 + 2000 = 13{,}000$$

Note that the exact sum is 13,488. Estimating is convenient when a calculator is not available. A baseline comparison can also provide piece of mind to determine if any operations completed by hand are on the right track. For example, the addition problem $877 + 946 = 1{,}823$ could be estimated as:

$$900 + 900 = 1{,}800$$

The set of integers consists of all whole numbers and their negatives. For instance, the set of integers are the following: ..., -4, -3, -2, -1, 0, 1, 2, 3, 4, ... The negative integers fall to the left of the positive integers on the number line. Note that the opposite of an integer is found by negating it. For example, the opposite of 5 is -5, and the opposite of -6 is 6. The addition of integers is not as straightforward as adding whole numbers and follows a few rules.

The sum of two positive integers is always positive. In order to add two negative integers, add the absolute value of each number and make the answer negative. Recall that the **absolute value** of a number is the distance from that number to 0 on the number line, and because it is measuring distance, it is never negative. The absolute value of a positive number is the number itself, and the absolute value of a negative number is its opposite. For instance, $|-6| = 6$ and $|6| = 6$. The addition of the two negative integers -9 and -4 is $-9 + (-4) = -(|-9| + |-4|) = -(9 + 4) = -13$. The sum of two negative numbers is always negative.

When a positive number is added to a negative number or a negative number is added to a positive number, the sign of the number with the larger absolute value is the sign of the result. Therefore, in this scenario, the answer can be either positive or negative. In order to find the sum, first, find the difference of the absolute values of the two numbers. If the negative integer has a larger absolute value, the sum is negative. For instance,

$$-9 + 6 = -(|-9| - |6|) = -(9 - 6) = -3$$

If the positive integer has a larger absolute value, the sum is positive. For instance,

$$-5 + 8 = (|8| - |-5|) = (8 - 5) = 3$$

If the two integers have the same absolute value, the result is 0. For instance, $-5 + 5 = 0$. In this example, -5 is known as the **additive inverse** of 5 because their sum is equal to 0. The sum of any number and its additive inverse, otherwise known as its **opposite**, is 0.

Adding decimals is comparable to adding whole numbers. If the sum of two decimals is to be found, the decimals should be lined up so that corresponding place values can be added. Zeros can always be added to missing place values on the right of a number if the two decimals do not have the same number of digits. Digits are first added in the furthest place value to the right, and then each sum is found on the other place values to the left just as is done with whole numbers. The following example outlines the process of the sum $65.183 + 14.65$.

First, the decimals are written vertically with decimal points lining up. Note that a 0 can be inserted in the thousandths place of 14.65 so that each decimal has values in the thousandths place. Also note that because addition follows the commutative property, it does not matter which decimal is written on top.

$$
\begin{array}{r}
65.183 \\
+14.650 \\
\hline
\end{array}
$$

Once the decimals are aligned, the values in the thousandths place are added. $3 + 0 = 3$, and 3 is written under the thousandths place.

$$
\begin{array}{r}
65.183 \\
+14.650 \\
\hline
3
\end{array}
$$

Next, the values in the hundredths place are added. $8 + 5 = 13$. This results in 13 hundredths, which is equivalent to 1 tenth and 3 hundredths. The 3 is written in the hundredths place, and the 1 is carried over the tenths place.

$$
\begin{array}{r}
1 \\
65.183 \\
+14.650 \\
\hline
33
\end{array}
$$

The values in the tenths place are added as $1 + 1 + 6 = 8$, and 8 is written under the tenths place.

$$
\begin{array}{r}
1 \\
65.183 \\
+14.650 \\
\hline
833
\end{array}
$$

Next, the values in the ones place are added. $5 + 4 = 9$, and 9 is written under the ones place.

$$
\begin{array}{r}
1 \\
65.183 \\
+14.650 \\
\hline
9.833
\end{array}
$$

Finally, the values in the tens place are added. $6 + 1 = 7$, and 7 is written under the tens place.

$$
\begin{array}{r}
1 \\
65.183 \\
+14.650 \\
\hline
79.833
\end{array}
$$

The result of the sum $65.183 + 14.65$ is 79.833. Note that estimating and rounding can also be helpful here. The same rounding rules for whole numbers applies to decimals. The values in the original problem can be rounded to the nearest ten to produce an estimate of $70 + 10 = 80$, which is extremely close to the exact answer. The values in the original problem can be rounded to the nearest one as $65 + 15 = 80$, which results in the same value. Estimating decimals is useful in the real world when dealing with money. For instance, at the grocery store, items can be rounded to the nearest dollar to estimate a total if someone has a specific amount of money needing to be spent.

Subtraction

Subtraction is equivalent to finding the difference between two numbers. Suppose that someone has 10 magazines, and she gives away 6 of them. She is left with 4 magazines in the end. This scenario is an example of subtraction and is written as $10 - 6 = 4$. The **minuend** is the value being subtracted from, which is 10 in this example. The **subtrahend** is the number being subtracted, which is 6 in this case. Finally, the result is known as the **difference**, which is the 4. Note that the difference, 4, plus the subtrahend, 6, is equal to the minuend, 10. This property is true for any subtraction problem, and it shows the relationship between subtraction and addition. Therefore, for any numbers a and b, the difference $a - b$ is equal to a unique value c such that $a = c + b$. This property is helpful when checking answers from a subtraction problem.

Just like addition, subtraction can be completed vertically for larger numbers. First, the ones digits are subtracted, then the tens digits, then the hundreds digits, etc. Consider the following example: $7653 - 4521$. The first value, 7653, is written on top of the other value vertically, 4521, so that all the digits align.

$$\begin{array}{r} 7653 \\ -4521 \\ \hline \end{array}$$

The ones digits are subtracted first. $3 - 1 = 2$, so the 2 is written under the ones place.

$$\begin{array}{r} 7653 \\ -4521 \\ \hline 2 \end{array}$$

Next, the tens digits are subtracted. $5 - 2 = 3$, so the 3 is written under the tens place.

$$\begin{array}{r} 7653 \\ -4521 \\ \hline 32 \end{array}$$

Then, the hundreds digits are subtracted. $6 - 5 = 1$, so the 1 is written under the hundreds place.

$$\begin{array}{r} 7653 \\ -4521 \\ \hline 132 \end{array}$$

Finally, the thousands digits are subtracted. $7 - 4 = 3$, so the 3 is written under the thousands place.

$$\begin{array}{r} 7653 \\ -4521 \\ \hline 3132 \end{array}$$

The difference is therefore 3,312. Because subtraction and addition relate, addition can be used to check this answer. It is true that $3312 + 4521 = 7653$. This problem was a particularly simple example because each digit in the first number was larger than each corresponding digit in the second number. If it is the case that a digit in the first value is less than a corresponding digit in the second value, a 1 must be "borrowed" from the next highest place value to allow for the subtraction to occur. For instance, consider the example $567 - 298$. First, 567 is placed above 298 vertically so that the place values align.

$$567$$
$$\underline{-298}$$

Next, the ones columns are subtracted. Notice that 8 cannot be subtracted from 7 because it is greater than 7. Therefore, 1 ten must be borrowed from the 6 tens to be regrouped with the 7 ones, making it 17. Therefore, the subtraction in the ones column is $17 - 8 = 9$. The 9 is written under the ones column.

$$17$$
$$56\cancel{7}$$
$$\underline{-298}$$
$$9$$

Then, the tens column is subtracted. Because 1 ten was borrowed in the previous step, there are 5 tens left over. However, 9 cannot be subtracted from 5, because it is larger. Therefore, 1 hundred must be borrowed from the 5 hundreds and regrouped with the 5 tens, making 15 tens. The subtraction in this column is therefore $15 - 9 = 6$. The 6 is written under the tens column.

$$15$$
$$\cancel{5}\,17$$
$$5\cancel{67}$$
$$\underline{-298}$$
$$69$$

Finally, the hundreds column is subtracted. Because 1 hundred was borrowed in the previous step, there are 4 hundreds left. $4 - 2 = 2$. The 2 is written under the hundreds column, resulting in the difference 269. Addition can be used to check the result. It is true that $269 + 298 = 567$, so the subtraction was computed correctly.

$$15$$
$$4\,\cancel{5}\,17$$
$$\cancel{567}$$
$$\underline{-298}$$
$$269$$

Subtraction does not adhere to the properties that addition does. For instance, order matters when subtracting. The same result is not obtained when the order of the two numbers is changed. For instance, $9 - 8$ is not equal to $8 - 9$. Therefore, subtraction is not commutative. Because order matters with subtraction, subtraction is not associative. Therefore, grouping symbols, such as parentheses, cannot be rearranged in a subtraction problem.

Estimating and rounding can also help in the subtraction process. For instance, the first example of $7,653 - 4,521$ can be rounded to the nearest thousand as $8,000 - 5,000$ to obtain the estimate 3,000, which is close to the actual value of 3,312. The second example of $567 - 298$ can be rounded to the nearest hundred to obtain $600 - 300$, which gives an estimate of 300. 300 is close to the exact difference of 298. Estimating is a quick way to check that the answer obtained by computing a mathematical operation by hand is on the right track.

An application of subtraction in the real-world is when two quantities are compared, and someone wants to know how much taller, how much longer, or how much more of something there is. For instance, if a building is 3,400 feet and another one is 2,300 feet, subtraction would be used to determine how much taller the first building is. The first building is $3,400 - 2,300 = 1,100$ feet taller. Notice that order is important in this operation, and the larger building is listed first in the problem.

The idea that subtraction and addition are related can also be seen in real-world scenarios. For instance, if it is known that a building is 800 feet taller than another building that is 2,500 feet tall, that means that the difference between the two buildings is 800 ft. Addition can be used to find the other building's height. Therefore, the other building is:

$$2,500 + 800 = 3,300 \text{ feet tall}$$

Subtracting decimals is comparable to subtracting whole numbers because they both can be done vertically. In order to subtract decimals, first the decimal points are aligned so that all of the place-values are lined up. If the two decimals are of different lengths, zeros can be added to ensure the same number of place values. Once the place values are lined up, the digits are subtracted starting from the right. If the decimals have the smallest place value in the thousandths place, this place value is the starting point. Then, the hundredths place values are subtracted, then the tenths, etc. Borrowing might be necessary if the number on top in a place value is smaller than the corresponding digit below. For example, consider the subtraction problem $45.832 - 23.94$. First the decimals are written vertically, lining up the decimal points, and a 0 is added to 23.94, making it 23.940.

$$\begin{array}{r} 45.832 \\ -23.940 \\ \hline \end{array}$$

The values in the thousandths place are subtracted first. $2 - 0 = 2$, and the 2 is written under the thousandths place.

$$\begin{array}{r} 45.832 \\ -23.940 \\ \hline 2 \end{array}$$

Next, the values in the hundredths place are subtracted. However, 3 is smaller than 4, so a 1 from the tenths place must be borrowed resulting in the subtraction $13 - 4 = 9$. The 9 is written under the hundredths place.

$$\begin{array}{r} {}^{13} \\ 45.8\cancel{3}2 \\ -23.940 \\ \hline 92 \end{array}$$

Because a 1 was borrowed from the tenths place, the next subtraction is $7 - 9$. 7 is smaller than 9, so a 1 is borrowed from the ones place resulting in $17 - 9 = 8$. The 8 is written under the tenths place.

$$\begin{array}{r} 17 \\ 7\ 13 \\ 45.\cancel{8}\cancel{3}2 \\ -23.940 \\ \hline .892 \end{array}$$

The last few steps involve subtraction on the left-hand side of the decimal point. Because 1 was borrowed previously, the subtraction in the ones column is $4 - 3 = 1$. The 1 is placed under the ones column.

$$\begin{array}{r} 17 \\ 4\ 7\ 13 \\ 45.\cancel{8}\cancel{3}2 \\ -23.940 \\ \hline 1.892 \end{array}$$

Finally, the tens place is subtracted resulting in $4 - 2 = 2$, giving the difference of 21.892. This answer can be checked through addition as $21.892 + 23.94 = 45.832$.

$$\begin{array}{r} 17 \\ 4\ 7\ 13 \\ 45.\cancel{8}\cancel{3}2 \\ -23.940 \\ \hline 21.892 \end{array}$$

The original problem can be estimated through rounding as well. If the original values in the problem are rounded to the nearest ten, $45.832 - 23.94$ turns into $50 - 20 = 30$. The original problem can also be rounded to the nearest one as $46 - 24 = 22$, which is closer to the actual difference of 21.892.

When subtracting integers, specifically when negative numbers are involved, rules similar to those given with adding integers must be followed. When subtracting integers, it can be helpful to think about subtraction as adding the opposite, or additive inverse, of the second number. For instance,
$$3 - 5 = 3 + (-5)$$

For any two integers a and b, $a - b$ can be rewritten as $a + (-b)$. Once the subtraction is turned into an addition problem, the rules of adding integers can be used. For this first example, the result of changing it to addition is:

$$3 - 5 = 3 + (-5) = -2$$

Notice that a larger positive number subtracted from a smaller positive number results in a negative number. Also, consider $-5 - 15$. This subtraction problem is turned into adding the opposite, which is $-5 + (-15) = -20$. A positive number subtracted from a negative number results in a negative number. Thirdly, consider $-4 - (-3)$. Again, the idea of adding the opposite is used. The opposite of a negative number is positive, so this problem turns into $-4 + 3 = -1$.

Therefore, whenever a negative number is subtracted, the "double negative" turns into addition. Real-world examples of subtracting negative numbers can involve finding differences in temperatures when

EXAM
PEDIA

negative temperatures are involved. For instance, the difference between 56 degrees Fahrenheit and -4 degrees Fahrenheit is $56 - (-4) = 56 + 4 = 60$ degrees Fahrenheit. This result could be checked by addition because:

$$60 + (-4) = 56$$

Multiplication

Multiplication is a quick way to compute repeated addition. For example, combining 8 sets of 5 through addition is equivalent to the multiplication of $8 \times 5 = 40$. Within this expression, the 8 and the 5 are referred to as the **factors** and the result, 40, is known as the **product**. A dot can also be used to denote multiplication as seen here:

$$8 \times 5 = 40$$

The relationship between repeated addition and multiplication can be seen using squares. For instance, the following 3 by 5 rectangle shows the multiplication of $3 \times 5 = 15$.

$$3 + 3 + 3 + 3 + 3 = 5 \times 3$$

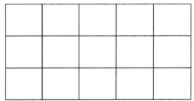

$$5 + 5 + 5 = 3 \times 5$$

There are three rows of 5 squares, and in total, there are 15 squares, which can be counted individually. Multiplication, rather than individual counting of squares, is a much quicker process. The number of rows times the number of columns results in:

$$3 \times 5 = 15$$

Because multiplication is repeated addition, it adheres to both the commutative and associative properties. The **commutative property of multiplication** states that multiplication can be processed in any order. For instance,

$$4 \times 2 = 2 \times 4 = 8$$

In generally, for any numbers a and b, $a \times b = b \times a$. The **associative property of multiplication** describes how grouping symbols play a role in multiplication. This property states that re-grouping products does not change the result of multiplication. For example, $(3 \times 2) \times 4$ is equivalent to $3 \times (2 \times 4)$. In both expressions, the multiplication in the grouping symbols, in this case the parentheses, is completed first. Therefore, equivalent expressions are 6×4 and 3×8, which are both equal to 24. Just like with addition, this property is useful because easier products can be grouped together first. Another item to note is that the product of 0 and any number is always 0. For example,

$$0 \times 5 = 5 \times 0 = 0$$

Finally, the number 1 is referred to as the **multiplicative identity** because a number times 1 is always itself. For instance,

$$14 \times 1 = 1 \times 14 = 14$$

Multiplication of larger whole numbers can be computed vertically. If one of the factors has more digits than the other factor, the longer number should be written above the number with fewer digits, aligning the place values. Starting out with a simple example, consider the multiplication problem 3476×5. First, 3456 is written above the 5, aligning the ones digits.

$$\begin{array}{r} 3476 \\ \times \quad 5 \\ \hline \end{array}$$

Then, the ones digits are multiplied. $6 \times 5 = 30$. Notice that a two-digit value cannot be written under the ones column, so the 0 is written in the ones column and the 3 is carried over to the tens column and written above the 7. This is because 30 is equivalent to 3 tens and 0 ones.

$$\begin{array}{r} 3 \\ 3476 \\ \times \quad 5 \\ \hline 0 \end{array}$$

Next, the tens digits are multiplied. $7 \times 5 = 35$. Then, the 3 tens that were carried over from the previous step are added to the 35, resulting in 38. The 8 is written below the tens column and the 3 is carried over to the hundreds column, written above the 4.

$$\begin{array}{r} 33 \\ 3476 \\ \times \quad 5 \\ \hline 80 \end{array}$$

The hundreds digits are then multiplied. $4 \times 5 = 20$. The 3 hundreds are added to 20, resulting in 23. Note that 23 hundreds is equivalent to 2 thousands and 3 hundreds. The 3 is written below the hundreds column and the 2 is carried over to the thousands column.

$$\begin{array}{r} 233 \\ 3476 \\ \times \quad 5 \\ \hline 380 \end{array}$$

Finally, the thousands digits are multiplied. $3 \times 5 = 15$, and the 2 carried over from the previous multiplication step is added, resulting in 17. 17 is written below the thousands column, which results in the final answer. The product of 3476 and 5 is 17,380.

$$\begin{array}{r} 233 \\ 3476 \\ \times \quad 5 \\ \hline 17,380 \end{array}$$

Multiplication, because it is based on repeated multiplication, helps define the distributive property. The **distributive property** states that multiplying a number times a sum of a group of numbers is equal to computing each multiplication separately and adding up those individual products. For instance, for any numbers a, b, and c, it is true that:

$$a \times (b + c) = (a \times b) + (a \times c)$$

The number a is said to be distributed throughout the expression in the parentheses $b + c$. Consider the specific example $2 \times (5 + 6)$. By following the order of operations, the expression within the parenthesis can be computed first as:

$$5 + 6 = 11$$

Then, the multiplication $2 \times 11 = 22$ is computed. Applying the distributive property allows for the 2 to be distributed first onto the values within the parentheses as $2 \times 5 + 2 \times 6$. Then, each product is found, and the final result is added as $10 + 12 = 22$, which is equal to the previous value.

The distributive property can allow for more difficult products to be evaluated. For instance, consider the product 43×24. Because $24 = 20 + 4$, the multiplication problem can be rewritten as $43 \times (20 + 4)$. Therefore, first, 43 is multiplied times 4. Then, 43 is multiplied times 20, and finally, the two products are added. This can all be done vertically. Writing 43 above 24, we have:

$$\begin{array}{r} 43 \\ \times\, 24 \\ \hline \end{array}$$

First, 43 is multiplied times 4, resulting in 172. This value, 172, is written in the first row under the 24, making sure all place values align.

$$\begin{array}{r} 43 \\ \times\, 24 \\ \hline 172 \end{array}$$

Then, 43 is multiplied by 20, resulting in 860. The 860 is written below the 172, making sure all digits align.

$$\begin{array}{r} 43 \\ \times\, 24 \\ \hline 172 \\ 860 \end{array}$$

Finally, the sum of 172 and 860 can be computed vertically, resulting in the final answer of 1,032.

$$\begin{array}{r} 43 \\ \times\, 24 \\ \hline 172 \\ +860 \\ \hline 1,032 \end{array}$$

A second way of thinking about vertical multiplication is to multiply the top value times each place value in the second value. Consider the same example and write 43 above 24:

$$\begin{array}{r} 43 \\ \times\, 24 \\ \hline \end{array}$$

First, $3 \times 4 = 12$ is evaluated. The 2 is written under the ones column and the 1 is carried over to the tens column. Then, $4 \times 4 = 16$ is evaluated, and the 1 from the previous multiplication is added, resulting in 17. 17 is then written under the tens column, resulting in the product of 43 and 4: 172.

$$
\begin{array}{r}
1 \\
43 \\
\times\ 24 \\
\hline
172
\end{array}
$$

Next, 43 is multiplied times 2. However, because the problem has now moved to the tens column, a 0 is written first in the ones column in a row below the 172. Then, $3 \times 2 = 6$ is written in the tens column, and $4 \times 2 = 8$ is written in the hundreds column. The product of 43 and 20 is 860.

$$
\begin{array}{r}
1 \\
43 \\
\times\ 24 \\
\hline
172 \\
860
\end{array}
$$

Finally, the answer to the original problem is found through vertical addition of 172 and 860, which results in the final product of 1,032.

$$
\begin{array}{r}
1 \\
43 \\
\times\ 24 \\
\hline
172 \\
+860 \\
\hline
1,032
\end{array}
$$

Estimating and rounding can also be helpful in multiplication, especially when dealing with large quantities. A quick estimate of the multiplication problem 1789×2901 involves computing the product after each number is rounded to the nearest thousand. The estimate would be:

$$2000 \times 3000 = 6,000,000$$

Multiplying numbers ending in zeros involves multiplying the nonzero digits together and then adding on the total number of zeros in the problem. For example, 2000×3000 is equal to 2×3 with 6 zeros. The exact answer to the original problem is 5,189,889.

A real-world application of multiplication is area. **Area** is equal to the number of square units that a two-dimensional shape occupies. For example, the area of a rectangle is equal to the product of its length, l, and its width, w. The formula for area of a rectangle is $A = l \times w$.

For instance, consider the following rectangle that has a length of 22 centimeters and a width of 8 centimeters:

22 cm

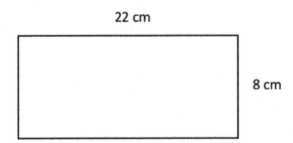

8 cm

Its area is $22 \times 8 = 176$ square centimeters, which can be abbreviated as 176 sq cm or 176 cm^2. Because a square has four equal sides, the area of a square is found by multiplying the length of its side times itself.

Multiplying decimals involves a pretty straightforward rule. When given two decimals to multiply, first ignore the decimal points and multiply as if there were no decimals. Then, a decimal point is placed in the result. The number of decimal places in the final answer is equal to the sum of the number of decimal points in both original factors. The number of decimal places is counted by starting at the digit in the far right and moving to the left. For example, consider 54.2×0.8. First, the decimal points are removed and the product $542 \times 8 = 4{,}336$ is found.

In the original problem, there are 2 total values in decimal places, so the final answer is found by moving the decimal point to the left 2 places, resulting in 43.36. Another example is 3.14×0.25. The decimals are removed first and the product $314 \times 25 = 7{,}850$ is obtained. The original problem has digits in 4 decimal places, so the decimal point is moved to the left four places, resulting in 0.785. Note that zeros can be inserted to the left of numbers, if necessary, in this last step.

Finally, the multiplication of integers is also straightforward. A positive integer times a positive integer is always positive. A negative integer times a negative integer is always positive because the two negatives cancel each other out. For example:

$$-5 \times (-7) = 35$$

In this scenario, because it is known that the answer is always positive, just multiply the absolute values of the original numbers. A positive integer times a negative integer, or a negative integer times a positive integer is always negative. For instance:

$$-8 \times 5 = 5 \times (-8) = -40$$

These rules can be helpful when multiplying more than two integers together. The product of an even number of negative integers is always positive. For instance:

$$(-2) \times (-2) \times (-2) \times (-2) = 16$$

Also, the product of an odd number of negative integers is always negative. For instance:

$$(-2) \times (-2) \times (-2) \times (-2) = -32$$

Finally, the integer -1 times any value just changes its sign, resulting in its opposite or additive inverse. For example, $(-1) \times 34 = -34$ and $(-1) \times -545 = 545$.

Fractions

Quantities such as the following: $\frac{2}{3}, -\frac{11}{12}$, and $\frac{5}{2}$ are referred to as **fractions**. The top number is known as the **numerator**, and the bottom number is known as the **denominator**. A fraction can be considered as a partition of a whole object that is divided into equal parts. For example, consider a pie divided into 6 equal parts as seen here:

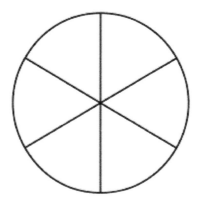

If 3 slices of the pie are removed, there are 3 out of 6 pieces left. The amount leftover can be written in fraction form as $\frac{3}{6}$. Note that one-half or $\frac{1}{2}$ of the pie is leftover in this case, so $\frac{3}{6}$ and $\frac{1}{2}$ are equivalent amounts. The numerator, 3, refers to how many of the equal parts we are referring to, and the denominator, 6, refers to how many equal parts the whole was originally divided into.

Here is a rectangle divided into 5 equal parts:

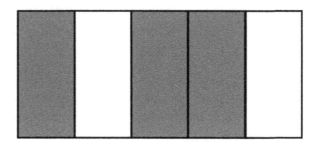

Note that 3 out of 5 parts are shaded, which is equivalent to the fraction $\frac{3}{5}$. Also, 2 out of the 5 parts are unshaded, which is equivalent to the fraction $\frac{2}{5}$. A fraction can also be thought of as a ratio because a ratio is a quotient of two quantities. The fraction $\frac{2}{5}$ is equivalent to the ratio $2:5$.

If the numerator and denominator are equal in a fraction, the fraction is equivalent to 1. For instance, $\frac{5}{5} = 1$. In other words, all 5 equal parts of the rectangle shown above are being referenced. This property is also true for negative numerators and denominators. For example, $\frac{-7}{-7} = 1$. Because 0 divided by any nonzero number is equal to 0, $\frac{0}{n} = 0$ for a nonzero value n. For instance $\frac{0}{12} = 0$. Recall that a number cannot be divided by 0, so a fraction of the form $\frac{n}{0}$ is always undefined. Finally, because any number divided by 1 is itself, the fraction $\frac{n}{1} = n$. For example, $\frac{-11}{1} = -11$.

In order to multiply two fractions, multiply the numerators together and multiply the denominators together. For instance,

$$\frac{2}{3} \times \frac{5}{11} = \frac{2 \times 5}{3 \times 11} = \frac{10}{33}$$

If a fraction is being multiplied by an integer, write the integer as a fraction with a denominator of 1 to place it in fraction form. For example,

$$5 \times \frac{1}{4} = \frac{5}{1} \times \frac{1}{4} = \frac{5 \times 1}{1 \times 4} = \frac{5}{4}$$

Multiplication with fractions is often seen in the real-world, and it is usually denoted with use of the word "of." For instance, if one-third of one quarter of a yard of fabric is needed for a quilting project, this amount would be equivalent to the product:

$$\frac{1}{3} \times \frac{1}{4} = \frac{1 \times 1}{3 \times 4} = \frac{1}{12}$$

Therefore, one-twelfth of a yard of fabric is needed for the project.

When computing operations with fractions, if the result is a fraction, it should always be written in simplest form. Simplest form is also referred to as **lowest terms**. A fraction in lowest terms has no common factors between the numerator and the denominator, other than 1. For instance, $\frac{1}{3}$ is in lowest terms, but $\frac{4}{12}$ is not because both the numerator and the denominator share a common factor of 4. If 4 is divided out of the numerator and the denominator, the fraction $\frac{1}{3}$ is obtained. Therefore, $\frac{1}{3}$ and $\frac{4}{12}$ are equivalent fractions. The equivalent fraction $\frac{4}{12}$ can be found by multiplying $\frac{1}{3}$ times $\frac{4}{4}$, which is a form of 1. The process of finding equivalent fractions will be helpful in both addition and subtraction of fractions.

In order to write a fraction in lowest terms, all common factors must be removed from both the numerator and the denominator. To complete this process, first, factor the numerator and denominator. Then, locate any common factors that appear in both the numerator and denominator and divide them out of both places. For instance, $\frac{75}{100}$ is not in lowest terms. Both the numerator and denominator share a common factor of 5. However, there might be more common factors as well. Factoring the numerator and denominator into prime numbers can be helpful. This process is known as computing a **prime factorization**. For instance, $75 = 5 \times 5 \times 3$ and $100 = 5 \times 5 \times 2 \times 2$. Therefore,

$$\frac{75}{100} = \frac{5 \times 5 \times \times 3}{5 \times 5 \times 2 \times 2}$$

The common factors of two 5's can be divided out in both the numerator and denominator, resulting in the fraction in simplest form $\frac{3}{2 \times 2} = \frac{3}{4}$. Note that if all factors are divided from either a numerator or denominator, a 1 is still there. Another way to place a fraction in lowest terms is by initially recognizing the greatest common factor between the numerator and denominator and dividing it out in one step.

For instance, 75 and 100 share a common factor of 25. Dividing this value from the numerator and the denominator results in:

$$\frac{75 \div 25}{100 \div 25} = \frac{3}{4}$$

The area of a triangle is an important application of multiplication with fractions. The formula for the area of a triangle with base b and height h is equal to $A = \frac{1}{2} \times b \times h$. For instance, consider the following triangle with base 18 and height 6.

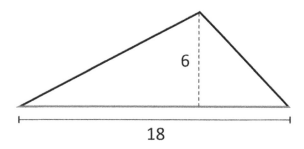

Its area is equal to $\frac{1}{2} \times 18 \times 6 = \frac{1}{2} \times \frac{18}{1} \times \frac{6}{1} = \frac{108}{2} = \frac{54 \times 2}{2} = 54$ square units.

The **reciprocal** of a fraction is found by interchanging its numerator and denominator. For example, the reciprocal of $\frac{2}{3}$ is $\frac{3}{2}$. It is always true that the product of a fraction and its reciprocal is equal to 1, and that the number 0 has no reciprocal due to division by 0. Division of fractions is defined in terms of multiplication. To divide a number by a fraction, multiply times its reciprocal. For example,

$$\frac{4}{5} \div \frac{2}{3} = \frac{4}{5} \times \frac{3}{2} = \frac{4 \times 3}{5 \times 2} = \frac{2 \times 2 \times 3}{5 \times 2} = \frac{2 \times 3}{5} = \frac{6}{5}$$

The **least common multiple (LCM)** of two numbers is equal to the smallest number that is a multiple of both numbers. The **least common denominator (LCD)** between two fractions with different denominators is equal to the LCM of the denominators. To find the LCM between two numbers, first check to see if the larger number is a multiple of the other number. If so, the larger number is the LCM. If not, then find the smallest multiple of the larger number that is a multiple of the other number. Once one is found, that value is the LCM. For instance, consider the fractions $\frac{1}{8}$ and $\frac{1}{15}$. 15 is not a multiple of 8, so multiples of 15 are analyzed in order to locate the LCD. The smallest multiple of 15 that is a multiple of 8 is the LCD. The multiples of 15 are 30, 45, 60, 75, 90, 105, 120, 135, 150, 165,... Notice that $8 \times 15 = 120$ is the smallest multiple of 8, so 120 is the LCD.

Addition of two fractions is simple if the denominators are the same. In that case, add the numerators, keep the denominators the same, and simplify if necessary. For instance,

$$\frac{2}{6} + \frac{3}{6} = \frac{2+3}{6} = \frac{5}{6}$$

If the denominators are different, the least common denominator must first be found. Then, each fraction is multiplied times a form of 1 to express them in equivalent fractions with the LCD as their denominator. If done correctly, the denominators will be the same. Therefore, add the numerators, keep the same denominator, and simplify if necessary. For instance, consider $\frac{1}{9} + \frac{5}{6}$. The denominators are different, and their LCD is 18. Each fraction is multiplied by a form of 1 to change them into equivalent fractions with 18 as their denominator as seen here:

$$\frac{1}{9} \times \frac{2}{2} + \frac{5}{6} \times \frac{3}{3} = \frac{2}{18} + \frac{15}{18}$$

The problem has now turned into one with the same denominators, and the sum is $\frac{17}{18}$.

Subtraction and addition are performed in a similar manner. If the denominators are the same, subtract the numerators and keep the denominators the same. For example,

$$\frac{6}{7} - \frac{5}{7} = \frac{6-5}{7} = \frac{1}{7}$$

If the denominators are different, the least common denominator approach is used. Consider the subtraction problem $\frac{7}{15} - \frac{3}{25}$. The denominators are different, and their LCD is 75. In order to compute the operation, each fraction is multiplied times a form of 1, changing them into equivalent fractions having 75 as their denominator. The problem turns into $\frac{7}{15} \times \frac{5}{5} - \frac{3}{25} \times \frac{3}{3} = \frac{35}{75} - \frac{9}{75}$, which is subtraction of two fractions with like denominators. The difference is $\frac{26}{75}$, which is a fraction in lowest terms.

A **mixed number** is a combination of an integer and a fraction. For instance, $2\frac{1}{3}$ is a mixed number and is read "two and one-third." The 2 is a whole number, so this mixed number refers to two whole quantities plus one-third, or $2 + \frac{1}{3}$. In order to complete operations such as addition, subtraction, multiplication, and division with whole numbers, they should be turned into improper fractions first. An **improper fraction** is a fraction in which the numerator is greater than the denominator. To turn a mixed number to an improper fraction, multiply the whole number by the denominator and add that value to the numerator. Then, write that result over the original denominator. For example, $2\frac{1}{3}$ is equivalent to:

$$\frac{2 \times 3 + 1}{3} = \frac{7}{3}$$

To turn an improper fraction into a mixed number, divide. The quotient is the whole number part of the mixed number, the remainder is the numerator, and the denominator stays the same. For example, $\frac{15}{2}$ is equal to $7\frac{1}{2}$ because $15 \div 2 = 7R1$.

When two fractions have a common denominator, the larger fraction is determined through a comparison of the numerators. The fraction with a larger numerator is the larger quantity. Therefore, $\frac{11}{5} > \frac{9}{5}$. If denominators are not the same, the fractions can be converted into equivalent fractions using the LCD and the same approach is used. For instance, in order to determine whether $\frac{2}{3}$ or $\frac{1}{2}$ is larger, they can be converted to fractions with 6, their LCD, as their denominator. The two equivalent fractions are $\frac{4}{6}$ and $\frac{3}{6}$ respectively. Because $\frac{4}{6} > \frac{3}{6}$, it is true that $\frac{2}{3} > \frac{1}{2}$.

Decimals

The set of **rational numbers** consists of all integers and fractions. Decimals can be used to represent all the rational numbers. For instance, the fraction $\frac{4}{5}$ is equivalent to the decimal 0.8, and the mixed number $5\frac{1}{4}$ is equivalent to the decimal 5.25. The word "decimal" is derived from the Latin word *decima*, which means a tenth of an amount. A real-world application of decimals involves money. For instance, $25.95 is equal to $25 and $\frac{95}{100}$ of a dollar and can be thought of as $25 + $0.95. The amount $0.95 is equal to 9 dimes and 5 pennies. A dime is one tenth of a dollar, and a penny is one hundredth of a dollar. Therefore, this monetary amount can be written in expanded form as:

$$\frac{9}{10} + \frac{5}{100} = \frac{95}{100}$$

Each single digit in a decimal corresponds to a place value. The digits to the left of the decimal point correspond to place values in the whole number portion such as ones, tens, hundreds, etc. The values to the right of the decimal point correspond to the tenths, hundredths, thousandths, ten thousandths, hundred thousandths, etc. Here is an example of a place-value chart:

Thousands	Hundreds	Tens	Units	Decimal Point	Tenths	Hundredths	Thousandths	Ten-Thousandths	Hundred Thousandths
				•					
				•					
				•					
				•					
				•					
				•					
				•					

A number can be entered in a place value chart to determine which digit is in each corresponding place value. For instance, consider the number 245.8901. The 2 is in the hundreds place. The 4 is in the tens place. The 5 is in the ones place. The 8 is in the tenths place. The 9 is in the thousandths place. The 0 is in the ten thousandths place, and the 1 is in the hundred thousandths place. In order to read a decimal verbally, the decimal point is stated as the word "and." The number to the left of the decimal point is read normally, and the number to the right of the decimal point is read as a whole number, attaching the name of the rightmost place value name. For instance, 245.8901 is read as two-hundred forty-five and eight thousand nine hundred one ten-thousandths. A common mistake is to use the word "and" in other places than the decimal, and this approach is incorrect. Therefore, when someone reads a decimal in words correctly, the word "and" corresponds to the decimal. For instance, ninety-eight and one hundred seventeen thousandths is written as 98.117.

A decimal can be converted to fraction form by first counting the number of decimal places, moving the decimal point that number of place values to the right, and writing this amount over a denominator of one plus that same number of zeros. For example, 0.9763 has four decimal places. Moving the decimal point to the right four places results in 9,763. Then, this amount is written over 1 plus 4 zeros, or 10,000. Therefore, the decimal in fraction form is $\frac{9763}{10000}$. A decimal that is larger than 1 can be written as a fraction as well, using the same rules. For instance, 5.983 has 3 decimals. Moving the decimal point over 3 place values results in 5983. Then, this amount is written over 1 plus 3 zeros, or 1,000. The decimal in fraction form is $\frac{5983}{1000}$. A decimal larger than 1 can also be written as a mixed number just by converting the decimal portion to a fraction and leaving the whole number alone.

In this same example, 0.983 is written in fraction form as $\frac{983}{1000}$. Therefore, 5.983 written as a mixed number is $5\frac{983}{1000}$. If a decimal is negative, the negative symbol is inserted before the fraction once converted. For instance, -0.9763 written as a fraction is $-\frac{9763}{10000}$. Any time a decimal is written as a fraction, the fraction must be written in simplified form, or in lowest terms. For example, 0.25 is equal to $\frac{25}{100}$. However, this fraction is not in lowest terms because both the numerator and the denominator share a common factor of 25. Dividing a 25 from both the numerator and the denominator results in the simplified form $\frac{1}{4}$.

All fractions can also be written as decimals. If the denominator of a fraction is a power of 10, the decimal is easily found by doing the opposite of writing a decimal as a fraction. First, count the number of zeros in the denominator. Then, move the decimal point that same number of places to the left. Finally, write the number as a decimal without any denominator. For example, consider the fraction $\frac{97}{100}$. The denominator has two zeros. Therefore, move the decimal two places to the left, resulting in 0.97. For another example, consider the fraction $\frac{898}{10}$.

Because this is an improper fraction, where the numerator is larger than the denominator, the decimal will include a whole number. There is one zero in the denominator, so moving the decimal one place value to the left results in 89.8. If a mixed number needs to be written as a decimal, the mixed number is first written as a sum of a whole number and a fraction, and the fraction is converted to decimal notation. For instance, $5\frac{99}{100}$ in decimal form is 5.99. Some zeros might need to be added in cases where there are more zeros in the denominator than place values in the numerator. For instance, consider the fraction $\frac{6}{1000}$. There are three zeros in the denominator, so in order to move the decimal three places to the left, two additional zeros must be added before the 6. Therefore, the corresponding decimal is 0.006.

If the denominator of a fraction is not a power of 10, its corresponding decimal can be found by using division (either long division or a calculator). For example, consider the fraction $\frac{5}{8}$. It is true that $5 \div 8 = 0.625$. This result is known as a terminal decimal because the decimal ends. Some decimals are not terminal, and therefore they must be rounded. For instance, $\frac{22}{7}$ is equal to $22 \div 7 = 3.142857143 \ldots$ For ease of use, this decimal can be rounded to the nearest thousandth place and written as 3.143.

Some decimals that are not terminal can show a pattern and are referred to as repeating decimals. For instance,

$$\frac{1}{9} = 1 \div 9 = 0.1111111$$

A repeated decimal is written with a bar over the portion that repeats. In this case, the decimal is written as $0.\overline{1}$. Common repeated decimals are $\frac{1}{3} = 0.\overline{3}$ and $\frac{2}{3} = 0.\overline{6}$. Repeated decimals can also be rounded. For example, $0.\overline{6}$ rounded to the nearest hundredths place is 0.67 and rounded to the nearest tenths place is 0.7.

Sometimes, it is difficult to determine if one decimal is larger than another because the number of decimal points does not determine its size. In order to compare two positive decimals, start at the leftmost digit and compare corresponding values in the same place value while moving from left to right. If place values differ, the decimal with the larger value is the larger of the two numbers. For instance, 2.145 is larger than 2.14. Note that a 0 can be added to 2.14 to make it 2.140.

The decimal 2.145 has a larger value in the thousandths place, making it the larger number. In order to compare two negative decimals, the same process is used, but the number with the first smaller digit while moving from left to right is the larger of the two decimals. For instance, -7.8934 is larger than -7.8939 because the 4 in the ten-thousands place in -7.8934 is smaller than the 9 in the ten-thousandths place of -7.8939.

Rounding decimals can be helpful when estimating. In order to round a decimal to a certain place value, first locate the value in the decimal that corresponds to that place value. Then look at the digit to its right. If the digit to the right is 5 or greater, increase the original digit by 1. If the digit to the right is 4 or less, leave the original digit alone. Finally, drop all digits to the right of the original digit. For example, rounding 6.783 to the nearest hundredth place results in 6.78. The 8 is in the hundredths place, and the value to its right, the 3, is 4 or less, so the original digit does not change. The same number 6.783 rounded to the nearest tenth place is 6.8. The 7 in the tenths place increases by 1 to become 9 because the value to its right is 5 or greater.

Estimating can be extremely helpful when dealing with money. Suppose someone goes to the store and wants to purchase items that cost the following amounts: $4.25, $5.65, $8.21, and $10.89. In this case, rounding each amount to the nearest dollar would help estimate the total: $4 + $6 + $8 + 11=$29, which is also the exact sum. Estimating can also be helpful when multiplying and dividing decimals, which are difficult operations to complete mentally. For instance, in order to estimate the product 7.79×4, round the decimal to the nearest whole number. Therefore, its estimate is $8 \times 4 = 32$. This value is close to the exact product of 31.16. Also, consider the quotient $90.267 \div 3.1$. If a calculator were not handy, this division could be easily estimated by rounding each value to the nearest whole number first. A good estimate is therefore,

$$90 \div 3 = 30$$

This result is close to the exact amount, which is 29.1183871.

Ratios and Proportions

A **ratio** is equal to the quotient of two different quantities. Specifically, the ratio of x to y can be written in fraction form as $\frac{x}{y}$ or in colon notation as $x: y$. Therefore, the ratio of 5 to 7 can be written as $\frac{5}{7}$ or $5: 7$. Typically in mathematics, ratios are written in fraction form so that they can be used in operations such as addition, subtraction, multiplication, and division. Ratios appear in everyday life. For example, a classroom might have 11 boys and 15 girls. The ratio of boys to girls could be written as $\frac{11}{15}$. Just as with all other types of fractions, ratios expressed as fractions should be written in simplified form. For instance, the ratio of 4 to 10 is expressed in simplified form as $\frac{4}{10} = \frac{2}{5}$, and the ratio of 15 to 100 is written in simplified form as:

$$\frac{15}{100} = \frac{3}{20}$$

Recall that simplified form, or lowest terms, means that the numerator and denominator do not share any common factors other than 1.

If a ratio compares two different types of amounts with two different measurements, the quantity is referred to as a **rate**. For instance, if an employee made $45 working 4 hours at his job, the rate is written in fraction form as $\frac{\$45}{4 \ hours}$. Notice that the units in the numerator are different than the units in the denominator. Sometimes it is helpful to convert the rate to a decimal by division, rounding if necessary. By dividing $45 by 4, the rate $11.25/hour is calculated. This quantity is the employee's hourly wage. Other common rates that appear in everyday situations include miles per gallon (mpg), miles per hour (mph), and dollars per pound ($/lb.).

A **unit price** is a type of ratio that describes the ratio of the cost of an item to the number of total units. For instance, if a 6-pack of soda is sold for $4.99, the cost of a single can of soda is its unit cost. In order to find the unit cost, divide the total cost by the number of units, which in the soda example is 6. Therefore, $\frac{\$4.99}{6 \ cans} = \$0.83$ per can, which is rounded to the nearest cent.

Problems that involve determining the best buy for different sizing and pricing options involve determining the unit cost for each option. For instance, if a medium pizza had 10 slices of pizza and was sold for $12, and a large pizza had 15 slices of pizza and was sold for $17, determining the cost per slice for each size would show which pizza was the better deal. The cost per slice in the medium pizza is $\frac{\$12}{10 \ slices} = \$1.20$ per slice, and the cost per slice in the large pizza is $\frac{\$17}{15 \ slices} = \$1.13$ per slice, rounded to the nearest cent.

Therefore, the large pizza is the better deal because the price per slice is lower.

When two sets of two numbers have the same ratio, they are proportional. For instance, the equation $\frac{5}{9} = \frac{15}{27}$ shows that the sets 5 & 9 and 15 & 27 are proportional. Notice that the fraction $\frac{15}{27}$ is equal to $\frac{5}{9}$ when it is written in simplified form. The equation is called a **proportion** and is read as "5 is to 9 as 15 is to 27." It is true that when two fractions are equal, their cross products are also equal. For this example, the cross products are 5×27 and 9×15, which are both equal to 135. Therefore, to determine if two pairs of numbers are proportional, show that their cross products are equal. For example, consider the two pairs of numbers 4.1 & 5.6 and 0.8 & 1.2.

If they were proportional, the following equation would be true:

$$\frac{4.1}{5.6} = \frac{0.8}{1.2}$$

The first cross product is $4.1(1.2) = 4.92$. The second cross product is $5.6(0.8) = 4.48$. Therefore, because their cross products are not equal, the pairs of numbers are not proportional.

Cross products can also be used to solve proportions that have missing values. If there is a variable in a proportion, such as an x, equate the cross products of the proportion and then divide by the number multiplied times the variable to find the solution. For instance, consider the proportion:

$$\frac{x}{14} = \frac{10}{6}$$

The variable x is the unknown quantity, and in order to solve the equation, first, find the cross products and set them equal. This step results in the equation $6x = 140$. Then, divide 140 by 6 to obtain the solution $\frac{140}{6}$, which is $\frac{70}{3}$ in lowest terms. In order to check the answer when solving a proportion, plug the solution back into the original proportion and see if the cross products are equal. For this example, $\frac{\frac{70}{3}}{14} = \frac{10}{6}$ is true because both cross products are equal to 140. Therefore, the solution is correct, and no mistakes were made when solving the original equation.

Proportions can also include decimals and fractions. In either case, the solution steps are the same. For instance, consider the proportion $\frac{0.15}{0.6} = \frac{t}{0.76}$, where the missing value is the variable t. Equating the cross products results in the equation $0.114 = 0.6t$. Then dividing 0.114 by 0.6 calculates the solution $t = 0.19$. For an example containing fractions, consider the proportion:

$$\frac{15}{\frac{1}{3}} = \frac{32}{x}$$

Equating the cross products results in the equation $15x = \frac{32}{3}$. Dividing by 15 gives the solution $x = \frac{32}{45}$.

Proportions have many applications in everyday life and in geometry, and they can also be used to make predictions. For instance, let's say a truck driver drove 4,638 miles in 4 days. A proportion could be used to determine approximately how many miles he would drive in 9 days. First, let m equal the approximate number of miles that he would drive in 9 days, which is the unknown quantity. Then, the problem is translated to a proportion. Each side of the proportion is the ratio of distance to time where the distance is in the numerator of the fraction and the time, in days, is in the denominator of the fraction.

Therefore, the corresponding proportion is:

$$\frac{4638}{4} = \frac{m}{9}$$

Next, the proportion is solved by equating the cross products. This step results in the equation $41742 = 4m$. Dividing by 4 calculates the solution $m = 10435.5$. Therefore, using the same ratio of miles driven per day, the truck driver is estimated to drive 10,435.5 miles in 9 days.

Proportions also have applications that relate to estimating populations. For instance, consider the scenario where a researcher wants to estimate how many deer are in a national park. One day, she goes to the forest and tags 150 deer. On another day, she locates 56 deer and sees that 14 of them have been tagged. She can use this rate to estimate how many total deer are in the forest by assuming the rate of tagged deer to untagged deer that she caught is equal to the rate of tagged deer to untagged deer in the forest. In order to build the proportion, let d = the number of total deer in the forest, which is the unknown quantity. Therefore, the proportion is:

$$\frac{14}{56} = \frac{150}{d}$$

Equating cross products results in the equation $14d = 8400$. Dividing by 14 gives the solution $d = 600$. Therefore, the researcher has used proportions to estimate that there are 600 deer in this forest.

A geometric application that uses proportions involves similar shapes. Two shapes that are similar have corresponding sides that have the same ratio. For instance, the following triangles are similar.

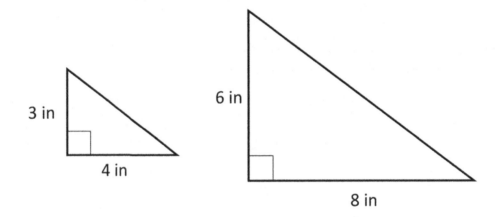

The sides with lengths 6 inches and 3 inches are known as **corresponding sides** because they are in the same place in both triangles. Also, the sides with lengths 8 inches and 4 inches are corresponding sides. Notice that the ratios between corresponding sides are equal:

$$\frac{8}{4} = \frac{6}{3} = 2$$

Proportions can be used to find missing side lengths if two figures are known to be **similar**. Consider the following example:

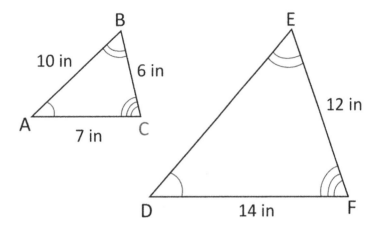

The two triangles are similar because the corresponding sides have equal ratios. Notice that for the given corresponding sides, $\frac{14}{7} = \frac{12}{6} = 2$. This ratio can be used to determine the missing side length. Because the corresponding side length to the unknown length in the smaller triangle is 10 inches, and the ratio of corresponding sides is 2, multiply 10 times 2 to determine that 20 inches is the missing side length in the larger triangle. A proportion can also be defined to determine this side length by using either set of corresponding sides. Let x be equal to the missing side length. Therefore,

$$\frac{10}{x} = \frac{6}{12}$$

Notice that the side lengths from the smaller triangle are in the numerator, and the side lengths from the larger triangle are in the denominator. Equating cross products results in the equation $120 \ inches = 6x$. Finally, dividing by 6 gives the solution $x = 20 \ inches$, which is the missing side length.

Household Measures

A common application of mathematics in everyday life is conversion between different units of measurement. The length of a line segment is commonly measured in inches (in), feet (ft), yards (yd), or miles (mi). There are 12 inches in 1 foot, 36 inches in 1 yard, 3 feet in 1 yard, and 5,280 feet in 1 mile.

Other symbols can be used to represent feet and inches. For example, 15 inches can be abbreviated as 15″ and 18 feet can be abbreviated as 15′. These units of length are known as American or English units because they are used in North America, and at one point, they were used in Great Britain. Most other countries use the metric system.

In order to convert between American units of length, one must recognize whether the conversion is from a longer to a shorter length or from a shorter to a longer length. If the conversion is from a longer to a shorter length, such as yards to inches, multiplication of the conversion factor is used. For example, let's convert 16 yards to inches. Because 36 inches = 1 yard, multiply 16 times 36 to obtain $16(36) = 576$ inches. Therefore, 16 yards are equal to 576 inches.

This process can also be thought of in terms of multiplying by a form of 1, known as a unit factor. There are two-unit factors that relate inches to yards:

$$\frac{1\ yard}{36\ inches} \text{ and } \frac{36\ inches}{1\ yard}$$

To convert yards to inches, multiply the original amount times the unit factor with the desired units in the numerator. Therefore,

$$16 \text{ yards } \left(\frac{36 \text{ inches}}{1 \text{ yard}}\right) = 16(36) \text{ inches} = 576 \text{ inches}$$

Notice that because there was a measurement of yards in both the numerator and denominator, both of those units cancelled out, and the length was left in terms of inches.

If the conversion is from a shorter length to a longer length, division is used. Let's convert 912 inches to feet. Because 12 inches = 1 ft, divide 912 by 12 to obtain $912 \div 12 = 76$ feet. Therefore, 912 inches is equal to 76 feet. A unit factor can also be used. There are two unit factors that relate inches to feet: $\frac{1\ feet}{12\ inches}$ and $\frac{12\ inches}{1\ feet}$. In order to convert inches to feet, multiply the original amount times the unit factor with feet in the numerator. Therefore,

$$912 \text{ inches } \left(\frac{1 \text{ feet}}{12 \text{ inches}}\right) = \frac{912 \text{ feet}}{12} = 76 \text{ feet}$$

The **metric system**, which is used in most countries across the globe, is based on powers of 10. Because of this fact, conversion between the different measurements is a somewhat simple process. In terms of length, the basic unit of measurement in the metric system is the meter (m), which is approximately equal to 1.09 yards. Other units of length in the metric system are multiples of a meter. For instance, one kilometer (km) is equal to 1,000 meters, one centimeter (cm) is equal to one $\frac{1}{100}$ of a meter, and one millimeter (mm) is equal to one $\frac{1}{1000}$ of a meter.

Miles are used the American system, and kilometers are used in the metric system; one kilometer is approximately equal to 0.6 of a mile. Inches are used in the American system, and centimeters are used in the metric system; one centimeter is approximately equal to 0.4 of an inch.

Conversions from one metric unit to another can be performed in a similar manner as discussed previously, with multiplication, division, or unit factors; however, the easiest method involves moving decimal places. Because the metric system is based on powers of ten, each place in the following table has a value one-tenth of the quantity to its left and 10 times the quantity to its right.

Length	Weight	Volume
1 km = 1,000 m	1 kg = 1,000 g	1 kL = 1,000 L
1 m = .001 km	1 g = .001 kg	1 L = .001 kL
1 m = 100 cm	1 g = 100 cg	1 L = 100 cL
1 cm = .01 m	1 cg = .01 g	1 cL = .01 L
1 m = 1,000 mm	1 g = 1,000 mg	1 L = 1,000 mL
1 mm = .001 m	1 mg = .001 g	1 mL = .001 L

Moving one place value either to the left or the right corresponds to moving one decimal place in the original measurement. Let's convert 50 meters (m) to decimeters (dm). Because a decimeter is one-tenth of a meter and is to the right of a meter on the chart, move the decimal one place to the right. Because there is only one zero in the original quantity, an additional zero must be added. Therefore, 50 m is equal to 500 dm. This process is the same as multiplying times 10. To convert 50 m to millimeters, move the decimal three place values to the right, resulting in 50,000 mm. The measurement of 50 m can also be converted to units with larger lengths. To convert 50 m to decameters (dam), move the decimal one digit to the left, resulting in 5 dam. To convert 50 m to km, move the decimal place three digits to the left, resulting in 0.05 km.

There are also conversions that allow American units to be converted to metric conversions and vice versa.

Measures of capacity answer the question how much of a liquid is in a container. In American units, common measures of capacity are those found in the kitchen, such as fluid ounces, cups, pints, and gallons. One gallon (gal) is equal to 4 quarts (qt). One quart is equal to 2 pints (pt.). One pint is equal to 2 cups, and it also equals to 16 fluid ounces (fl oz). Therefore, one cup is equal to 8 fluid ounces. Fluid ounces are often shortened to just ounces, or oz. Conversions are completed in the same manner as units of length. Unit fractions can be used, or sometimes it is easier just to multiply or divide.

For instance, let's convert 18 gallons to ounces. There is not a direct conversion between gallons and ounces. Therefore, intermediate steps must be used. One gallon is equal to 4 quarts, so 18 gallons are equal to $18 \times 4 = 72$ quarts. One quart is equal to 2 pints, so 72 quarts are equal to $72 \times 2 = 144$ pints. One pint is equal to 2 cups, so 144 pints are equal to $144 \times 2 = 288$ cups. Finally, 1 cup is equal to 8 oz, so 288 cups are equal to:

$$288 \times 8 = 2,304 \text{ oz}$$

In metric units, volume in terms of capacity is measured in liters (L). Just as with meters, the same metric prefixes are used with liters. In addition to liters, milliliters (mL) are also a commonly used measure of capacity. To convert from liters to milliliters, move the decimal point three places to the right. To convert from milliliters to liters, move the decimal point three places to the left.

One liter is equal to 1,000 cubic centimeters (cm^3), which is a measure of volume. The following relationships are helpful when working with drug dosages: 1 L = 1,000 mL = 1,000 cm^3 and 0.001 L = 1 mL = 1 cm^3. In the medical community, cubic centimeters are often abbreviated as cc.

American units of weight are measured in pounds (lbs.), ounces (oz), and tons (T). The amount of 1 pound is equal to 16 ounces, and 1 ton is equal to 2,000 pounds. Therefore, to convert pounds to ounces, multiply the number of pounds by 16. To convert ounces to pounds, divide the number of ounces by 16. To convert tons to pounds, multiply the number of tons times 2,000, and to convert pounds to tons, divide the number of pounds by 2,000. Metric units of weight are normally referred to as units of **mass**, where *weight* and *mass* are used interchangeably. However, they do not exactly mean the same thing because the **mass** of an item never changes, but an item's **weight** changes depending on how close it is to the earth's center of gravity.

The gram (g) is the basic unit of mass in the metric system, and it has a mass of 1 cm^3 of water. Just like with liters and meters, the metric prefixes are used with grams. The most commonly used metric units of mass are kilogram (kg), gram (g), and milligram (mg). Converting back and forth between metric units of mass involves moving decimal places in the same manner as with liters and meters.

To convert to a smaller unit of mass, move the decimal place to the right. To convert to a larger unit of mass, move the decimal place to the left. For example, to convert 4,500 mg to g, move the decimal place three places to the left. Therefore, 4,500 mg is equal to 4.5 g.

Finally, temperature is a commonly used household measure. In America, Fahrenheit is used to measure temperature while in most other countries, Celsius is used. Celsius is also utilized in science applications. To convert a quantity in Celsius to Fahrenheit, use the formula $F = \frac{9}{5}C + 32$, where C represents the temperature in Celsius, and F represents the temperature in Fahrenheit. To convert a quantity in Fahrenheit to Celsius, use the formula:

$$C = \frac{5}{9}(F - 32)$$

The boiling point of water in Fahrenheit is 212°, and the boiling point of water in Celsius is 100°.

General Math Facts

Roman numerals are a system of numbers stemming from the ancient Roman numeric system. The symbols used in this system are I, V, X, L, C, D, and M, and they stand for 1, 5, 10, 50, 100, 500, and 1,000, respectively. All the symbols and the numbers that they represent can be seen in the following table.

Roman Numeral	Numerical Value
I	1
V	5
X	10
L	50
C	100
D	500
M	1000

When Roman numerals are combined, in some instances, they are added. For instance, III is equal to 3, VI is equal to 6, XX is equal to 20, and DCI is equal to 601. Therefore, when a smaller symbol appears after a larger symbol, the symbols are added. However, if a smaller symbol appears before a larger symbol, the smaller value is subtracted from the larger value. For instance, IV is equal to 4, and IX is equal to 9. As a rule, no more than three symbols can be used in a row. For example, IIII is a case where the Roman numerals are used incorrectly, and the proper way to express the number 4 is IV.

Large numbers can be converted to Roman numerals by breaking the number up into thousands, hundreds, tens, and ones, and writing each number in its equivalent form using the Roman numeral system. For instance, consider the number 2,789. It is broken up into 2,000 + 700 + 80 + 9. The number 2,000 is represented in Roman numerals as MM, while 700 is represented in Roman numerals as DCC. 80 in Roman numerals is LXXX. Finally, 9 is represented in Roman numerals as IX. Combining them in order results in 2,789 = MMDCCLXXXIX.

Typically, time is given in **standard time**, especially if a watch is used to read the time. With standard time, the hours range from 1 to 12, and either a.m. or p.m. is attached if the time is before noon or after noon, respectively. However, another way to express time is by using **military time**, which is a 24-hour clock. With this system, the hours run from 0 to 24, and attaching a.m. or p.m. is unnecessary. The hours 1:00 a.m. to 12:00 p.m. correspond to 01:00 to 12:00 in military time, and the hours 1:00 p.m. to 12:00 a.m. correspond to 13:00 to 0:00 in military time. Therefore, 9:30 am in standard time is 09:30 in military time, and 9:30 p.m. is 21:30 in military time.

Note that a 0 is placed before any hour that is a single digit, which is different from standard time. Any time before noon in standard time is the same numerical value in military time, but the a.m. or p.m. is taken off and the 0 is added. To find the military time for any time after noon in standard time, add 12 hours to the numerical value and drop the a.m. or p.m. Also, sometimes times in military time are written without the colon. Therefore, 9:30 a.m. can be written as 0930, and 3:30 p.m. can be written as 1530.

Calculating drug dosages and solutions is another useful type of conversion process. The ratio and proportion method is a way that allows one to calculate both dosages and solutions. Recall that a **ratio** is equal to a fraction of two quantities with the same units, and a **proportion** is formed when two ratios are set equal. To solve a proportion, use cross-multiplication. Therefore, let's say that a doctor's order to a patient is for them to receive 300 mg of an oral medication one time a day. On this medication label, it states that one tablet of this medication is equal to 75 mg. To find out how many tablets this patient needs daily, use cross-products. Let x be the number of tablets. Therefore,

$$75 \text{ mg} \times x = 300 \text{ mg}$$

Dividing by 75 results in:

$$x = \frac{300}{75} = 4$$

Therefore, 4 tablets need to be given to this patient daily. This ratio and proportion method can also be used when working with liquid oral medications. Let's say that a doctor's order to a patient is for her to receive 75 mg of a cough syrup p.o. once a day. The abbreviation p.o. refers to *per os*, which denotes that the medicine is to be taken orally. In this example, the label on the medicine states that the syrup is 25 mg/ml. To determine how many ml she receives each day, cross-products can be used again. Let x be the unknown quantity of cough syrup. Therefore,

$$25 \frac{\text{mg}}{\text{ml}} \times x = 75 \text{ mg}$$

Dividing both sides by $25 \frac{\text{mg}}{\text{ml}}$ results in $x = 3$ ml. Therefore, 3 ml of the cough syrup need to be administered once daily, orally, to this patient.

Percentages appear in everyday life, and it is important to be able to work with them. A **percentage** is a quantity per hundred. For example, the percentage 65% refers to 65 out of 100, and if 65 out of 100 people voted yes for a levy, one could say that 65% voted yes. Percentages can be converted to decimals by moving the decimal point two digits to the left in the percentage and dropping the percent symbol. For example, 65% is equal to 0.65. Converting a decimal to a percentage involves moving the decimal point two digits to the right. For example, 0.92 is equal to 92%.

Problems that involve percentages typically involve a missing quantity: either the percent, the part, or the whole. For instance, consider the following problem: What is 80% of 110? To determine the answer, convert 80% to decimal form: 0.8. Then, multiply 0.8 times 110 to obtain 88. Therefore 80% of 110 is equal to 88. In this case, the part is 88 and the whole is 110. The part was the missing value. Sometimes the whole can be missing. For instance, consider the following problem: 65% of what number is 39? In this case, the part is 39 and the whole is missing. To find the whole, divide 39 by 0.65, the decimal form of 65%, to obtain 60. Finally, there are problems where the percentage is missing. Consider the following problem: 18 is what percent of 120? To find the percentage, divide 18 by 120 and convert the decimal to a percentage. Therefore,

$$18 \div 120 = 0.15 = 15\%$$

A variable is a symbol for a number that is unknown. Common variables used in mathematics are x and y. Combinations of variables with integers and operations such as addition, subtraction, multiplication, and division are known as algebraic expressions. Examples of algebraic expressions are $2x + 7$, $4x^2 - 9$, and $6x^4 - 9y^2$. Variables can be substituted into algebraic expressions in order to evaluate them. For example, if $x = 2$ and $y = 3$, $6x^4 - 9y^2$ can be evaluated. Substituting 2 for x and 3 for y results in:

$$6(2)^4 - 9(3)^2$$

The order of operations is used to obtain:

$$6(16) - 9(9) = 96 - 81 = 15$$

The order of operations is a set of rules that defines the order in which to complete mathematical operations correctly. **PEMDAS** is the mnemonic device attached to the order of operations, which adheres to the following precedence: Parentheses (or other grouping symbols), Exponents, Multiplication and Division (from left to right), and Addition and Subtraction (from left to right). In the previous example, the exponents were evaluated first, then the multiplication, then the subtraction.

An equation is different than an expression. An **equation** consists of a combination of variables and integers, basically an algebraic expression, plus an equals sign. Some examples of equations are $4x + 7 = 1$, $y = 5x + 2$, $4(x + 9) = y$, and:

$$3x - 8y - 9 = 0$$

An equation in one variable can be solved. A solution to an equation in one variable is comprised of the value that when plugged into the variable, makes the equation true. A true equation has values that are equal on both sides of the equals sign. The goal in solving an equation is to isolate the variable on one side of the equals sign, resulting in a real number on the other side of the equals sign. Basically, whatever operations exist in the expression, the opposite needs to be completed on both sides in order to isolate the variable. Consider the equation:

$$5x + 20 = 100$$

In order to isolate the variable x, subtract 20 from both sides. Therefore, $5x + 20 - 20 = 100 - 20$, or $5x = 80$. Then, divide both sides by 5, resulting in $\frac{5}{5}x = \frac{80}{5}$, or $x = 14$. The solution can be checked by substituting it into the original equation to see if it makes a true equation as follows:

$$5(14) + 20 = 80 + 20 = 100$$

If there are parentheses in the equation, they must first be cleared in order to solve the equation. They can be cleared by using the distributive property. Consider the following expression: $4(x + 3)$. In order to remove the parentheses, "distribute" the 4 throughout the parentheses, meaning multiply it times each term inside the parentheses. Therefore, an equivalent expression is $4x + 12$. Now, consider the equation:

$$10(x - 6) = 90$$

In order to solve for x, first distribute the 10 to clear the parentheses. This step results in:

$$10x - 30 = 90$$

Then, add 30 to both sides, resulting in $10x - 30 + 30 = 90 + 30$, or $10x = 120$. Finally, divide both sides by 10 to obtain $\frac{10}{10}x = \frac{120}{10}$, or $x = 12$. Again, this solution can be plugged in to the original equation to see if it makes a true equation in order to check the answer.

Reading Comprehension

Identifying the Main Idea

When identifying the **main idea** of a passage or paragraph, readers should look for not just the **topic** of the paragraph (what the paragraph is about), but also what is being written about the topic itself. In short, the **topic** is the who or what. Who is being discussed? What is being discussed? Both the topic *and* what is being said about it are the **main idea**.

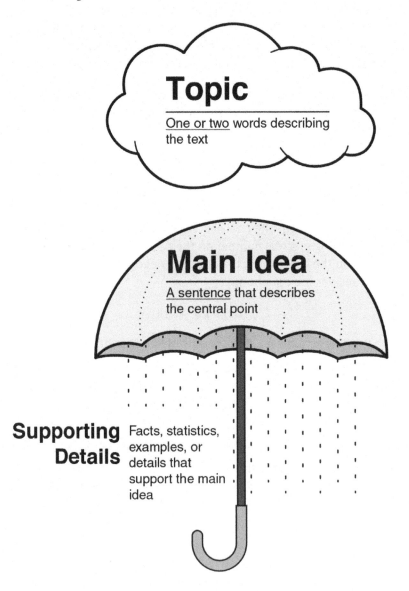

Let's look at an example:

John is incredibly tall and is, therefore, an exceptional basketball player.

In that sentence, John is the subject or topic, but the main idea, what the sentence is really about, is that he is an exceptional basketball player. From this example, it's clear that the main idea of a sentence, paragraph, or passage, is about more than who or what (the topic); it's also why the topic is being discussed. What is the writer trying to communicate? The main idea is provided through the details.

So, to identify the main idea of a passage or paragraph, readers must look for both the topic *and* the **supporting details**, which tell us more about the topic. The main idea answers "Why is this important?"

Supporting details provide readers with facts or information about the topic. In the example above, one supporting detail is that *John is incredibly tall*. From that detail, readers are led to the detail regarding his athletic ability.

Supporting details can also include examples or comparisons as well as reasons and other logical connections between the topic and main idea. In instances like this, it can be more difficult to identify the subject and main idea because it may not be stated clearly. Instead, it is implied. So, the reader must be able to identify the supporting details and deduce the main idea of the paragraph based on the information provided. Fortunately, finding the topic and main idea should be easy. There are a few tricks to identifying both.

First, the topic is usually brought up in the first sentence of a passage. To communicate clearly, the writer should announce the subject to a reader from the start. The first paragraph of a passage is often one of the best places to begin determining the topic and main idea of a piece of writing. The same information can also typically be found in the closing paragraph, where a writer is likely summarizing the points and main idea. Throughout the passage, supporting details may repeat the main idea or the writer's point. What conclusions can a reader draw throughout the piece based on the supporting details? Does the writer use repetition throughout to emphasize their main point?

If a reader can summarize the passage in a way that reflects its meaning and agrees with the writer's own thoughts, then the main idea is likely clear. Another trick to test comprehension is to imagine a question that would be answered by the paragraph. For example, if the paragraph is about the history of baseball (that's the topic), and the supporting details reveal facts, milestones, and anecdotes about baseball's importance during difficult times in U.S. history, one could say the paragraph answers the question "How did baseball become known as America's pastime?"

This is the beginning of Shirley Chisolm's Presidential Candidacy Announcement in 1972:

> I stand before you today as a candidate for the Democratic nomination for the presidency of the United States of America.
> I am not the candidate of Black America, although I am Black and proud.
> I am not the candidate of the women's movement of this country, although I am a woman and I'm equally proud of that.
> I am not the candidate of any political bosses or fat cats or special interests.
> I stand here now without endorsements from many big-name politicians or celebrities or any other kind of prop. I do not intend to offer to you the tired and glib clichés, which for too long have been [an] accepted part of our political life.
> I am the candidate of the people of America.

One reason this is a great example is that, in the very first sentence, we see the **topic**, that she is a *Democratic candidate*. However, we also see other methods used to reveal the main idea and the focus of the rest of her speech. We get **supporting details** about who she is (a Black woman not beholden to political party or donors) and how she has been identified both in the press and within the party.

Further, the repetition of these ideas reinforces her main point. In other words, she says I am not just these things (the supporting details) which instead tell listeners who she is. The **main idea** of this passage (and of her speech) is how she is a candidate for *all* Americans. If we look back at the strategies discussed, one could ask "Who was Shirley Chisolm?" and this paragraph, in part, answers that. We see the topic come up in the first sentence. Repetition emphasizes her main point. She concludes by stating the main point.

Finding Meaning of Words using Context Clues

Very often, in the course of reading articles, research papers, and textbooks, readers come across unfamiliar words. Conventional wisdom suggests using a dictionary to learn the definition, but most readers are able to figure out what a word means simply by the context within the text. In other words, the sentences, phrases, and words that come before and after the unknown word help readers know what the unknown word means. These are referred to as **context clues**, and there are several types that are beneficial to improving one's reading comprehension and fluency.

- **Definition/Restatement**: Simply put, this means that immediately following the word in question, the writer includes a definition of the word or restates the idea using different vocabulary. For example: *The surgery would require placement of multiple hemostats, a tool used to control bleeding, prior to ligation.* In this case, the word *hemostat* is defined, or its meaning is restated, immediately following its use.

- **Example:** Sometimes a writer will provide an example of the word in the same, or in a nearby, sentence to clarify the meaning. For example: *Sanitoriums, such the Maryland Tuberculosis Sanitorium, were a popular medical mitigation strategy for nearly one hundred years.* In this example, readers may be unfamiliar with *sanitoriums*, but the example, especially because it includes Tuberculosis in the title, provides information for the reader regarding what type of facility it was.

- **Synonym:** Synonyms are words that share the same meaning. Thus, this strategy relies upon the inclusion of a word that means the same thing as the unknown word but used elsewhere in the text. It is similar to the definition/restatement strategy. For example: *People with alopecia, or baldness, may first exhibit symptoms in childhood, but many don't see hair loss until their thirties.* In this example, the initial word *alopecia*, is replaced with a synonym almost immediately afterwards, which should inform a reader that it means baldness.

- **Comparison:** These types of context clues, much like the others, use words or phrases that have a similar meaning, but readers should also look for comparison words/phrases such as: *similar to, like, as, also, resembling, much like*, etc. Essentially, readers should look for words/phrases that indicate one thing is being compared to another. For example: *Otolaryngologists, like all ENT doctors, can diagnosis and treat for head and neck issues as well.* In this example, the word *like* indicates a comparison between otolaryngologists and ear, nose, and throat doctors.

- **Contrast/Antonym**: Contrast, or antonym, clues appear when the writer uses a word that means the opposite of the word in question or is vastly different in an essential way, allowing a reader to determine the meaning of the unfamiliar word. For example: *One of the side effects of the medication was listed as halitosis; however, George kept his breath fresh with peppermint gum.* In this example, readers should be clued in by the word *however,* which suggests contrast. Because what follows that key word is the opposite of the meaning of halitosis, readers can surmise that halitosis means bad breath.

- **Cause and Effect:** In this type of context clue, readers will be able to define the unknown word through its relationship to other words in the text, specifically a **cause** (what happens) and **effect** (the result). For example: *When the patient's head hit the windshield during a car accident, it resulted in severe injury, including a subdural hematoma, which required the patient to undergo a brain CT scan.* In this example, even if readers are unfamiliar with the term *subdural hematoma*, they should be able to determine that the accident caused a severe head injury, and this further necessitated a scan.

- **Inference**: This is, perhaps, the strategy readers think of most often when they think of context clues. An **inference** is an educated guess the reader makes based on other descriptors or clues elsewhere in the text. Sometimes, this means a reader may need to read a few sentences prior to being able to define the unfamiliar word. For example: *Though no one was certain how the altercation in the lobby started, hospital staff had to call security. Prior to the arrival of the guards, the two men had destroyed a chair, broken a window, and bloodied each other's faces.* In this example, a reader might be unfamiliar with the world *altercation*. The sentence after describes a fight, so the reader can infer that *altercation* means fight.

- **Lists/Categorization**: This type of context clue includes the unknown word in a list or category of similar words so that a reader can determine meaning. For example: *The doctor mentioned that narcotics were likely going to be prescribed for the patient and might include one of the following: Oxycodone, Tramadol, or Hydrocodone.* In this example, a reader might be unfamiliar with how the term *narcotic* is used in the medical profession. The list that follows includes regulated pain killers that are prescribed for patients, which clarifies the meaning/intent of narcotics in this context.

- **Mood/Tone:** In this case, the unknown word must match the tone the writer exhibits. For example: *The nursery staff was jubilant at the news of a safe delivery of a healthy baby to a fellow nurse after a high-risk pregnancy.* In the example, words like *safe* and *healthy* convey a positive tone/mood in that these would be things to celebrate and feel happy and excited about, which is what *jubilant* means.

- **Experience:** Sometimes, in the course of reading, a word's meaning is clear only because, in the reader's own life, there has been a similar experience or feeling. Because a reader can relate to the experience, the meaning of an unfamiliar word becomes clear. For example: *On his first day of nursing school, Mitchell was discombobulated. There were books and scrubs and instruments to buy, classes to find, names to remember, homework, schedules, and on top of all that were his responsibilities at home.* For some readers, the experiences of day one of nursing school may remind them of how they felt on a first day of school, which can help them understand that *discombobulated* means confused and disoriented.

- **Structure/Analysis:** This type of context clue is more useful in certain fields. In particular, the medical field, which relies fairly heavily upon the use of Latin language roots. In this type of context clue, the structure of the word itself provides its own context clue. For example: *The patient was scheduled for a cholecystectomy after multiple surgeries to remove gallstones.* In this example, analysis of the structure of the word *cholecystectomy* reveals the -ectomy root, which means to remove something, as in mastectomy, appendectomy, etc. The analysis and other contextual clues (*gallstones*) enable a reader to figure out that *cholecystectomy* is the removal of the gallbladder.

Passage Comprehension

One goal of written text is to convey a message, so the reader is as much a critical component of the text as the writer. This is because the message is unsuccessful if the recipient fails to understand the main idea, interpret the tone, grasp the main points, and understand how and why a conclusion was drawn. In other words, a reader must comprehend the text.

Using Logic and Reason

One of the first steps of comprehension is the use of logic and reason in writing, sometimes called **critical thinking skills**. The flow of a text is established by rules of argumentation, which require a writer to make a claim (**thesis**) and support that claim with data and information. For readers, the goal is to be able to identify the claim being made as well as the key data points (called **grounds**), and any reasoning behind them (sometimes called **warrants**), so that a reader can determine if the argument being made is valid.

Let's look at an example:

Claim: The hospital will close soon.

Grounds (evidence):

- The hospital is no longer accepting new patients.
- Surgeries were transferred.
- The fifth floor was completely shut down due to disrepair.

Warrant (reasoning): To stay open, a hospital needs to admit new patients, to perform its role in the community, and to be kept up to code.

Based on the evidence and the reasoning, it is logical to conclude that the hospital will close soon. This is how logic and reason should work in an argument. However, a reader should be aware that the organization of the argument may not always be linear. A writer may have multiple claims, each with its own evidence. Further, each piece of evidence may include multiple data points or sources for support, and the claim may not be stated clearly or explicitly. It is the reader's job to bring their own comprehension skills to understand and analyze the text.

Analyzing the Passage

As noted above, reading is not passive. Readers have a responsibility to engage with a text, and often that involves analyzing what the passage means, why it is significant, and how it impacts a reader's life, work, or even the world at large. This is sometimes also called **textual analysis**.

One of the first steps in analysis is just to read the passage. Oftentimes, readers want to jump right in and start taking notes, answering questions, and applying information, but each of these activities only allows the reader to address small sections of the text rather than the text as a whole. The other advantage of reading the entire passage through first is that confusing or complicated portions or ideas in the passage may become clearer as more information is provided. Therefore, the first strategy is to read the full text.

The next step would be to mark up the text or take notes. This may include underlining important information; noting claims, evidence, and warrants in the margins; asking questions in the margins; connecting ideas, claims, or information to one's own experiences; and making connections to the text in general, which may even involve physically drawing arrows or lines between connected ideas or themes.

Once these items have been identified, the reader can establish the main idea, claim, and evidence, and analyze them for sound reasoning. If there are questions that seem unanswered, perhaps the answer is elsewhere in the text. Reader should draw their own conclusions and ideas about the text. Often, this is also where readers develop their own questions for further research or exploration.

It's important to remember that reading this way, especially at first, isn't a fast process. In the case of test taking, one tip is to read the passage, then read the questions, and on a second read through, keep the questions in mind. This way a reader can more easily identify some of the information being sought, identify key points, and read with a deeper purpose. Alternatively, the questions can be skimmed prior to reading the passage initially.

Reading Speed

The best way to improve one's reading speed is to read more. Barring that option, there are a few tips and tricks to help test takers read faster without compromising comprehension.

1. *Try scanning.* This technique should be used regardless of whether one is trying to read quickly or not. This involves previewing the text and scanning for headings, sub-headings, words in bold, numbers or statistics, abbreviations, etc. In a textbook, this process might also include looking at any pictures or diagrams. Remember, the key here is not reading every word but to scan in the same way someone would skim a menu at a new restaurant.

2. *Read phrases rather than words.* One of the ways we can speed up reading is by not reading each and every word on the page, but instead, reading phrases or, in some cases, reading beyond the small words (*the, and, an, is, of*, etc.). Our brains have the capacity to fill in the blanks for us by using pattern recognition. Learn to recognize phrasing patterns and reading by phrases becomes easier.

3. *Avoid sub-vocalization.* Students often learn to read by reading aloud, so the habit becomes to continue this silently by saying or mouthing the words as we read. Learning to avoid this will also increase reading speed.

4. *Read with purpose and focus.* One of the primary causes of slow reading is needing to go back and re-read portions because the reader lost focus or didn't know what information was needed from the text. As discussed above, this is why reading (or better yet, scanning) the questions after a first read through is helpful when taking a test.

Author's Purpose and Tone

One great way to help a reader understand a passage is to answer the question "Why did the writer write this?" There are many reasons a writer may write: to entertain, inform, persuade, self-express, or even a combination of two or more of these. Understanding which of these motives is the primary goal informs the reading process and helps a reader identify main ideas, claims, and the organizational structure that reveals that information.

Tone often reveals purpose. **Tone** is the attitude the writer has towards the subject and how that is conveyed. Tone is often revealed through language choices (formal, descriptive, factual, sarcastic, detailed, vague, abstract) and the details the writer chooses to include.

Mood also reveals purpose. **Mood** is how the reader feels as they read the passage.

Informative texts are often detailed and written in plain language (or the language of the specific field/industry). The mood of an informative text is usually rather serious and typically lacks other emotions. That's not to say that informative writing can't be entertaining. Many nonfiction books and documentary films rely on the crossover appeal, but as noted above, there may be more than one purpose. Persuasive or entertaining writing will often rely on evoking one or multiple emotions in a reader.

While reading a passage, ask questions about tone and mood, as the answers will reveal quite a bit about purpose. Once a reader understands why a writer is delivering a message, it becomes easier to discover what the writer hopes a reader will take from it.

Remembering Important Information

One of the biggest struggles readers report is an inability to remember or retain the information needed. Some of the strategies already discussed will certainly help, but below are a few other tips to consider. One of those tips, of course, is to read more. Reading is a skill and, like all others, requires practice. The more one reads, the better they get at it. If a reader struggles with comprehending informative texts, that's where they should focus their effort.

1. *Create connections.* Students who make connections to the text they are reading are more likely to remember what they read. These connections don't need to be academic in nature. A reader can choose to remember something personal or to make a connection to a personal experience or their prior knowledge. Such connections create a pathway in the brain that makes the new information easier to remember.

2. *Use repetition.* This can take the form of writing notes or re-reading passages, sentences, or phrases. If something is repeated (for example, a favorite song), it is easier to remember, and the same is true for text. Readers may want to mark sections to revisit.

3. *Take notes.* There's no wrong way to take notes. What works for one reader or learner may not work for another. Notes can be as simple as one word to trigger a connection or a full sentence that summarizes the point one is trying to remember. The simple act of writing out the idea strengthens the chance of remembering it and/or the connection.

Making Logical Inferences

One key strategy strong readers use to aid comprehension is making inferences. **Inferences** require readers to make connections between pieces of information that may or may not be clearly connected. It's a logical leap with a safety net. That is, it's a leap based on data or information presented and available, rather than a wild guess made without considering any information; thus, it is a *logical* inference. It's important to note that making inferences is process, much like a math problem. A reader observes 1 + 1. A reader infers, based on the data (1 + 1) and the process, even without the equal sign, that the answer is 2. In other words, a conclusion (2) is based on data (1 + 1), our background knowledge (+ means add), and reasoning (put all of it together: 1 + 1 = 2).

One of the most important parts of making this kind of connection is that a reader can also support the conclusion or inference. That is, one can point to the information or data that informs the conclusion. Let's look at an example:

> A man is handed a piece of paper while at the reception desk in a doctor's office. He looks around the desk, pats his coat pocket, and then peers over the reception counter.

Even without him asking for a pen, one can make a logical inference from his behavior that he is looking for a pen. We can do this based on the information gathered from observed behavior and what is already known about that behavior from one's own experience.

First, because people are often asked to complete or sign forms at a doctor's office, we can infer that a similar request was made to the man at the counter. Next, because he appears to be looking for something, we get visual data. Both the visual information and being handed the paper help to inform a conclusion. We take the data presented, add it to what we already know, and draw a conclusion. This is logical inference.

In the example, the pen was never mentioned. The same can happen in a reading or in a text. As a reader, one will be presented with pieces of information and be asked to make connections without explicitly being given all of the information. Inference relies on logic, existing knowledge, and the information or data presented.

When reading, readers should use all the available information presented to help draw conclusions and make connections. They should examine titles, headings, subheadings. They should look for transitional words and phrases that help establish connections between ideas and should look for key words, data, and what conclusions the writer draws. All of these tricks help readers draw conclusions and infer ideas, the hallmark of advanced reading skills.

Vocabulary

The following vocabulary words are official terms for the HESI exam. Test takers should become familiar with their meaning and usage.

- **Abstain (verb):** to not partake or participate in something
  Example: During finals week, Joe abstained from all social activities.

- **Accountable (adjective):** responsible for behavior, choices, or actions
  Example: The OR nurses are accountable to the surgeon.

- **Adhere (verb):** to stick, as in an object or belief system
  Example: Julia adheres to all the rules posted in the staff room and is irritated when others do not.

- **Adverse (adjective):** negative, as in the impact of an action
  Example: Low staff morale has had an adverse effect on patient outcomes.

- **Aegis (noun):** under the protection or with support
  Example: The hospital's latest research program was initiated under the aegis of the affiliated university's institutional review board.

- **Ambivalent (adjective):** having mixed, uncertain, or wavering feelings
  Example: When asked about his preferred nursing focus, Louis was ambivalent.

- **Apply (verb):** to put something forward (often as in a skill or oneself); to exert
  Example: After watching Fiona apply quick thinking to a medical emergency, the EMT asked if she'd considered applying to nursing school.

- **Assent (noun):** agreement or approval
  Example: When the professor asked if all the students understood the expectations, they nodded in assent.

- **Audible (adjective):** able to be sensed through hearing
  Example: At the first incision, the new students watching the operation made an audible gasp.

- **Bacteria (noun):** singular-celled microorganism, some of which can be responsible for various diseases
  Example: It's fairly well known that kitchen sponges are teeming with bacteria, some of which can be dangerous.

- **Bilateral (adjective):** having two sides; derived from *bi,* which means "two" and *lateral* meaning "sides"
  Example: The patient had bilateral knee pain.

- **Cardiac (adjective):** related to the heart
  Example: After an abnormal ECG, Richard was transferred to the cardiac unit.

- **Cavity (noun):** a hollow space surrounded by solid matter
  Example: The dentist told Sarah that failure to fill the cavity in her tooth might result in further decay.

- **Cease (verb):** to stop
  Example: The nurse asked that we cease celebrating the good news, as patients were trying to rest.

- **Chronology (noun):** the arrangement of events or dates in the order of their occurrence
  Example: The doctors were able to create a chronology of the patient's symptoms by backtracking from the current visit.

- **Compensatory (adjective):** designed to offer relief from unwelcome or unpleasant effects of something
- *Example*: The child's medical bills were paid through a compensatory fund provided by the negligent toy company.

- **Concave (adjective):** having hollow or depressed physical characteristics
  Example: The malnourished child's belly was concave.

- **Concise (adjective):** brief and to the point
  Example: Though he needed to cover a lot of information, the presenter was concise.

- **Consistency (noun):** uniformity, often to create equity or stability
  Example: The efficacy of this medication is impacted by the consistency of delivery and dosage.

- **Constrict (verb):** to tighten or restrict
  Example: Anaphylactic shock is extremely dangerous as it causes the throat to constrict, impeding breathing.

- **Contingent (adjective):** dependent on variables or chance
  Example: Shift changes are contingent upon staffing needs and availability.

- **Contraindication (noun):** action (e.g., medical choice) that should be avoided as it will likely cause harm
- *Example*: Due to the patient's heart issues, any surgery is a contraindication despite the reported leg pain.

- **Convulsive (adjective):** creating spasms or seizures
  Example: One of the dangerous side effects of the new drug is that some patients may become convulsive.

- **Cursory (adjective):** quickly, and therefore poorly, executed or examined
  Example: The patient was dissatisfied with what appeared to be a cursory examination.

- **Defecate (verb):** the act of emptying one's bowels
  Example: Post-operative concerns included potential blockages, so nurses were required to monitor the patient's ability to defecate.

- **Deficit (noun):** the amount by which something falls short, whether funds or other measurement
  Example: The hospital faced a deficit resulting in the termination of some services.

- **Depress (verb):** to reduce or lower
  Example: The goal of the team meeting was to depress resistance to the changes.

- **Depth (noun):** measurement of distance often in terms of volume or from top to bottom
  Example: Because they were unsure of the water's depth, the kids were told not to dive off the boat.

- **Deteriorating (adjective):** falling apart; worsening condition
  Example: Despite the doctor's best efforts, the patient's health was deteriorating.

- **Device (noun):** an object designed for a specific purpose, job, or task
  Example: Our hospital was selected as the test facility for Stryker's new device used in dialysis.

- **Diagnosis (noun):** the identified illness or medical issue based on the patient's symptoms or presentation
  Example: After a thorough examination and considerable testing, the doctors were finally able to offer a diagnosis.

- **Dilate (verb):** to open wider or become more open
  Example: To examine one's eyes properly, an ophthalmologist must dilate the patient's pupils.

- **Dilute (verb):** to weaken or reduce strength
  Example: The medication was concentrated, so the instructions told the patient to dilute it with water.

- **Discrete (adjective):** individually detached or separated
  Example: The centrifuge was used to isolate discrete particles so they could be examined individually.

- **Distal (adjective):** anatomically decentralized location or located away from the point of anatomical attachment
  Example: The pain was localized at the distal end of the muscle rather than the point of insertion.

- **Dysfunction (noun):** does not work as intended, whether a system or singular part
  Example: When the patient walked, the doctor noted a limp likely caused by hip dysfunction.

- **Empathy (noun):** one's ability to connect with and understand someone else's feelings
  Example: When delivering bad news to the family, the nurse showed great empathy.

- **Equilibrium (noun):** a state of being balanced
  Example: After surgery, it took the patient quite some time to be able to walk and maintain equilibrium.

- **Etiology (noun):** the root cause of a medical condition
  Example: Once the etiology is determined, the doctors will be better able to create a treatment plan for the patient.

- **Exacerbate (verb):** to amplify a negative situation
  Example: The doctor warned Joseph that continuing to run would exacerbate his knee injury.

- **Expand (verb):** to grow bigger
  Example: Next year, the hospital will be expanding and will include a pediatric oncology unit.

- **Exposure (noun):** having come into contact with something
  Example: Because of the patient's condition, he was told to limit his exposure to cold temperatures.

- **Extension (noun):** an addition to an existing object; to add length or enlarge
  Example: The grabber tool acts as an extension to a patient's arm for items that may be out of reach.

- **External (adjective):** on the outside
  Example: The only remaining injuries from the accident were purely external.

- **Fatal (adjective):** deadly
  Example: The accident left the driver in the hospital and was fatal for the passenger.

- **Fatigue (noun):** exhaustion
  Example: The doctor warned that even if the fever broke, the fatigue would likely continue.

- **Flexion (noun):** the ability to bend, as with appendages of the body
  Example: After the collision on the ice, the player had limited flexion in his knee.

- **Flushed (adjective):** warm to the touch and red in appearance
  Example: The young child had a fever, and his face was flushed.

- **Gastrointestinal (adjective):** involving the stomach and intestines
  Example: Many foodborne illnesses result in gastrointestinal discomfort.

- **Hematologic (adjective):** related to blood
  Example: Anemia and sickle cell disease are hematologic conditions.

- **Hydration (noun):** water absorption to the body or other living system
  Example: Athletes, especially those in warmer climates, need to be mindful of hydration to maintain performance levels.

- **Hygiene (noun):** cleanliness practices that help maintain health and prevent the spread of disease.
  Example: Hand washing is the simplest form of personal hygiene we can practice to maintain health.

- **Impaired (adjective):** limited function
  Example: Those who drive under the influence of alcohol have impaired reaction times.

- **Impending (adjective):** will happen in the near future
  Example: The nurses were quite excited about their impending graduation.

- **Impervious (adjective):** unaffected or unbothered
  Example: While everyone else was nervous, Luther seemed impervious to the pressure of the moment.

- **Imply (verb):** to suggest through insinuation rather than direct communication
  Example: When Alex gave an answer, the look on the instructor's face seemed to imply it was incorrect.

- **Incidence (noun):** prevalence of, often, negative events
  Example: The incidence of infection or even sepsis is of significant concern to hospitals.

- **Infer (verb):** to draw a conclusion through information and reasoning rather than a clear statement
  Example: From the look on the patient's face, the nurse could infer that her level of pain was greater than she let on.

- **Inflamed (adjective):** agitated, as with temperament or appearance; red or swollen
  Example: As a result of the infection, her skin was inflamed.

- **Ingest (verb):** to consume, whether liquid or solid
  Example: After an intestinal blockage, the patient was reluctant to ingest solid foods.

- **Initiate (verb):** to begin
  Example: Upon their arrival, the EMTs were required to initiate live-saving measures.

- **Insidious (adjective):** slow moving, but often nefarious or dangerous
  Example: Lyme disease is insidious, with symptoms gradually growing worse over time.

- **Intact (adjective):** unbroken; complete
  Example: Despite the collision, the car's windshield stayed intact.

- **Internal (adjective):** inside
  Example: The bruising on her skin suggested significant internal bleeding.

- **Invasive (adjective):** non-native and often insidious
  Example: Because of the size of the incision, the surgery was not considered invasive.

- **Kinetic (adjective):** in motion or moving
  Example: Kinetic energy is created through movement, such as running, and can be converted into other types of energy.

- **Labile (adjective):** subject to change
  Example: The patient's mental condition was labile and affected her physical therapy efforts and successes.

- **Laceration (noun):** a significant cut or gash on the skin
  Example: The wound most prominent after the accident was a laceration that stretched from forehead to chin.

- **Latent (adjective):** undeveloped or unused
  Example: Being that they caught the disease early, it was still in the latent stage and no symptoms were currently present.

- **Lateral (adjective):** related to the sides
  Example: Due to his knee injury, lateral movement proved difficult.

- **Lethargic (adjective):** slow or inactive
  Example: Even when the medications wore off, the patient remained lethargic.

- **Manifestation (noun):** the appearance of an abstract idea or the indication of an illness
  Example: Lyme disease symptoms vary in their manifestation and may include anything from fatigue and fever to Bell's Palsy.

- **Musculoskeletal (adjective):** relating to the muscular and skeletal systems together
  Example: Carpal tunnel syndrome is among the disorders that impact the musculoskeletal system.

- **Neurologic (adjective):** referring to the nervous system, including the anatomy and function
  Example: Neurologic disorders include a wide variety of sub-groups, like Down Syndrome and Muscular Dystrophy, each with different causes and manifestations.

- **Neurovascular (adjective):** condition related to the blood vessels of the brain
  Example: It's important to recognize the symptoms of neurovascular conditions, like a stroke, so that care can be delivered quickly.

- **Nutrient (noun):** dietary component vital for wellbeing and health
  Example: Including a lot of fruits, vegetables, and whole grains is important for a nutrient-rich diet.

- **Occluded (verb):** to block or cover
  Example: Eye exams typically begin by reading an eye chart with one eye occluded.

- **Ongoing (adjective):** continuous or in progress
  Example: As the hospital continued to expand, hiring new staff was ongoing.

- **Oral (adjective):** related to the mouth
  Example: The patient was given the choice between a shot and an oral medication.

- **Otic (adjective):** related to the ear
  Example: Patients complaining of hearing loss should have a complete otic exam.

- **Parameter (noun):** a measurable variable that helps define boundaries
  Example: The patient's testing numbers were outside the parameters for normal liver function.

- **Patent (noun):** government license establishing ownership of an invention to its creator
  Example: Pharmaceutical companies often try to expedite the research and development of drugs to file for the patent first.

- **Pathogenic (adjective):** related to disease-causing microorganisms
  Example: Covid-19 has proven to be a highly pathogenic virus.

- **Pathology (noun):** branch of medical science that studies the origin and effects of diseases
  Example: Doctors can now diagnose Alzheimer's disease via a brain scan due to better understanding of the pathology.

- **Posterior (adjective):** the back or near to the backside
  Example: A posterior tear in the ligaments of the knee is likely to end a young athlete's sports career.

- **Potent (adjective):** powerful
  Example: The doctors prescribed a potent mix of prescriptions to control and minimize the patient's pain.

- **Potential (adjective):** possessing the ability to grow into something
  Example: The early drug trials suggested significant potential for treating the disease.

- **Precaution (noun):** defensive steps taken to prevent something bad from happening
  Example: Prior to her procedure, the doctors requested she take antibiotics as a precaution.

- **Precipitous (adjective):** abrupt, sudden, or rushed
  Example: The patient's mother blamed his injuries on his precipitous actions.

- **Predispose (verb):** to lean towards a specific belief, action, or state
  Example: Exposure to certain chemicals may predispose someone to developing cancer.

- **Preexisting (adjective):** a condition or belief that is present from an earlier date
  Example: One of the primary arguments about the ACA is ensuring that individuals with preexisting conditions can secure health insurance.

- **Primary (adjective):** first in importance or order
  Example: Her primary symptom was extreme fatigue.

- **Priority (noun):** positioned or treated as the most important
  Example: In the emergency room, patients with significant blood loss are treated as a priority.

- **Rationale (noun):** the logical grounds for a decision or course of action
  Example: The doctor was able to provide that patient with the rationale behind the dietary recommendations.

- **Recur (verb):** happens again or over and over
  Example: Once Rachel was symptom-free, she asked the doctor if there was a chance those symptoms would recur.

- **Renal (adjective):** related to the kidneys
  Example: Without the help of dialysis, the patient would likely suffer renal failure.

- **Restrict (verb):** to constrain or limit
  Example: In order to control blood sugar levels, the doctor asked Michael to restrict his consumption of sweets.

- **Retain (verb):** to keep
  Example: The patient's low activity level and obesity led her to retain water in her legs and ankles.

- **Serene (adjective):** tranquil; composed
  Example: In order to help with her recovery and allow her to rest, the hospital staff worked to create a serene environment.

- **Status (noun):** the condition of a person or thing at a given time
  Example: The family asked the nurse to update them on their uncle's post-surgery status.

- **Sublingual (adjective):** under the tongue, as with the delivery of medication or liquid
  Example: Vitamin B is said to be most effective when administered sublingually.

- **Supplement (noun):** substance that, as an additive, complements or strengthens that to which it is added
  Example: Despite having a fairly balanced diet, the doctor recommended Sarah take a calcium supplement.

- **Suppress (verb):** to hold back
  Example: In order to prevent chest pain, the doctor recommended a medication to help suppress David's cough.

- **Symmetrical (adjective):** composed of the exact same parts or components directly across a common axis
  Example: Essentially, both sides of a face are symmetrical, though sometimes there are small, barely noticeable variations.

- **Symptom (noun):** a physical or noticeable manifestation of an illness or disease
  Example: When discussing her illness with the doctor, Monica was unsure whether her headaches were a symptom or from the stress of the diagnosis.

- **Syndrome (noun):** a collection of symptoms that appear together and mark a specific condition
  Example: Epstein-Barr Syndrome is marked mostly by fatigue and weakness.

- **Therapeutic (adjective):** having curative or healing properties
  Example: The doctor recommended a therapeutic massage as a way of managing muscle pain associated with her treatment.

- **Toxic (adjective):** poisonous
  Example: Most household cleaners are toxic if ingested.

- **Transdermal (adjective):** through the skin
  Example: In effort to quit smoking, Michael purchased transdermal nicotine patches.

- **Transmission (noun):** the act of sending or transferring something
  Example: The doctors expected no further transmission of the disease among community members.

- **Trauma (noun):** a psychologically or physically damaging incident
  Example: Car accidents are likely to result in significant injuries and trauma.

- **Triage (noun):** the prioritization of patients and injuries within a medical center
  Example: Severe winter weather, which caused a multi-car pile-up on the highway, made the triage area of the hospital very busy.

- **Ubiquitous (adjective):** omnipresent; everywhere
  Example: Hand sanitizing stations at the hospital are ubiquitous.

- **Urinate (verb):** the act of passing liquids from the body
  Example: The doctor warned that the diuretic would likely mean the patient would need to urinate more frequently.

- **Vascular (adjective):** related to the system of capillaries, arteries, and veins within the body; the system that carries blood
  Example: Varicose veins are considered a vascular disease that can often be treated through surgical procedures.

- **Verbal (adjective):** oral or spoken
  Example: The doctor assured Amanda that, in addition to verbal instructions, she'd provide documentation as well.

- **Virulent (adjective):** toxic or extremely dangerous; hostile
  Example: Sepsis is a particularly virulent infection that can lead to death.

- **Vital (adjective):** essential or necessary
  Example: The doctor insisted that physical therapy would be a vital part of the patient's recovery.

- **Volume (noun):** the space available or filled by, typically, a liquid; noise level
  Example: Perhaps one of the biggest complaints in double occupancy rooms is the television volume.

Grammar

Parts of Speech

Nouns

A **noun** is a word that names a person (e.g., nurse), an animal (e.g., dog), a place (e.g., hospital), a thing (e.g., car), or an abstract idea (e.g., compassion).

Types of Nouns

There are different types of nouns, but the most important ones to remember are:

- **Proper nouns** are nouns that represent a specific person (e.g., *Dr. Smith*), place (e.g., *St. Anthony's Hospital*), or thing (e.g., *Porsche*). Proper nouns are capitalized.

- **Common Nouns** are nouns that refer to any person, place, or thing (abstract or concrete) that is not specific. For example, *dog* (common) vs. *Rover* (proper), *the city* (common) vs. *New York City* (proper), *month* (common) vs. *June* (proper).

- **Abstract Nouns** are nouns that denote non-tangible things that cannot be seen, heard, felt, touched, or tasted. They are often concepts, qualities, or ideas such as *equality, love, care*, etc.

- **Collective Nouns** are nouns that define a group of things, animals, or people, such as *flock, jury, committee,* or *class*.

While there are other categories of nouns, these aforementioned ones will be the most frequently used. It's important to note that some nouns may be classified in two different groups. There are times, such as in mottos, where a noun can be both proper and abstract. For example, Delaware's state motto is Liberty and Independence. It is a proper noun because it is the state's motto, even though they are also abstract nouns.

Pronouns

A **pronoun** is a word that replaces a noun or another pronoun. Pronouns are used in sentences to keep them concise and non-repetitive. The word a pronoun replaces is called the **antecedent**. In the example sentence *Jim didn't think he was late to school*, the word *Jim* is the antecedent and the word *he* is the pronoun.

Types of Pronouns

- **Personal Pronouns** is a type of pronoun that takes the place of a person's name (e.g., *she, her, he, him, I, me, you, we, us, they, them, it*).

- **Possessive Pronouns** are pronouns that show ownership, or possession (e.g., *my, mine, our, ours, your, yours, his, hers, its, their, and theirs*). Note that unlike other possessives, these do not utilize an apostrophe.

- **Indefinite Pronouns** are non-specific and are often vague. They can be collective (e.g., *everyone*), or they can be singular, (e.g., *someone*).

- **Demonstrative Pronouns** are pronouns that identify something specific, often by space and time, and they can be either singular or plural. The four demonstrative pronouns are *this*, *that*, *these*, and *those*.

    - **This** indicates proximity and replaces a singular subject. (e.g., This is a cozy house.)

    - **That** indicates a farther distance and replaces a singular subject. (e.g., That is my new house on the corner lot.)

    - **These** also indicates proximity but replaces a plural subject. (e.g., These are very smart dogs.)

    - **Those** indicates a farther distance and replaces a plural subject. (e.g., Those are my children.)

There is one other way to distinguish pronouns, and this determines how they are used in a sentence. Deciding which pronouns are appropriate to use depends on whether they are subject or object pronouns.

Subject Pronouns

The **subject pronouns** such as *I, you, he, she, it, we, they* are used whenever the pronoun is the subject of the sentence. In other words, if the pronoun answers the question *who* or *what* in relation to the verb in the sentence, use a subject verb. Here are some examples:

I would love to go to nursing school.

The verb phrase is *would love to go*...who would love to go? *I would*, so use the subject pronoun *I*.

He was late to class on the first day.

Who was late? *He* was, so use the subject pronoun *he*.

They both transferred into the class at the same time.

Who transferred? *They* did. Again, use the subject pronoun.

She and I went to the bookstore to purchase our textbooks.

Who went to the bookstore? *She and I* did. One great way to hack this kind of sentence is to separate the pronouns and try the sentence with each pronoun independently: *She went to the bookstore* and *I went to the bookstore.*

Object Pronouns

The object pronouns are: *me, you, him, her, it, us,* and *them*. You'll likely notice here that *it* and *you* appear on both lists. They can be used as either subject or object pronouns. Use object pronouns whenever the pronouns are **not** the subject of the sentence. In other words, if the verb is describing who or what, and the pronoun does not answer that question, it should be an object pronoun.

As an object in a sentence: *Susan loaned her textbook to me. Susan* is the subject of this sentence because she's the one who did the loaning. *Me* is the object because it's the person to whom Susan loaned the book.

Verbs

A **verb** is a word that shows an action or a state of being.

Types of Verbs

Action Verbs: Action verbs are words that show action (e.g., dig, run, talk), though they can also show ownership (e.g., I own this car). Action verbs also often describe what the subject of a sentence is doing (e.g., I ran).

Helping Verbs: Helping verbs help the main verb (usually an action verb) complete verb phrases and help convey time (e.g., *will be* going).

Linking Verbs*: Linking verbs connect a subject to more information about that subject (e.g., John *is* tall).

Adjectives

Adjectives modify nouns. *Modify* means to change with the inclusion of more information. In the case of adjectives, that can be a quality (e.g., giant), state of being (e.g., green), or a quantity (e.g., thousands). These are referred to as **descriptive adjectives**. Much like nouns, there are different types of adjectives. Some of these types offer degrees of modification, often for the purposes of comparison. They are the following:

Positive/Absolute Adjectives simply offer a description. For example, *Allison is funny*. The adjective here is the word *funny,* which describes Allison.

Comparative Adjectives compare two things. For example, *Allison is funnier than Matt*. The adjective here is the word *funnier,* which describes Allison in comparison to Matt. The word *than* is often used with a comparative adjective.

Superlative Adjectives compare three or more things. Sometimes, the objects of comparison are not mentioned in the sentence when it is implied to be superlative among many things. For example, *Allison is the funniest.* The adjective here is the word *funniest,* which describes Allison in comparison to many others (including Matt!). Notice the use of the article "the" which accompanies the superlative to mark it as the definitive.

Possessive Adjectives

The key piece to identifying adjectives is remembering that they describe the noun. They provide more information about the noun. Therefore, in the case of possessive adjectives, this means they show us the ownership of a specific noun. These adjectives include the possessive pronouns such as *my, your, our, his, her, its,* and *their.* Notice the following example:

> You left *your* stethoscope in Room 125.

In this sentence, the word *your* modifies the noun stethoscope and acts as an adjective.

Demonstrative Adjectives

Much like possessive adjectives, **demonstrative adjectives** help us answer the question *which thing.* They tell us more about the noun being referred to. *This, that, those, these,* and *what* are examples of demonstrative adjectives. The following is an example of their usage:

> *This* patient has been waiting for over an hour.

In this sentence, the word *this* modifies the noun *patient* and acts as an adjective.

Interrogative Adjectives

Interrogative adjectives go right along with the demonstrative adjectives. They ask the questions that demonstrative adjectives answer. Interrogative adjectives include *which* and *what.*

> *Which* patient has been waiting for over an hour?

Nouns that Act as Adjectives

These are tricky in such a way that they look like nouns, but they act like adjectives describing a noun. *We went to the hospital training program.* In this case, the word *hospital*, normally a noun, is acting as an adjective as it describes the training program.

Adverbs

Adverbs are like adjectives in the manner that they are both descriptive. However, while adjectives describe nouns, adverbs describe verbs, adjectives, or other adverbs. Adverbs often answer *how, why, when, where, or what* about a verb, an adjective, or another adverb. Often, they end with the letters *ly* (e.g., quickly, slowly, lazily). However, it is important to remember their role, more than relying on the *ly* ending as some adjectives end in *ly* like *friendly.*

Types of Adverbs

Adverbs of frequency provide information about an event's rate of occurrence. They include words such as *always, never, sometimes, occasionally, rarely, often,* etc. The following is an example:

> Change of shift *normally* includes a brief overview of what happened on the earlier shift.

In this sentence, the adverb tells us how often the brief is included. The word *normally* appears just before the verb it modifies and just after the subject of the sentence *change of shift.* Here is another example:

> I *always* keep a change of scrubs in my bag.

Adverbs of manner answer the question *how*. They include words like *quickly, happily, angrily, easily, poorly* among many others. Here is a usage example:

The patient *easily* completed the PT tasks.

In this sentence, the adverb comments on how easily the task was completed. Note that it is placed just before the verb and after the subject.

Unlike adverbs of frequency which tell us "how often," **adverbs of time** tell us *when* something will happen. They include words like *now, yesterday, tonight, tomorrow, today*. Here is an example of how they are used:

I'm picking up an extra shift *tomorrow*.

In this sentence, the adverb does not appear immediately before or after the verb it modifies. However, the word *tomorrow* answers the question *when* and modifies the verb.

Adverbs of place tell us where something happened or where something is. They typically come right after the main verb or the clause they modify. This includes *abroad, everywhere, towards, anywhere* among others. The key piece here is that the word modifies the verb; it answers where something happens. It is different from prepositions as the latter specify the position of an object or subject. Here is an example:

You'll need to go *towards* the elevator and make a right turn to find cardiology.

Adverbs of degree come before the adjective or the adverb they modify, to either amplify (e.g., very) or diminish (e.g., barely) them. This includes words like *too, really, fully, just, terribly*, etc. The following is an example:

It was clear the patient had a white coat phobia as she appeared *extremely* nervous.

In this sentence, the word *extremely* modifies (and amplifies the degree of) the adjective *nervous*, which describes the state of the patient. Here is another example:

She was in so much pain that she *hardly* noticed the doctor enter the room.

In this sentence, the word *hardly* modifies the verb *noticed* to suggest that she *almost did not*, so *hardly* diminishes the degree.

Adverbs of evaluation tell a reader/listener how the writer/speaker feels about the entire clause that follows. This type of adverb is usually at the beginning of the sentence (as an introductory element) and includes a comma directly afterwards. Here is an example:

Hopefully, she will recover quickly.

Notice how the adverb, *hopefully*, here modifies the entire clause where the writer hopes the person will recover quickly. The word *quickly* is also an adverb here which modifies the verb *recover*.

Adverbs of certainty, as the name implies, are adverbs that suggest how sure the speaker or writer is about something (word being modified). This includes the words *obviously, certainly, definitely, clearly,* etc. An example follows:

> She was *clearly* upset about the demotion.

The adverb *clearly* here states certainty about the subject (she) being upset. However, this type of adverb doesn't always need to come right before the word it modifies. Here is another example:

> *Obviously*, we won't be admitting new patients while on auxiliary power.

Here the adverb starts the sentence, modifying the clause.

Prepositions

Prepositions are the words in a sentence that state position, placement, and time in relation to other words in the sentence. They tell us where one noun is in relation to another noun. However, prepositions do not stand on their own. They are a part of prepositional phrases or a group of words that provide the information. For instance, when one asks where something is, the answer "on" is not enough. The rest of the prepositional phrase is needed to complete the idea such as *on the table*.

There are four types of prepositions. Those that determine direction, time, location, and space.

Direction: *The testing lab is to your left.* In this sentence, *to your left* is the prepositional phrase, while *to* is the actual preposition.

Time: *Because the surgery is at 11am, we will need to prep the patient at 8am.* In this sentence, *at* is the preposition while *8am* and *11am* complete the phrase.

Location: *While the doctor's office is here, the labs are in another wing.* In this sentence, *in another wing* is the prepositional phrase while *in* is the preposition.

Space: *The doctor is waiting just outside the exam room.* In this sentence, *outside the exam room* is the prepositional phrase while *outside* is the preposition.

Conjunctions

Conjunctions are the networkers of the word world. They make connections, particularly between words, phrases, and other parts of the sentence. There are three primary types of conjunctions.

Coordinating conjunctions are the ones that are most commonly used. A great way to remember them is to remember the mnemonic *FANBOYS*, where F stands for the conjunction *for*, A for *and*, N for *nor*, B for *but*, O for *or*, Y for *yet*, and S for *so*. Coordinating conjunctions are used to connect words, phrases, and clauses. Here is an example of one in context:

> Doug hated going to the doctor, *yet* he went yearly for his flu shot.

In this example, *yet*, the coordinating conjunction connects two independent clauses *Doug hated going to the doctor* and *he went yearly for his flu shot.* Without the conjunction, you have either two sentences or a run on. The use of the conjunction allows formation of a compound sentence, which adds a variety of ideas.

Correlative conjunctions work in pairs, meaning if you see one, you must see the other. They work together to connect one part of a sentence to another. The pairs include, but are not limited to, the following:

- As - *adjective* -as
    - Rotations in pediatrics are not *as bad as* rotations in oncology.
- Either/or
    - *Either* we get the vaccinations now *or* we do it on our next visit.
- Both/and
    - We will need *both* an x-ray *and* an MRI.
- Not only/but also
    - *Not only* will she need stitches, *but also* a cast.
- Neither/nor:
    - The doctor offered the young girl a treat after her visit, but she wanted *neither* the lollipop *nor* the small toy.

The most important thing to remember about **subordinate conjunctions** is that their use will likely make the clause dependent. In this case, the dependent clause will need to be paired with an independent clause, otherwise, it is just a fragment. Subordinate conjunctions include the words *although, because, since, unless, when, and while*. Consider the following example of usage:

> *Because* I wanted to go into nursing from a young age, I've been familiarizing myself with potential programs for years.

Note that if *Because I wanted to go into nursing school from a young age* is left off the sentence, it would be a sentence fragment because the subordinate conjunction creates the dependent clause. Here is another example of a subordinate clause at work:

> The patient will not heal quickly or properly *unless* he does the PT exercises at home.

In this simple sentence structure, there is a main clause and a subordinate clause, so no comma is necessary.

Interjections

Interjections are a bit like salutations (e.g., *hello, hi*) or closings (e.g., *see you, goodbye*) in that they come at the start or end of a sentence, and they insert the author's presence directly into the text. Although they are typically not complete sentences on their own, they can stand alone. They are often quick expressions of a feeling or a response to something. Here is an example:

> *Whoa!* Slowdown in the hallways please.

In this sentence, *whoa* is the interjection. Here is another example:

> *Hmmm*, I don't know the answer to that. Let me consult with someone.

The interjection here is *Hmmm*. As noted above, they can stand alone as well:

> *Congratulations!*

Note that most interjections are followed by an exclamation point (!). As discussed in the section on punctuation, exclamation points are used primarily for expressing emotions.

Articles

Articles are essentially adjectives such that they modify a noun. They add specificity to a noun by helping a reader determine how many or which one of a thing. Articles include *a*, *an*, and *the*.

The is referred to as a **definite article** because it means something specific. Here is an example:

> The patient was given *the* form.

In this case, it's a very specific form.

A/an are **indefinite articles**. We can slightly alter the previous example—*The patient was handed a form*. This time around, the *form* is not nearly as specific. It could be *any* form, hence the term *indefinite articles*. The following scenarios differentiate the usage of each of them.

Use *a* when:

- A singular noun begins with a consonant letter (e.g., *a* doctor, *a* nurse, *a* procedure)

- A singular noun begins with a consonant sound (e.g., *a* uniformed person, *a* university-affiliated hospital)

- A noun starts with an *H* (e.g., *a* hospital, *a* hotel)

Use the article *an* when:

- A singular noun begins with a vowel (*a, e, i, o, u*) (e.g., *an* injury, *an* exam)

- A word starts with a silent *h* (e.g., *an* hour, *an* honor)

Usage

Clauses and Sentences

A **complete sentenc**e requires two parts—a subject and a predicate. The **subject** denotes who or what the sentence is about, and the **predicate** reveals more about the subject. A complete sentence is also called an **independent clause** and can stand on its own. Dependent clauses cannot stand on their own because they are typically providing more information about something in the sentence. They depend on the subject and predicate to make sense. The following are examples of independent and dependent clauses.

Dependent Clause: *While John and Maria waited.* So naturally one might ask, *what happened while they waited?* The thought is incomplete. It depends on more information.

Independent Clause: *The radiologist looked at the x-rays.* This is a complete idea. There is a subject, *Radiologist*, and predicate (what he or she did) *looked at the x-rays.* Thus, the following sentence constitutes a combination of independent and dependent clauses to create a complete sentence. *The radiologist looked at the x-rays while John and Maria waited.*

Types of Sentences

Declarative sentences make a statement or state an opinion. Here are some examples:

I hate broccoli.

Blue is my favorite color.

Imperative sentences are commands or requests. Here are some examples:

Close the door, please.

Get on the bus.

Interrogative sentences ask a question and usually begin with *who, what, where, why, when, how, or do.* Here are some examples:

Do you know what time that store closes?

How are you feeling today?

Exclamatory sentences express extreme emotion (e.g., excitement, anger, surprise, fear). Here are some examples:

I aced my final exams!

We're going on vacation!

Run-Ons and Fragments

Two of the most common sentence errors are run-on sentences and sentence fragments.

Run-on sentences happen when two independent clauses are put together. When a comma is used to connect them, it's called a **comma splice**. When there is no comma, the clauses are **fused**. Either one of these actions creates a run-on sentence.

Sentence fragments are incomplete ideas; either the subject or the predicate is missing.

Run on sentences can be fixed by doing one of the following:

- Adding a period between the sentences
- Adding semicolon between the sentences
- Adding a comma and a coordinating conjunction
- Adding a subordinating conjunction or a dependent word

Below is an example of a run-on sentence, followed by the four ways to fix it.

Tamara and Rachel love spicy food Michael does not.

- Fix #1: Tamara and Rachel love spicy food. Michael does not.
- Fix #2: Tamara and Rachel love spicy food; Michael does not.
- Fix #3: Tamara and Rachel love spicy food, but Michael does not.
- Fix #4: While Tamara and Rachel love spicy food, Michael does not.

Sentence fragments are incomplete sentences. Often, they are easy to spot because they are missing either a subject or a verb, or both. They become more difficult to spot when they have both the subject and the predicate but do not have the complete idea. For example, the sentence fragment *because he went to the store* has a subject (he) and a verb (went), so it may seem complete. However, the dependent word (because) at the beginning suggests that something else happened. This is a dependent clause, as it depends on the rest of the sentence to make complete sense.

Sentence Structures

A **simple sentence** is a sentence that contains only one independent clause. An example of a simple sentence is *John likes to run.*

A **compound sentence** takes two independent clauses and joins them either via a semicolon or a coordinating conjunction. Consider the following examples:

John likes to run; he also likes to cycle.

John likes to run, and he likes to cycle.

Complex sentences include an independent clause and a dependent clause. *Mary was going to be late to the party* is an independent clause. *Mary was going to be late to the party because she missed the bus* is a complex sentence where *because she missed the bus* is the subordinate clause.

Complex-compound sentences are a combination of the last two sentence types discussed. They take two independent clauses and a subordinate clause and put them together. An example is, *Mary was going to be late to the party because she missed the bus, so I offered her a ride.* Both the sections *Mary was going to be late to the party* and *I offered her a ride* are independent clauses. The section *because she missed the bus* is the subordinate clause, and *so* is a coordinating conjunction that connects the independent clauses.

Modifiers

Modifiers are words, phrases, or clauses that provide more information, like a definition or description, about something in the sentence. Single word modifiers are typically adjectives and adverbs while clauses are usually separated from the independent clause by a comma.

If one takes a simple sentence—*Curtis was worried about the test*—and adds modifiers, one can not only add more information, but also make the sentence more interesting. *Curtis, who was late in starting the program, diligently studied in the library, but was still worried about the test.* Modifiers here (about Curtis and his actions) make the sentence far more detailed.

However, when one adds in modifiers, sentences run the risk of having two errors: **misplaced modifiers** and **dangling modifiers**.

Misplaced Modifier

As modifiers typically modify (i.e., provide more information) about a noun, any modifier that is placed too far from the noun it modifies can create a lot of confusion, making the sentence hard to follow. For example, if one takes the independent clause *The girl ordered coffee at the café* and adds in a modifier about the girl (*in the red dress*), the sentence might erroneously become *The girl ordered coffee at the café in the red dress.* The modifier in this sentence is misplaced because it makes it seem that the café is in the red dress, rather than the girl. To fix this, the modifier needs to be closer to Andrea, not at the end of the sentence: *The girl in the red dress ordered coffee at the café.*

Dangling Modifier

Dangling modifiers are a bit different in that the proximity to the word being modified is not the issue but its existence in the sentence is. In other words, the modifier doesn't appear connected to a clear subject in the sentence. Consider the following example:

Not having read the instructions, the table was put together improperly.

It is not clear *who* it was that did not read the instructions and so the modifier *Not having read the instructions* is dangling. One can fix it easily by including a clearly defined subject in the sentence.

Not having read the instructions, I put the table together improperly.

Phrases

As much as all the elements act independently within a sentence, many of them still act as a single unit called a phrase. **Phrases** are words that, altogether, express a single concept. There are eight different kinds of phrases.

A **noun phrase** includes the noun and any of its adjective modifiers. Here is an example:

The small brown puppy was being trained.

In this example sentence, *the small brown puppy* is a noun phrase.

A **verb phrase** includes the verb and any of its modifiers, including adverbs and objects. An example follows:

Antonio *walked quickly down the hall.*

In the above sentence, *walked quickly down the hall* is the verb phrase. *Walked* is the verb, *quickly* is the adverb, and *down the hall* tells us where the walking was taking place.

A **gerund phrase** is a noun phrase that begins with a gerund as the noun. **Gerunds** are typically verbs that are acting as nouns. They are easily recognized because they typically end in *-ing*. For example, *swimming* can be a verb as in *I went swimming,* or it can be used as a noun (a gerund) as in *Swimming is one of my favorite sports*. An example of a gerund phrase is as follows:

Sailing lessons start next Saturday.

In this example sentence, *sailing lessons* is the gerund phrase.

An **infinitive phrase** is a noun phrase that begins with an infinitive verb (to + verb). An example follows:

> Nick made an appointment *to see the doctor*.

In that sentence, *to see the doctor* is the infinitive phrase.

An **appositive phrase** modifies nouns by renaming or defining them more specifically. An example would be:

> Dr. Nelson, my favorite in the practice, was never late to appointments.

In that sentence, *my favorite in the practice* is the appositive phrase.

A **participial phrase** is a verb that acts as an adjective and begins or ends with a past or present participle of a verb. In other words, participial phrases start or end with verbs that are either in past tense or present continuous tense.

> Leaving the semester behind, Darla headed home for summer.

In this sentence, the participial phrase is *Leaving the semester behind.* Note that it is NOT a gerund phrase because *leaving* is not a gerund in this sentence.

A **prepositional phrase** begins with a preposition and can act as multiple parts of speech such as *nouns, adjectives, and adverbs*.

> The nurse placed the vials on the table.

In this sentence, *on the table* is the prepositional phrase acting as an adverb pertaining to where the vials were placed.

An **absolute phrase** is a non-essential phrase attached to an independent clause with a comma. It is non-essential in the sense that if the phrase were removed from the sentence, the meaning of the sentence would not change. However, the presence of an absolute phrase adds depth to the sentence itself.

> The nurses clocked out at the end of their shift, *emotionally spent.*

In this sentence, *emotionally spent* is the absolute phrase.

Punctuation

End punctuation comes at the end of a sentence. As a quick review, end punctuation includes *periods, question marks, and exclamation points*. All sentences need some form of end punctuation.

Commas

Commas indicate a pause between parts of a sentence. However, commas are not simply added in any part where one would take a breath, nor are they necessarily used anytime a sentence starts to appear too long. The following is a list of where commas are properly placed.

- **Use a comma after introductory elements**. This can include words such as transitions (e.g., *furthermore*), phrases, and clauses.

- **Use a comma before coordinating conjunctions that join two independent clauses**. It is important to remember the independent clauses portion of this rule. Although *and* is a coordinating conjunction, a comma cannot be placed before *and* as in *I made myself a peanut butter and jelly sandwich*. On the other hand, a comma is necessary between two independent clauses within a sentence like in *I made myself a peanut butter and jelly sandwich, and I poured a glass of milk.*

- **Use a comma between items in a list**. When listing three or more items in a sentence, a comma should be placed in between the items. For example: *Paul purchased scrubs in black, blue, and green.*

- **Use a comma between descriptive words not joined by a conjunction.** This rule is a lot like the previous rule regarding listing descriptive words. For example: *Lisa described the new scrubs as itchy, stiff, and generally uncomfortable.*

- **Use a comma between non-essential clauses/modifiers.** These are clauses/modifiers that do not change the meaning of a sentence when removed. They are offset with commas to allow readers to follow the main idea of the independent clause.

- **Use a comma to set off clauses at the end of a sentence.** This can be for subordinate clauses/modifiers that do not create a misplaced modifier when placed at the end of a sentence. For example: *John dislikes the new doctor, especially when he is condescending.*

- **Use a comma between cities and states and in dates.** Commas are used to help make reading places/locations and dates a bit easier as in the following sentences. *Anna was born in Memphis, Tennessee* and *My family has a barbecue planned for July 4, 2021.*

Semicolon

There are only three instances when a **semicolon** is necessary.

- **Use a semicolon to combine independent clauses that are related to one another**. This is one of the ways mentioned to fix run-on sentences. *Tony and Maria work quite well together; however, they are rarely scheduled for the same shifts.*

- **Use a semicolon in addresses written without line breaks.** The semicolon would be placed where line breaks would be. For example: *Museum of Arts and Crafts; Dr. Smith; 3500 5th Ave North; Dayton, NJ 08810*

- **Use a semicolon in complicated lists where commas are already used.** An example would be *Nurses traveled from Tucson, Arizona; Bellingham, Washington; Kalamazoo, Michigan; and Bangor, Maine.*

Colons

There are four scenarios where **colons** can be used, though it is likely to observe one usage more than others.

- **Colons can be used in business letter greetings.** Colons can be used in place of a comma when writing a formal business letter. For example: *Dear Mr. Smith:*

- **Colons can be used to separate a title and subtitle.** This applies to books and movies and the like. For example: *Speed 2: Cruise Control*

- **Colons can be used to introduce a list.** This is generally how colons are most frequently used. A rule to remember here is that the colon should never interrupt the main clause of the sentence. *The instructor told us that every student should have: pens, a stethoscope, a notebook, and the course text.* This use of the colon is incorrect because it interrupts the sentence. Colons almost act as an introduction to the list. *The instructor told us that all students should have the following items: pens, a stethoscope, a notebook, and the course text.* This sentence uses the colon correctly as it introduces the list without interrupting the sentence.

- **Colons can be used to introduce a quote.** This only applies after a complete clause. For example: *In talking to his students, the instructor wanted to encourage them to follow their passions and, therefore, shared with them this quote:* Then, the colon here would introduce the quote.

Quotation Marks

Quotation marks ("") always appear as a set. Oftentimes, quotation marks are used when stating a person's exact words. This is referred to as a **direct quote** as it captures word-for-word what the speaker said rather than summarizing. Sometimes, quotation marks are also used in titles. The following sentence is an example of a direct quote.

"Could you please show the patient to the exam room?"

However, there are a few things to look at in this example. First, note that the initial quotation mark (") comes at the very start of the sentence, followed by a capital letter. Next, note that the clause is a question; therefore, a question mark needs to end the sentence before using the final quotation mark (").

On some occasions, speech tags precede quotation marks. **Speech tags** are phrases that punctuate a dialogue and can provide more information about the speaker. In one example *Sally asked, "Could you please show the patient to the exam room?"*, the speech tag is *Sally asked*. Keep in mind that speech tags can come at the end of the sentence, as in this example, *"Could you please show the patient to the exam room?" she asked the nurse*. Here, the speech tag is *she asked the nurse*. Notice here that the word *she* is not capitalized even though it comes after the question mark in the quote. In this structure, the quote and the tag are one sentence together.

In some cases where the quotation is a declarative sentence and not an interrogative one, the quoted statement is ended with a comma right before the final quotation mark, followed by a speech tag. An example is as follows: *"Show the patient to the exam room," she told the nurse.*

Finally, quotation marks are sometimes used in titles of short works. **Short works** are defined as songs (e.g., "Little Red Corvette"), poems (e.g., "The Raven"), short stories (e.g., "The Legend of

Sleepy Hollow"), articles that appear in print like magazines, newspapers, websites, book chapters (rather than the title of the book, which is handled differently), and television episodes (rather than the show).

To summarize, remember the following important points:

- Quotation marks come in pairs. They are used to open and end a direct quote.
- Punctuation marks like commas and end sentence punctuations are placed within the quotes.
- Speech tags can be either at the start or the end of the quotation.
- Quotation marks are also used in titles of shorter works.

Apostrophes

Apostrophes are used in two main occasions. Firstly, they are used when suggesting ownership or possession. (e.g., Mary's book, The Smiths' house, the men's room). Secondly, they are used in contractions (e.g., *don't* to shorten do not, and *won't* to shorten will not).

Possessive Nouns

Add *'s* to a singular noun to show ownership even if the noun ends in *s*. Here are some examples:

Mary's textbook or Charles's textbook.

If a noun is plural and ends in s, just add an apostrophe.

The nurses' lounge.

If the noun is plural but does not end in *s*, add *'s*.

The children's waiting room.

An apostrophe may also be used with measurements of time that suggest possession.

Last semester's course load was much heavier.

Apostrophes are **never** used to make a plural version of a noun. Furthermore, they may not be used with possessive pronouns. *That book is hers* is correct. *That books is her's* is incorrect.

Capitalization

The following are the most common rules of capitalization:

- Always capitalize the first word in a sentence.

  o *The* doctor will be in later.

- Capitalize the first word in a direct quote.

  o After the exam, the doctor asked, "*Do* you have any questions?"

- The personal pronoun *I* is always capitalized, regardless of where it appears in a sentence.

  o She's going later, but *I* am leaving now.

- Proper nouns are always capitalized. Remember they name a specific person, place, or thing. These include people's names, cities/locations, ships, planets, monuments, and geographic names.

    o The stethoscope was invented by *René Laennec*.

    o She will be relocating to *Cincinnati* after graduation.

    o Despite only living a few states away, she has never seen the *Atlantic Ocean*.

- Holidays, special events, and historical events are also capitalized.

    o If you worked on *Thanksgiving*, you'll likely have *Christmas* off.

    o As a historian with interest in the *Revolutionary War*, Charlie was one of the most fascinating patients to visit.

- Capitalize the names of races, religions, languages, and nationalities.

    o Of the three women in the waiting room, one is *Canadian*, one is *American*, and one is *Japanese*.

    o They were looking for an RN who was fluent in *Spanish*.

    o The hospital chaplain is trained to minister to all faiths, whether the patient or family is *Jewish, Catholic,* or *Muslim*.

    o The form required patients to enter demographic information and asked how they identified racially: *Caucasian, African American, Asian, Hispanic or Latino, American Indian* or *Alaskan Native*, or *Native Hawaiian* or *Pacific Islander*.

- Organizations, businesses, institutions, and government bodies are all capitalized.

    o I'm not sure who the patient is, but the *Federal Bureau of Investigation (FBI)* has an agent outside his room.

    o Most of our hospital beds are made by *Stryker*.

    o During our staff meeting, we learned that half of the nurses were involved with the *Girl Scouts of America*.

- The names of specific branded products are capitalized.

    o I prefer *Coke* to *Pepsi*.

    o If you look out in the lot today, you'll notice a lot of *Subarus* and *Hondas*.

- The important words in titles of books, movies, songs/albums are all capitalized.

    o Textbook of *Basic Nursing*

    o *One Flew Over the Cuckoo's Nest*

Some common capitalizing mistakes include capitalizing the following words, which do not require it:

- Names of seasons: spring, fall, winter, summer

- Generic directions: north, south, east, west (unless you are referring to a specific region as in: *We are traveling to the Northeast to see family.*)

- Names of school subjects (unless a language or specific title): history, math, science. However, do capitalize course names like Advanced Spanish or Biology 101.

Commonly Confused Words

The English language is notoriously difficult to learn for a few reasons, but one big reason is the number of words that sound similar but are spelled differently and have different meanings; they're called **homophones**. Here is a list of a few of the more common ones:

They're/Their/There

There is a contraction of the words *they* and *are*. *Their* shows ownership. *There* pertains to a direction or an existence of something. Here are some examples:

> If you're looking for the sample vials, they're in the lab.

> A guest from the health department is visiting their class.

> If you find the vials I'm looking for, can you please put them over there?

You're/Your

You're is a contraction of the words *you* and *are*. *Your* shows ownership. Here are some examples:

> *You're* going to take the exam next month, aren't you?

> Did you forget *your* notes?

It's/Its

It's is a contraction of the words *it and is*, and *it and has*. *Its* shows ownership.

> *It's* about time that they updated the classrooms.

> The hospital bed is broken; *its* rear right wheel has fallen off.

Who's/Whose

Who's is a contraction of the words *who is* or *who has*. *Whose* shows ownership. Here are some examples:

> *Who's* interested in forming a study group?

> I don't know *whose* hand sanitizer this is, but I'm going to use some.

Our/Are

Our shows ownership before a noun. *Are* is a conjugation of the verb to be. Here are some examples:

> *Our* class is doing a site visit at an urgent care facility.

> *Are* you going on that trip?

Than/Then

Than is used to make a comparison. *Then* is an adverb of time telling when something is happening. It can also be used to suggest *next,* usually in a step-by-step instruction.

> I like geriatrics more *than* I like pediatrics.

> I went down to the ER first, *then* I went to radiology.

To/Too/Two

To is a preposition or part of an infinitive (to + verb, such as: to swim, to test). *Too* is an adverb meaning also or very. *Two* is the number and can be used as an adjective.

> Are you going to be able *to* swap shifts with me?

> I was *too* tired to focus in class today.

> There are *two* open shifts; can you take one?

Choose/Chose

Choose is a verb which means to select. *Chose* is the past tense of the same verb.

> I don't know which rotation I'll *choose* next.

> I *chose* my own lab partner, but I regret it.

Which/Witch

Which can be a pronoun that suggests choice or an adverb that introduces a clause. *Witch* is a noun that means sorceress (as in the Wicked Witch of the West). Here are some examples:

> *Which* classes are you signing up for first semester?

> I'm eligible for a scholarship if I get my grades up, *which* looks likely.

> The pediatrics team dresses for Halloween, so I'm going as a *witch*.

Loose/Lose/Loss

Loose is an adjective that means unrestrained or not tight. *Lose* is a verb that means to not win or not be able to find/keep. *Loss* is a noun that means defeat, death, or the opposite of victory or gain, or the experience of losing something. Consider the following examples:

The experiment was a failure when all the testing animals got *loose*.

Did you *lose* your keys?

The doctor expressed condolences for the family's *loss*.

Where/Wear/Were

Where is an adverb referring to a place. *Wear* is a verb that means to put on or exhaust, or a noun that means weakened or compromised. *Were* is the plural past tense conjugation of the verb *to be*.

Where will you be going to nursing school?

Be sure to *wear* your scrubs on the first day!

We *were* the last ones to finish the exam.

Affect/Effect

Affect is a verb that means to change, create an emotional impact, or imitate. *Effect* is a noun that means the consequences (as in cause and effect).

I'm not sure how this quiz score will *affect* my grade.

This medication has significant side *effects*.

Quite/Quit/Quiet

Quite is an adverb that means very, completely, or acutely. *Quit* is a verb that means to stop or a noun pertaining to peaceful. *Quiet* is an adjective that means silent or without noise.

I was *quite* surprised at my test score.

Our overall goal is to get all smoker-residents to *quit*.

The patient was put in a single room as he needs a lot of *quiet*.

Threw/Through/Thru

Threw is the past tense of the verb throw. *Through* can either be an adverb or a preposition that means traveling into one end and out the other. *Thru* is slang for *through* and should not be used in any formal writing.

He *threw* me the keys, so I could open the door.

If you go *through* that door, you'll see a map of the campus on the wall.

Passed/Past

Passed is the past tense of the verb *pass*, meaning transferred, went by, or is over. *Past* is a noun that refers to history. It is also an adjective that means former.

I *passed* the clipboard to the nurse at the station.

In the *past*, I did not know what I wanted to do for my career, but now I'm sure I want to be a nurse.

Weather/Whether

Weather is a word that refers to the condition of the atmosphere. *Whether* is an adverb that suggests possibility or options.

When the *weather* is bad, we see an increase in activity due to accidents.

I don't know *whether* I want to focus on physical or occupational therapy.

Cite/Site/Sight

Cite means to quote or attribute. *Site* refers to a place (physical or virtual). *Sight* means something one might see.

I failed the paper because I forgot to *cite* my sources.

They are preparing the *site* for a new hospital wing.

Watching the child walk for the first time after the surgery was a heartwarming *sight*.

By/Buy/Bye

By is a preposition that suggests proximity or provides attribution. *Buy* is a verb that means to purchase, or it can be used as a noun to suggest a bargain. *Bye* is an interjection and is the shortened version of *goodbye*.

The doctor stopped *by* the patient's room to check on his progress.

After a long day, my feet are killing me, so I won't *buy* these shoes again.

It was hard to leave so I stopped to say *bye* to everyone.

Advice/Advise

Advice is a noun that refers to guidance, suggestion, or recommendation. *Advise* is a verb that signifies the act of giving a suggestion.

The best *advice* I got before starting school was to not overload my schedule.

She *advised* me to avoid working with a specific practice in town.

Accept/Except

Accept is a verb that means to approve or take (as in a gift). *Except* is a preposition that means to leave out.

I was happy to *accept* a position at Bayfront.

I liked all my classes *except* phlebotomy.

Common word confusion issues also include some words that are commonly misspelled or misused. Those words include, but are not limited to, the following:

Should've/Should of

The contraction *'ve* (could've, would've etc.) is short for *should have*, so the correct usage, without the contraction, is *should have*, not *should of*.

All right

This is the only form of these two words. Though *alright* is often used in casual and informal writing, it is not correct. In other words, *alright* is acceptable in informal settings like in messaging or social media, but not acceptable in formal writing.

A lot

Even though it is said, and sometimes written, as one word, the correct usage is with two words.

Adverse/Averse

Adverse means bad, like in the sentence: *This medication has adverse effects. Averse*, on the other hand, means to have opposition to, like in the sentence: *I am not averse to drawing blood.*

Biology

Biology Basics

The scientific study of life and the scientific inquiry about the living world is called **biology**. Life is organized and characterized by several processes and properties. Some of these properties include order, energy processing, growth and development, evolutionary adaptation, environment response, regulation, and reproduction, which are shown in the figure below. The five main unifying themes that embody the properties of life are biological organization, information, energy and matter, interactions, and evolution.

Themes in Biology 1: Organization

There are generally ten levels of biological organization. From a global to a microscopic scale, they are called the biosphere, ecosystems, communities, populations, organisms, organs, tissues, cells, organelles, and molecules and atoms.

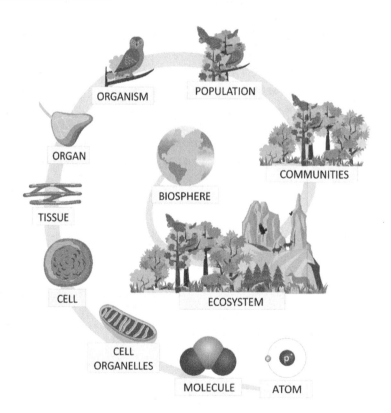

Atoms are the main building blocks of all known matter. Each atom is made up of subatomic particles called the neutron, proton, and electron. Atoms bond and combine to create **molecules**. Biological organization involves the structure and function of cells. The **cell** is the most basic unit of life and is made up of larger nonliving molecules. Some organisms, such as the paramecium, are **unicellular**, meaning "single-celled." Many organisms are **multicellular**, meaning they have more than one cell. Similar cells can combine to form **tissues**. The groups of cells within a given tissue work together to perform a specific function. **Organs** are made up of several tissues and work with one another to create an **organ system**. An **organism** is a single-cell life form or plant/animal made up of several organ systems. A **population** is composed of one species within a particular area that is similar and can interbreed with one another. A **community** is comprised of a population of many plants and animals within an ecosystem. Within a physical environment, the **ecosystem** contains the community of populations that interact with the land, water, and climate. All of the ecosystems found on planet Earth make up the **biosphere**.

Themes in Biology 2: Transmission of Genetic Information
Every form of life can **reproduce**. Reproduction is a process where an organism makes a new organism similar to itself. Through reproduction, all living organisms pass on genetic information as they create new offspring. Organisms can produce offspring identical to themselves because they pass on hereditary information such as genes and DNA. All cells are enclosed by a membrane and have genetic information. Single-cell organisms such as bacteria can split in two, whereas multicellular organisms undergo a reproductive process that involves the union of sperm and an egg. In human fertilization, the male transfers sperm to the female reproductive system. After the eggs are released into the fallopian tubes of the female, the sperm and egg combine within the ampulla of the fallopian tube

Shortly after, cell division occurs and proceeds to various developmental stages. For both single and multicellular organisms that undergo reproduction, genetic instructions called **genes** are passed from one generation to the next. All organisms have genes that contain long twisted molecules called **deoxyribonucleic acid (DNA)**. DNA is a double helix made up of two long chains (left) or two complementary strands (right) containing nucleotides. Genetic information is stored in sequences of four nucleotides that carry bases called adenine (A), thymine (T), guanine (G), and cytosine (C). DNA provides the instructions for the metabolism and organization of specific organisms. **Mutations** cause inheritable changes in the organism's genetic information, which then result in unique members of a particular species. The diversity found in living organisms is due to mutations, which allow organisms to acquire specific traits to adapt to their environment.

Themes in Biology 3: Transformation of Energy and Matter
The organization of matter and energy is essential for many organisms. Organisms maintain organization by consuming nutrients and an outside source of energy. Plants are **autotrophs (producers)** since they produce their food, and animals are **heterotrophs (consumers)** since they consume organisms for food. During photosynthesis, organisms such as plants can absorb solar energy and transform it into chemical energy stored in organic molecules as sugar. Cells in an organism use nutrient molecules to produce products through a series of chemical reactions, as shown in the image below. Nutrient molecules (food) provide energy to consumer organisms, such as animals. Consumers will use food for chemical energy to perform work. The amount of work an organism can perform depends on the amount of energy available. **Metabolism** refers to all chemical reactions that take place in the cell. Organisms are dependent on one another and continuously interact. In an environmental community, called an **ecosystem**, animals consume food from plants or other animals. When animals die, insects and fungi break down the animal's organic matter, and nutrients are returned to Earth. In an ecosystem, energy flow is one-way, but chemicals will cycle within organisms and the environment.

Themes in Biology 4: Interactions in Biological Systems
Organisms must be able to respond to their environment and other organisms accordingly. The response typically results in a movement. For instance, some organisms will initiate beating of their microscopic hairs, called cilia, to move towards or away from a light source. The response from an organism allows it to perform its daily activities that are collectively referred to as the organism's

behavior. Living organisms must also maintain biological balance known as **homeostasis**. The existence of life on Earth will depend on the organism's ability to maintain a tolerable range regarding physiological factors such as acidity, moisture level, and temperature. Organisms must have systems that manage and monitor their internal conditions. Feedback and control mechanisms (**regulation**) within an organism are needed to make routine adjustments. For example, in negative feedback regulation, if a person forgets to eat or is fasting, the liver releases stored sugar to keep the sugar (glucose) levels in the blood within a normal range.

Themes in Biology 5: Evolution and the Diversity of Life

Evolution is the core concept in biology that explains how living organisms developed from a single ancestor. In a process called **adaptation**, living organisms can undergo modifications or changes that allow them to function better in a specific environment. For example, to keep warm in cold water, penguins developed a type of fat called blubber underneath their skin. These adaptations allow for **evolutionary change**, a process whereby populations of organisms change and adapt to their environments throughout many generations. When descent occurs from a similar ancestor, the adaptation can be passed down so that the offspring are already better suited to the environment and have a better chance of survival. Biologist and naturalist Charles Darwin developed the theory of **natural selection** that explains how adaptation occurs. Darwin described three main observations from nature that suggested common descent with modification.

> 1. Individuals within a population vary in traits, and some of these traits are passed from the parent to offspring. These traits are **heritable**.

> 2. A population will produce more offspring than are needed to survive. Competition can result since there are more individuals within the environment.

> 3. Species can become suited to their environment by adapting to new circumstances.

Based on these three observations, Darwin concluded that individuals that acquired traits suited to their local environment would increase the likelihood of survival and reproduction. Over time, a larger proportion of individuals will have the advantageous traits. Darwin reasoned that in natural selection, evolutionary adaptation occurs because the natural environment consistently selects the movement of more apt traits, among variant traits in the population, from one generation to the next. Mutations will trigger natural selection since mutations introduce variations among members within a population. Natural selection is driven by **evolution**, whereby organisms with traits better suited to the environment have a higher chance of survival and reproduction.

The Tree of Life

Natural selection results in the formation of diverse species. The diversity of life can be organized into three main domains: **Bacteria**, **Archaea**, and **Eukarya**. The identification and grouping of organisms based on specific rules is called **taxonomy**, and the study of evolutionary relationships among various organisms is called **systematics**. Taxa are the basic classification categories among organisms and are, from most to least inclusive, **domain**, **kingdom**, **phylum**, **class**, **order**, **family**, **genus**, and **species**. A species is a group of interbreeding individuals.

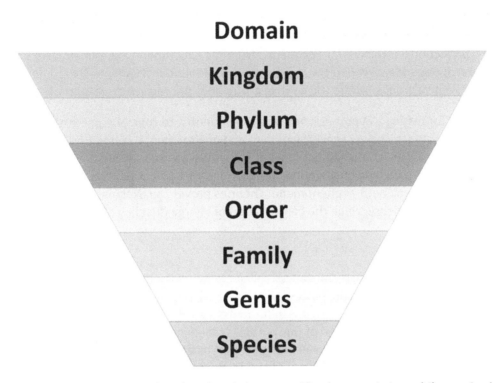

Species in the same genus are closely related and share specific characteristics, while species in the same kingdom share general features. Species are less related when placed in a different domain. Domain **Bacteria** and **Archaea** contain **prokaryotes**, a type of simple organism that lacks a nuclear membrane. Archaea are the least evolved; they live in aquatic settings that lack oxygen but can live in a salty or acidic environment. For example, bacteria can live in our skin, intestine, water, and soil. Domain **Eukarya** contains **eukaryotes**, which are organisms that contain a nuclear membrane and organelles. Eukaryotes have features similar to archaea, which both have similar cell walls and membranes.

Therefore, Eukarya are descendants of the Archaea. Domain Eukarya consist of four main groups called Protists, Fungi, Plantae, and Animalia. **Protists** consist of many kingdoms that can have single cellular and multicellular forms of life. Some examples include algae, protozoans, and water molds. Some protists are photosynthesizers. Kingdom **Fungi** have specialized and complex cells that help decompose dead organisms. Some types include mushrooms, molds, yeasts, and ringworms. **Plantae** organisms are multicellular and photosynthetic with specialized tissues. Some examples include specific algae, mosses, ferns, and flowering plants. **Animalia** consists of multicellular organisms that consume and process food. Some common examples include jellyfish, zebras, mammals, and insects.

Binomial nomenclature is used by scientists to assign living organisms a two-part scientific name. For instance, the scientific name for the wolf is *Canis lupus*. The first word (Canis) is the genus, and the second word (lupus) is designated as the species within the genus. The scientific name (genus) can be abbreviated as *C. lupus*.

The Scientific Method

Through **observations**, scientists can understand a natural event or phenomenon by watching or seeing what takes place. Understanding comes through our senses. Instruments extend our ability to observe a phenomenon, and scientists discuss their experiences through scientific literature and seminars. A scientist typically proposes a **hypothesis**, a possible explanation for an observed phenomenon. The hypothesis is an informed statement that can be tested using the scientific method. Scientists carry out a series of procedures, called **experiments**, to test the hypothesis. They often use deductive reasoning and provide a prediction based on their knowledge from the experiment. Experiments are designed with an experimental (**independent**) variable and a responding (**dependent**) variable. Experiments contain test groups and control groups, where the **control group** does not receive the experimental variable.

Models are useful for testing a hypothesis and allow the scientist to control aspects of the experiment. For example, a scientist can change specific variables and environmental conditions. Scientists present **scientific theories**, which are combined concepts of supported and related hypotheses, to understand the world. Experiments, data, and observations support theories. **Scientific laws** are statements based on observations that predict natural phenomena. **Theories** provide an explanation of a phenomenon. Evolution is considered a theory, while the conservation of energy (first law of thermodynamics) is a law.

Water

All known matter is made up of basic substances called elements. An **element** is a type of substance that can't be broken down into simpler substances through chemical means. Elements such as carbon, hydrogen, nitrogen, oxygen, phosphorus, and sulfur make up 95% of our body weight and, therefore, are basic to life. Elements are composed of tiny particles called atoms. **Atoms** are the smallest component of an element that still retain all of the properties of the element. **Atomic symbols** are one- or two-letter symbols used to designate the name of an element. Positively-charged **protons**, neutrally-charged **neutrons**, and negatively-charged **electrons** are the subatomic particles that make up the atoms.

A **molecule** contains a group of two or more atoms that are bonded together. A **compound** contains two or more elements in a fixed proportion that are united chemically. Salt (NaCl) is only a compound, and water is both a molecule and a compound (molecular compound). All compounds are molecules; however, not all molecules are compounds, such as hydrogen gas (H_2, a molecular element).

The Chemistry of Water

Water is composed of water molecules, and each water molecule is made up of two atoms of hydrogen and one atom of oxygen. The molecular formula for water is H_2O. Each hydrogen atom is covalently bonded (single-bonded) to the oxygen atom. **Covalent bonding** involves the sharing of valence electrons between two atoms such that each atom contains a complete octet of electrons in its valence shell. Single covalent bonds share two electrons, double bonds share four electrons, and triple bonds share six electrons. There are two single covalent bonds in water.

The image below shows the electron model, ball and stick model, and space filling model of water. Oxygen shares two electrons with each hydrogen atom. The ball and stick model shows the number of covalent bonds between oxygen and hydrogen. Electrons are not shared equally between the oxygen and hydrogen atom; this bond type is called a **polar covalent bond**. Chemicals bonds where electrons are shared equally between two atoms are called **nonpolar covalent bonds**.

The shape of the molecule can determine whether the entire molecule is polar or nonpolar. When considering the positions of the atoms in space, water has a bent molecular geometry. If the electron space is considered, then the electron geometry is tetrahedral, due to the two lone electron pairs from oxygen. Since oxygen has more electrons and lone pair electrons, it is more electronegative than hydrogen. Oxygen is slightly negative (δ^-), and hydrogen is slightly positive (δ^+). The electron density is pulled towards the oxygen atom, and because the shape of water is nonsymmetrical, the water molecule is polar. The space-filling model shows the 3-D shape and polarity.

Here are the three model types for the structure of water:

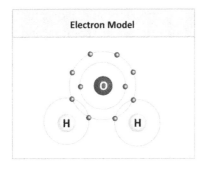

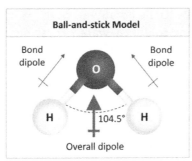

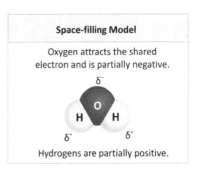

The polarity of water can influence its interaction with other molecules. The intermolecular interaction occurs through hydrogen bonding. A **hydrogen bond** results from the attraction of a slightly positive (δ^+) hydrogen atom to a slightly negative (δ^-) atom. The slightly negative atoms are typically nitrogen, oxygen, and fluorine. Hydrogen bonding occurs with polar molecules such as water and is indicated by dotted lines between hydrogen atoms in one molecule to the oxygen atoms of another water molecule (as shown in the graphic below).

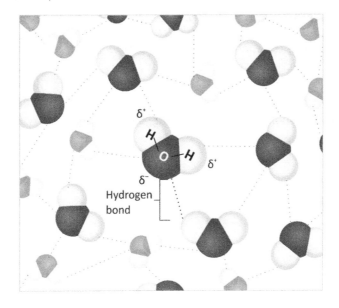

Properties of Water

Hydrogen bonding allows water to stick together and provides water with its unique properties. Without hydrogen bonding, water would freeze and boil at a temperature below -90°C. Water remains a liquid on the Earth's surface between 0°C (freezing) and 100°C (boiling). The **heat capacity** of a substance (C_s) is the amount of heat energy (Joules or calories) needed to create a unit change in temperature. Water has a relatively high heat capacity compared to many substances on Earth.

Consequently, water captures heat, and its temperature falls slowly compared to other substances. Biological aquatic organisms can maintain their average internal temperatures due to water's high heat capacity, which protects them from rapid temperatures changes in the environment. Hydrogen bonding also allows water to have a high heat of evaporation, and hydrogen bonds must be broken before water boils. In hot environments, an animal will begin sweating, and the body heat from the animal will allow the water to vaporize. As water evaporates from a surface, it removes a relatively large amount of heat from the body, thereby cooling it. Due to the polarity of water, water acts as a solvent and allows for a large number of polar substances to be soluble in water. These dissolved substances are **solutes**, and the combination of these solutes in water makeup a **solution**.

The polarity of water facilitates chemical reactions within living systems. Ions and polar molecules that disperse in water collide, allowing a reaction to occur. Ionic compound salts, such as sodium chloride, dissolve when added to water. An ionic compound is held together by an **ionic bond**, a strong attractive force between the positively and negatively charged ions. Due to the attraction of water to sodium chloride, the ionic compound separates into positively-charged sodium ions and negatively-charged chloride ions. The negative ends of water (oxygen) will be attracted to the sodium ions, and the positive ends of water (hydrogen) will align to the chloride ions. Polar molecules such as ammonia (NH_3) will also dissolve in water.

Polar molecules, such as ammonia and glucose, are **hydrophilic** since they are attracted to water and can dissolve in water. Hydrophilic means 'water loving.' Hydrophilic molecules will also attract other polar molecules. **Hydrophobic** molecules are 'water fearing.' Hydrophobic molecules, such as oil and hydrocarbons, tend to be nonionized and nonpolar; therefore, they cannot attract water. Gasoline (octane) is another example of a nonpolar molecule that is hydrophobic and cannot mix with water.

The survival and function of plants depends on **capillary action**, a phenomenon where liquid flows through a thin tube without opposition to forces such as gravity. Capillary action occurs because water molecules portray cohesive and adhesive forces. The **cohesive forces** are the result of intermolecular hydrogen bonding with other water molecules. The adhesive forces are the result of weak intermolecular forces (dipole-dipole, hydrogen bonding, London dispersion) between the water molecules and the polar surfaces.

As seen below, when water evaporates from leaves on a tree, the column of water moves upward due to the cohesive forces in water molecules with one another and the adhesive forces of water to the polar substances along the tubular vessel.

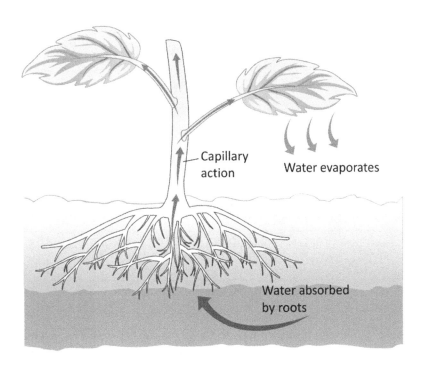

Biological Molecules

Organic chemistry is the chemical study of living organisms. The term **organic** refers to compounds and molecules that contain carbon and hydrogen. In a living organism, there are four types of organic molecules called carbohydrates, lipids, proteins, and nucleic acids. These four types of organic molecules are collectively called **biomolecules**, and each type has a specific cell function. The diverse set of biomolecules is due to the presence of carbon, which has unique chemical properties and is the basis of life.

Carbon

The carbon atom always forms four covalent bonds and has a total of four valence electrons and two first shell electrons. The shape and function of a biomolecule depends on how carbon shares electrons with other carbon atoms. **Hydrocarbons**, such as octane, are long hydrocarbon chains made up of C-H bonds. Hydrocarbons can form ring structures, long branch structures, and may consist of single $C - C$, double $C = C$, and triple $C \equiv C$ bonds. Double and triple bonds are less flexible than single bonds and restrict the motion of bonded atoms. These bond types will affect the shape of a molecule and influence its function. For instance, double bonds are present in saturated and unsaturated fats (lipids). Lipids can store energy because they contain $C = C$. Flexibility of a carbon structure is ideal for biomolecules.

The backbone of a carbon chain in an organic molecule, known as the **skeleton**, accounts for the shape of the molecule. Organic molecules are diverse because they contain various type of functional groups attached to the skeleton.

These **functional groups** contain a specific combination of bonded atoms that always react in a certain way, even if attached to a different carbon skeleton. The carbon skeleton in a biomolecule acts to position the functional groups for a chemical reaction. Most of the chemical reactivity of a biomolecule is due to its bonded functional groups. The chemical properties of functional groups always stay the same. The image below shows three common functional groups. The letter R refers to the place where the functional group attaches to the carbon skeleton.

Functional Group	Structure	Properties
Hydroxyl	O / R \ H	Polar
Methyl	R ——— CH_3	Nonpolar
Carbonyl	O ‖ C / R \ R`	Polar

The type of functional group present determines the biomolecule's properties, such as its chemical reactivity. Functional groups also determine the polarity of the organic molecule. For instance, carbon skeletons with a **hydroxyl group** (-OH) makes the organic molecule an **alcohol**. Alcohol groups are present in sugars and some proteins. **Amino acids** are present in proteins, and they contain **carboxyl groups** (-COOH). **Carboxylic acids** are highly polar groups that act as acids by releasing protons into water or an aqueous environment, in a process termed **ionization**. During protein formation, the carboxyl group in an amino acid will react with an amino group located on a second amino acid.

Some organic molecules, called **isomers**, have the same molecular formulas but have a different arrangement of atoms on the carbon skeleton. These isomers can have different functional groups that will change the properties and chemical reactivity. For example, the plant-fruit sugars called fructose and glucose are isomers that have the same molecular formula $C_6H_{12}O_2$ as shown below.

Glucose   ### Fructose

All four biomolecule classes (carbohydrates, proteins, nucleic acids, and lipids) are generally called **macromolecules** because they consist of smaller subunits that are connected. Nucleic acids, proteins, and carbohydrates are known as **polymers** since these biomolecules are constructed by linking a larger number of similar subunits called **monomers**. Polymers can vary in length. Lipids such as fatty acids and glycerol are not polymers since they are composed of two subunits. Some carbohydrates are **polysaccharides**, a type of polymer that consists of monosaccharide subunits. Proteins consist of polypeptide polymers that contain **amino acid** monomers.

DNA and RNA are types of polymers that consist of **nucleotide** monomers and are both types of nucleic acids. Macromolecules are typically produced by **condensation reactions** (dehydration reactions) since a hydroxyl (-OH) and a hydrogen atom (-H) are removed as a subunit is connected. The equivalent of one water molecule is removed in a condensation reaction.

When biomolecules are broken down, a **hydrolysis reaction** occurs, where an -H attaches to one monomer, and an -OH group attaches to another monomer. Therefore, hydrolysis reactions break down polymers through the addition of water and are the opposite of condensation reactions. Condensation and hydrolysis reactions are typically initiated by special catalyst molecules called **enzymes**. Catalysts increase the rate of reactions.

Carbohydrates

Carbohydrates include chains of sugars (polymers) and simple sugar molecules. **Monosaccharides**, the monomer subunits, are connected into long polymer chains of complex carbohydrates called **polysaccharides**. Polysaccharides act as short-term, energy-storage molecules and can be broken down into sugar molecules. Plants store glucose as **starch**, and animals store glucose as **glycogen**. Starch, found in potatoes for example, can be unbranched (amylose) and branched (amylopectin).

Monosaccharides are simple sugars that consist of one sugar molecule and have a carbon backbone of three to seven carbons. **Pentoses** are monosaccharides that contain five carbons, and **hexoses** have six carbons. Glucose is a hexose that is a major cellular fuel source and can be broken down into chemical energy called ATP. **Disaccharides** contain two monosaccharides joined together and are created during a dehydration reaction. Sucrose is an example of a disaccharide and is a known sugar in plants (sugarcane) used to sweeten food.

Lipids

Because lipids contain relatively long hydrocarbon chains (C-H), they are insoluble in water. Fats called **triglycerides** are the main lipid used by animals for long-term energy storage and insulation. In plants, triglycerides are called **oils**. A triglyceride contains two subunits: fatty acids and glycerol. The fatty acid contains a long hydrocarbon chain and a carboxyl group (-COOH) at the end. Fatty acids are either **saturated**, meaning C=C bonds are absent or **unsaturated**; C=C bonds are present along the chain. There are fewer hydrogen bonds in unsaturated fatty acids. **Glycerol** contains three carbon atoms with three hydroxyl groups (-OH). Glycerol is soluble in water. Through a dehydration reaction, the -COOH groups of fatty acids can react with the -OH group of glycerol to produce a fat molecule and three molecules of water, as shown in the image below.

The diagram at the top shows the formation of a fat molecule:

Glycerol (with three H-C-OH groups) **+** **3 fatty acids** ⟷ **3 water molecules** (3H₂O) and a **Fat molecule**, via a **Dehydration reaction** (forward) and **Hydrolysis reaction** (reverse). One fatty acid shows a "kink".

$$Glycerol + 3\ fatty\ acids \underset{Hydrolysis\ reaction}{\overset{Dehydration\ reaction}{\rightleftharpoons}} 3H_2O + Fat\ molecule$$

Metabolism

Organisms undergo several reactions within their cells. A **cell** can be thought of as a miniature chemical factory where thousands of reactions can take place. For instance, sugars can be converted to amino acids. These amino acids make up the structure of a protein. When we consume and digest food, proteins are broken down into amino acids and converted to sugars. The sum of all the chemical reactions within an organism is known as its **metabolism**. An organism's metabolism is an important property of life that involves the interactions between molecules. Within the cell, there are thousands of chemical reactions that have intersecting metabolic pathways. A **metabolic pathway** can begin with a specific molecule, and through a series of steps, a product is formed.

A unique enzyme will catalyze each step of the pathway. Each enzyme is regulated so the metabolic supply and demand are balanced. The cell's metabolism manages the energy resources of the cell and its materials. Within the metabolic landscape, there is an "uphill" or catabolic process, and a "downhill" or anabolic process. **Catabolic pathways** refer to degradative processes whereby complex molecules are broken down into simple molecules and energy is produced. **Energy** can be defined as the organism's ability to perform work. Energy can be used to rearrange matter. Cellular respiration is an example of a catabolic process where glucose (sugar) is broken down in the presence of oxygen to produce carbon dioxide and water. Therefore, energy stored in organic molecules can be broken down to perform work within the cell. **Anabolic pathways** use energy and take simple molecules, such as amino acids, to synthesize larger molecules, like proteins. As energy is released from a catabolic process, it can be stored and used to drive an anabolic process.

Bioenergetics is the study of how energy moves within a living organism. There are many forms of energy such as kinetic, potential, and thermal energy. **Kinetic energy** is associated with the relative motion of objects, and **potential energy** is related to energy possessed within an object based on its relative location. Water flowing over a waterfall is an example of kinetic energy, and a ball placed on top of a hill contains stored potential energy. Food is a type of potential energy known as **chemical energy** since it's made up of biomolecules. Chemical energy is stored within chemical bonds. The greater the number of chemical bonds in a biomolecule, the more chemical energy that is stored. As a person moves or walks, chemical energy is converted into a type of kinetic energy known as **mechanical energy**. Mechanical energy is the sum of the potential (chemical) energy and kinetic energy that the person does to perform work.

Within an ecosystem, the flow of energy into an organism will result in the dissipation of heat. **Thermal energy** is attributed to the kinetic energy possessed by the random motion of molecules and atoms. **Heat** is the transfer of thermal energy from one object to another. Heat flows from hot to cold objects. The **first law of thermodynamics** explains that energy is always transferred and transformed but never destroyed. When an animal consumes food from a plant, some of that chemical energy is converted into mechanical energy and heat, as shown in the figure below. In photosynthesis, as a plant absorbs light energy, it transforms it into chemical energy (carbohydrates) but also dissipates heat in the process.

The **second law of thermodynamics** states that as energy is transformed, there is a loss of usable energy in the form of heat, thereby increasing the entropy of the universe. **Entropy** is a measure of randomness of a collection of matter. For example, as a bear runs, it releases heat and products such as carbon dioxide (exhaling) and water (sweating). The products are a form of molecular disorder called entropy.

Organisms take in complex molecules and replace them with simple but less ordered types of matter. For instance, a bear eats fish and increases the entropy of the surroundings when exhaling carbon dioxide and sweating. Such biochemical reactions are called **spontaneous** because they are energetically favorable and do not require energy input. Chemical reactions that are **nonspontaneous** decrease the entropy of the system and require an input of energy. Nonspontaneous reactions are not energetically favorable unless energy is supplied. The **Gibbs free energy change (ΔG)** is the amount of energy in a system that performs work. The value of free energy tells us whether a reaction is spontaneous. A negative ΔG indicates a spontaneous process, and a positive or zero ΔG indicates a nonspontaneous process. When a chemical reaction approaches equilibrium, ΔG approaches zero. A process is spontaneous and performs work when it moves towards equilibrium.

Chemical reactions are **exergonic** if the forward reaction results in the net release of free energy. Energy leaves the system, and the reaction is spontaneous, $-\Delta G$. **Endergonic** reactions are nonspontaneous, $+\Delta G$, and absorb free energy from the surroundings into the chemical system, as illustrated below.

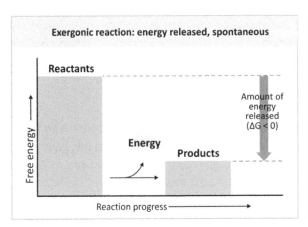
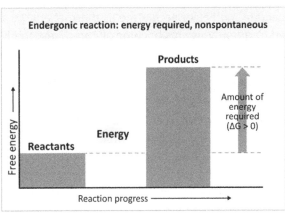

Within a cell, the metabolism never reaches equilibrium because materials (glucose) are moving in while waste (carbon dioxide/water) is moving out of the cells. The cell needs to continuously perform work to survive. To avoid equilibrium, the product of a reaction within a cell does not accumulate but becomes a reactant in the next step. In a catabolic process such as cellular respiration, the reaction proceeds due to the large free energy difference maintained between glucose/oxygen (top of the hill) and water/carbon dioxide (bottom of the hill).

ATP (adenosine triphosphate) will fuel cellular work by **energy coupling** where exergonic reactions are used to drive endergonic reactions. Hydrolysis of ATP is exergonic:

$$ATP + H_2O \rightarrow ADP + P_i \, , \Delta G = -7.3 \; kcal/mol$$

Chemical, transport, and mechanical are types of work performed by the cell. If the absolute value of ΔG for an endergonic reaction is less than the energy released by ATP hydrolysis, then energy coupling can occur, as shown below.

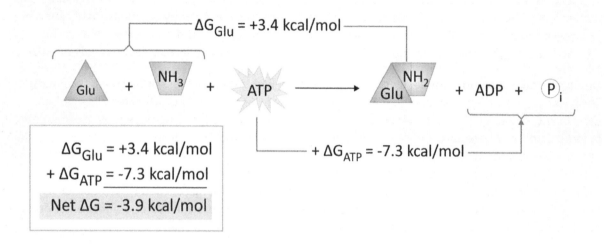

An **enzyme** is a type of macromolecule—typically a protein—that serves as a catalyst. **Catalysts** are chemical agents that increase the rate of a reaction without being destroyed. These catalysts can speed up metabolic reactions because they lower the activation energy barrier. The **activation barrier** (E_a) is the amount of energy needed to contort the reactants so bonds can be broken to form product molecules. Energy to surmount the barrier typically is supplied by heat through thermal energy. Reactant molecules accelerate as thermal energy and are absorbed so that they collide more forcefully and frequently. Atoms become agitated, and the likelihood of bond breakage increases. When enough energy is absorbed, the reactants reach an unstable structure called the **transition state**.

Cells

The cell is the most basic and functional unit of all organisms. **Visible light microscopes** are often used to view cells (4 mm (4x) to 25-micrometer diameter), and the **electron microscope (EM)** has given biologists the necessary resolution to observe the organelles of cells. A light microscope uses visible light to penetrate the specimen. Light is then refracted (bent) off a glass lens towards our eyes allowing us to observe the microscopic specimen. Electron microscopes focus a beam of electrons onto a specimen. The resolution is controlled by adjusting a relatively short wavelength of light. The **scanning electron microscope (SEM)** has allowed scientists to see the topography or a 3-D image of the specimen's surface. To study the internal structure within the cell, scientists have employed the **transmission electron microscope (TEM)**.

There are two unique types of cells: prokaryotic and eukaryotic cells. The domains Archaea and Bacteria contain prokaryotic cells, and the domain Eukarya (plants, fungi, animals, and protists) consists of eukaryotic cells. All cells are bound by a selective barrier called a **plasma membrane**. The **cytosol** is a jelly-like, semi-fluid substance found in the cell that suspends subcellular components, such as organelles.

In **eukaryotic cells**, most DNA is located within an organelle called the **nucleus**. The nucleus in eukaryotes is bound by a double membrane. In contrast, a **prokaryotic cell** contains DNA concentrated in an area called the **nucleoid**, which is not bound by a membrane.

In eukaryotes, the **cytoplasm** is the region between the plasma membrane and the nucleus. Unlike prokaryotes, eukaryotes contain many organelles that have specialized functions. Eukaryotes typically have a cell size ranging from 10-100 micrometers in diameter, whereas prokaryotes are about 0.1 to 1 micrometer. The **plasma membrane**, present in eukaryotes and prokaryotes, functions as a selective barrier that allows the passage of nutrients, oxygen, and waste. The membrane is a **phospholipid bilayer**, where the **hydrophobic** parts of the lipids and embedded proteins are located in the interior of the membrane. The **hydrophilic** regions of the phospholipids point toward the aqueous layer and contain carbohydrates attached to the protein. The larger the organism, the greater the number of cells. A high ratio of surface-to-volume is important for the efficient exchange of materials into and out of the cell. The eukaryotic cell contains elaborately arranged internal membranes that divide the cell into various compartments. The compartmentalization of the cell into organelles is crucial since it allows incompatible metabolic reactions to occur simultaneously.

Eukaryotic Cells

While some genes in the eukaryotic cell are located in mitochondria and chloroplasts (plants), most of them are found inside the **nucleus**, which is approximately 5 micrometers in diameter. **The nuclear envelope**, as depicted below, is a double membrane that encloses the nucleus and separates it from the cytoplasm. The nuclear envelope contains pores, which are roughly 100 nanometers in diameter. A **pore complex** allows RNA and proteins to enter and exit these pores. A netlike array of protein filaments called the **nuclear lamina** lines the nuclear side of the envelope (except the pores) and provides support to help shape the nucleus. DNA is organized into compact units called **chromosomes** and is located within the nucleus.

Chromatin is a complex of DNA and proteins that makes up chromosomes. There are 46 chromosomes in a human cell, although sex cells (sperm and eggs) contain 23 chromosomes. Each chromosome contains a long strand of DNA that wraps around specific proteins. The nucleus contains a dense mass of granules and fibers called the **nucleolus**. Ribosomal RNA is produced within the nucleolus, with instructions given by DNA.

Proteins and ribosomal DNA complexes make up cellular components called **ribosomes**, which are responsible for producing proteins. Ribosomes are not organelles and generally contain large and small subunits. Some ribosomes are not membrane-bound but are suspended in the cytosol. These free ribosomes create enzymes that function in the cytosol, such as enzymes that break down sugars. Bound ribosomes create proteins that specialize in packaging, secretion, and insertion into the membranes. Ribosomes are also found on the cytoplasmic side of the nuclear envelope.

The cell contains an extensive network of membranous tubules and sacs called the **endoplasmic reticulum (ER)** shown in the image below. The ER separates the **ER lumen**, the cavity or internal component of the ER, from the cytosol. There are two types of ER called the smooth and rough ER. **Smooth ER** lacks ribosomes while the **rough ER** is studded with ribosomes on its outer membrane surface. The smooth ER is responsible for metabolic processes such as carbohydrate metabolism, lipid synthesis, calcium ion storage, and detoxification of poisons.

In eukaryotic cells, chloroplasts and mitochondria are types of organelles that produce energy (ATP). Plants and algae contain **chloroplasts**, which are organelles that are involved in photosynthesis and are approximately 3-6 micrometers long. In animals, the **mitochondria** (1-10 micrometer long) are cellular respiration sites where oxygen is utilized to produce ATP by extracting energy from fats and sugars. Chloroplasts and mitochondria have similar evolutionary paths and are believed to have been engulfed by ancestor eukaryotic cells. **Endosymbiont theory** explains that these early eukaryotic cells engulfed a type of oxygen-based, non-photosynthetic, prokaryotic cell. The prokaryote became a living cell within another (**endosymbiont**) and formed a relationship with the host cell.

As evolution progressed, both the host and endosymbiont became a single cell. This eukaryotic cell, containing mitochondria, eventually took up a photosynthetic prokaryote and evolved into a eukaryotic cell with a chloroplast. The theory is widely accepted because mitochondria and chloroplast contain double membranes, ribosomes, and circular DNA molecules; and the DNA from both organelles are similar to bacterial DNA. Another fact supporting the endosymbiont theory is that chloroplasts and mitochondria are slightly independent because they can grow and reproduce inside the cell.

The double membranes of the mitochondria are made up of a phospholipid bilayer with embedded proteins. The outer mitochondrial membrane is smooth, while the inner membrane is convoluted and contains an inner folding called **cristae**. This folding greatly increases the surface area and enhances the productivity of cellular respiration. The inner membrane divides the mitochondria into two internal compartments called the **intermembrane space** and the **mitochondrial matrix**. The matrix contains proteins, DNA, and enzymes that function as catalysts in cellular respiration for ATP production.

Found in plant cells, the green pigment in chloroplasts is **chlorophyll**. Chloroplasts contain a narrow intermembrane space located between the double membrane. **Thylakoids** are another type of membranous system that contains flat interconnected sacs that resemble flat poker chips. Each stack is referred to as a **granum**, and the **stroma** is the fluid outside the thylakoids. The stroma contains DNA, ribosomes, and enzymes. There are three compartments called the thylakoid space, the stroma, and the intermembrane space. These compartments allow for the conversion of light to chemical energy.

Cellular respiration

Cellular respiration is a catabolic process where complex molecules are broken down into simpler molecules and energy is released. Electron transfer from the fuel molecules (glucose) to other molecules plays an important role in this process. Glucose is rich in potential energy and is broken down to produce energy and heat. The stored energy from fuel biomolecules (carbohydrates, fats, and proteins) can be used to perform cellular work. Cellular respiration involves aerobic (with oxygen) and anaerobic (without oxygen) processes. **Aerobic respiration** is the most efficient catabolic process where oxygen is consumed along with the organic fuel. **Fermentation** is less efficient since it partially degrades sugars and occurs without oxygen. Cellular respiration is often associated with aerobic conditions since most eukaryotes (animals) and prokaryotes carry out aerobic respiration. Aerobic respiration is similar to gasoline combustion in an automobile since oxygen is mixed with an organic fuel. For example, glucose found in food acts as a fuel in cellular respiration and gasoline (hydrocarbons) acts as the fuel in combustion. Both processes result in the production of water, carbon dioxide, and energy. Gasoline combustion, unlike cellular respiration, can result in the production of carbon monoxide. The energy created in cellular respiration is in the form of ATP and heat. ATP must be produced by the cell continuously to perform cellular work.

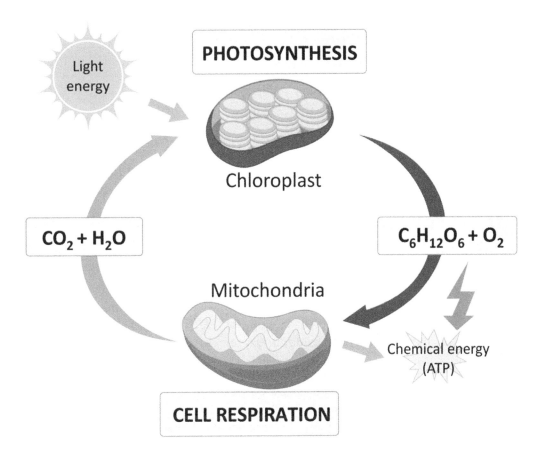

To create ATP, electrons must be relocated by carrying out oxidation-reduction reactions to release energy stored in organic fuels. **Redox reactions**, short for **oxidation-reduction reactions**, are chemical reactions where one or more electrons are transferred from one reactant to another molecule. The oxidation and reduction of chemical reactions are co-occurring in a redox reaction. **Oxidation** refers to the loss of electrons from one species to another. **Reduction** is when one chemical species gains electrons transferred from another. In oxidation, removing electrons from a species increases the overall positive charge and oxidation state. In reduction, adding electrons decreases the positive charge because negatively-charged electrons are added.

The simplest example of a redox reaction is the addition of sodium to chlorine to form sodium chloride (table salt). Sodium loses an electron to chlorine and becomes oxidized. Chlorine gains an electron from sodium and becomes reduced. Sodium acts as an electron donor, which is also termed the **reducing agent**. Sodium will reduce chlorine, and chlorine will accept the donated electron. Chlorine acts as the electron acceptor, and is known as the **oxidizing agent**. Chlorine oxidizes sodium by removing an electron from sodium.

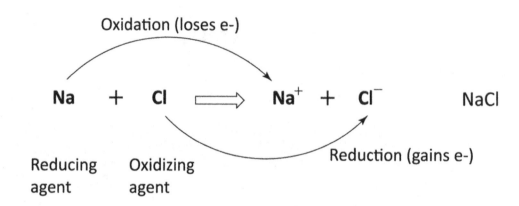

Oxidation (loses e-)

$$Na \ + \ Cl \implies Na^+ \ + \ Cl^- \qquad NaCl$$

Reducing agent   Oxidizing agent

Reduction (gains e-)

In biological substances, redox reactions will alter the degree of electron sharing within a covalent bond. In methane (CH_4), the electron affinity, for the valence electrons, is about the same between carbon and hydrogen. Both elements have similar electronegativity values. When methane reacts with oxygen gas in a combustion reaction to form carbon dioxide CO_2, the electrons are shared less equally because oxygen is more electronegative. Since carbon has slightly lost electrons and become more positive when forming carbon dioxide, methane has been oxidized. Oxygen gas (O_2) shares electrons equally between each atom.

However, when water H_2O is formed, oxygen is now bonded with two hydrogen atoms. Since oxygen is more electronegative, the electrons in each O-H will gravitate towards oxygen. Since oxygen has partially gained more electrons (meaning it is now more negative) in water, oxygen gas has been reduced. Oxygen gas is typically an oxidizing agent since oxygen is electronegative. When an electron travels from a less electronegative atom to a more electronegative one, there is a loss in potential energy. The burning of methane or breakdown of biofuels in cellular respiration moves electrons towards oxygen. The released chemical energy can then be used for work (to create ATP). Organic molecules are a source of hilltop electrons, and as electrons are transferred to oxygen, they "fall" down an energy gradient.

As glucose breaks down through several steps, electrons are removed. A specific enzyme catalyzes each step. In redox reactions, electrons are passed to a coenzyme electron carrier called **nicotinamide adenine dinucleotide (NAD)**. The oxidized form of the coenzyme is called NAD^+ and is an electron acceptor (oxidizing agent) during cellular respiration. Enzymes called **dehydrogenases** remove two protons and two electrons from a glucose substrate and deliver two electrons and one proton to NAD^+. The coenzyme reduces to NADH, and the remaining proton stays in solution.

The electrons transferred to NADH will eventually move to oxygen in a series of steps. Eventually, hydrogen will combine with oxygen to form water, but this does not occur in one explosive step. Instead, cellular respiration uses an electron transport chain to facilitate the fall of electrons to oxygen in a series of energy-releasing steps. In eukaryotes, the electron transport chain (ETC) contains many proteins/molecules within the inner mitochondrial membrane.

At the lower energy end, oxygen will capture the electrons by combining with two protons to form water. The ETC process is exergonic and releases -53 kcal/mol of energy; however, as electrons cascade down the chain, energy is released in small steps. Each step results in electrons being transferred downhill to a more electronegative carrier.

Three major metabolic stages in cellular respiration are glycolysis, pyruvate oxidation/citric acid cycle, and oxidative phosphorylation. These are depicted below. Glycolysis takes place in the cytosol and consists of a series of ten reactions. The first step involves the breakdown of one 6-carbon glucose into two 3-carbon pyruvate molecules. In eukaryotes, pyruvate enters the mitochondria and is oxidized to acetyl CoA. When one molecule of acetyl CoA enters the citric acid cycle, two molecules of carbon dioxide are created. In oxidative phosphorylation, electrons from NADH pass electrons down the chain, where they combine with molecular oxygen and protons to form water. The redox reactions of the ETC release energy, which is stored and used to produce ATP.

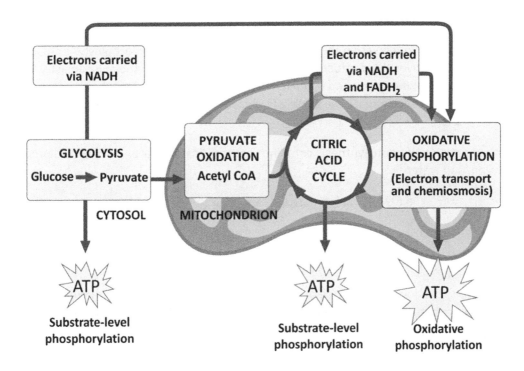

The total inputs in glycolysis include one 6-carbon glucose, two NAD+, two ATP, four ADP, and four phosphate groups (Pi). The total outputs in glycolysis are two 3-carbon pyruvate molecules, two NADH, two ADP, and four ATP. Therefore, the net gain is 2 ATP molecules. In glycolysis, only two out of the possible 36-38 ATP molecules from glucose have been produced.

A preparatory reaction occurs when the two pyruvate molecules are converted to an acetyl group and two molecules of carbon dioxide. Two molecules of NAD^+ are converted to NADH.

In step one of the citric acid cycle, acetyl-CoA will combine with oxaloacetate to form the 6-carbon citrate. The total inputs in the cycle are two 2-carbon acetyl groups, six NAD^+, two FAD, two ADP, and two phosphates (P_i). The total outputs are four carbon dioxides, six NADH, two $FADH_2$, and two ATPs.

NADH and $FADH_2$ carry electrons to the ETC. As electrons travel from one protein to another, through redox reactions, protons from the mitochondrial matrix are pumped into the intermembrane space. As the protons flow down a concentration gradient, from the intermembrane space to the matrix, ATP is created. Each electron pair that enters through NADH creates three ATP, and each electron pair that enters through $FADH_2$ creates two ATP. The formation of a total of 34 ATP molecules is possible. Water is the final byproduct, and the oxygen in water is the final electron acceptor.

Photosynthesis

Most plants are organisms called **autotrophs** since they can create organic molecules from carbon dioxide without consuming other living things. Plants are specifically called photoautotrophs since they use light to produce organic substances and fuel for themselves through a process called **photosynthesis**. In most plants, the leaves are the primary site of photosynthesis. The **mesophyll** is a tissue located in the interior of the leaf that contains mesophyll cells. Each mesophyll cell contains about 30–40 chloroplasts. Microscopic pores called **stomata** allow for the entry of carbon dioxide and the release of oxygen. Most green portions of the plant contain a green pigment called **chlorophyll**, which gives leaves their color.

Chlorophyll is a molecule found within the thylakoid membranes of the chloroplast. As chlorophyll absorbs light energy, it drives the production of organic molecules within the chloroplasts. The two membranes of the chloroplasts surround a dense fluid called the **stroma**. **Thylakoids** are membranous sacs within the stroma that segregate the stroma from the thylakoid space. The sacs are stacked into columns called **grana**.

The general net reaction of photosynthesis combines carbon dioxide, water, and light to produce glucose, oxygen, and water.

$$6\,CO_2 + 12H_2O + light \rightarrow C_6H_{12}O_6 + 6O_2 + 6H_2O$$

Or

$$6\,CO_2 + 6H_2O + light \rightarrow C_6H_{12}O_6 + 6O_2$$

The photosynthesis reaction is the reverse of cellular respiration. Photosynthesis involves redox reactions and water splitting, whereby electrons are transferred with protons from water and carbon dioxide to a reduced sugar. Photosynthesis is an endergonic process since the electrons increase in potential energy as they move from water to sugar. Energy is provided by light.

There are two main phases in photosynthesis, and each phase contains multiple steps. Chloroplasts use light energy to make sugar by managing both phases in photosynthesis. The first phase is called the **light reactions** (*photo* part), and the second phase is called the **dark reactions** or the **Calvin cycle** (*synthesis* part).

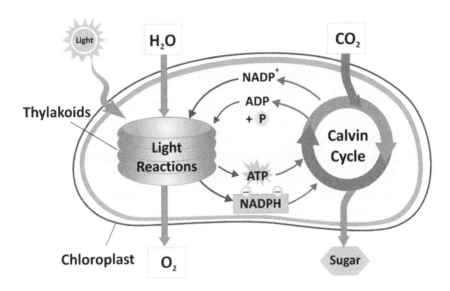

The light reactions occurring in chloroplasts convert solar energy into chemical energy. The sites of the light reactions are the thylakoids of the chloroplasts. As water is split apart, it creates a source of protons, electrons, and oxygen. Within the cycle, oxygen gas is produced as a byproduct. Chlorophyll absorbs light and initiates the transfer of electrons/protons from water. These electrons are stored to an electron acceptor called nicotinamide adenine dinucleotide phosphate ($NADP^+$)). With solar energy, two electrons and one proton are added to $NADP^+$, which reduces it to NADPH. The reduction takes place outside the thylakoid. In a process called **photophosphorylation**, ADP is combined with a phosphate (P_i) to produce ATP through chemiosmosis.

With direct light and the help of NADPH and ATP, sugars are produced in the Calvin cycle within the stroma. The Calvin cycle begins by adding carbon dioxide captured from the air to organic molecules that are present in the chloroplasts. The process of adding carbon into organic compounds is called **carbon fixation**. Using chemical energy from ATP and NADPH, carbon dioxide is reduced to a carbohydrate by the addition of electrons.

The Light Cycle

Light is a type of electromagnetic energy released by the sun. The sun emits various wavelengths of light. The length of each crest on a light wave is called a **wavelength**. Visible light includes colors that we can see and has a wavelength ranging from 380 (violet) to 750 (red) nanometers. Photosynthesis is driven by visible light energy. Light has wave-like properties in addition to particle characteristics. **Photons** are discrete particles of light. Light can be absorbed by pigments found in plants. Plants contain pigments such as chlorophyll *a* and *b*. The main photosynthetic pigment is chlorophyll *a*. Violet blue and red light are optimal for photosynthesis. Chlorophyll *b* and accessory pigments called **carotenoids** absorb specific wavelengths of light and transfer some energy to chlorophyll *a*. Carotenoids function in photoprotection by absorbing and dissipating excessive light energy without causing damage to chlorophyll.

Chlorophyll *a* and *b* are structurally identical and differ by one functional group. Each pigment is made up of a light-absorbing "head" molecule called a **porphyrin ring** and a hydrocarbon tail that interacts with proteins within the thylakoid membranes. When chlorophyll absorbs a light particle (photon), it causes an electron within the chlorophyll to transition from a ground state orbital to an excited state orbital. The electron acquires more potential energy in the unstable excited state and then releases energy as heat (and fluorescent light) when it drops to the ground state.

A **photosystem** makes up special proteins found in the membrane of the thylakoid. These proteins are composed of a photosystem that contains a reaction center complex surrounded by light-harvesting complexes. **Light-harvesting complexes** contain various pigments such as chlorophyll *a* and *b* that channel photon energy toward the reaction center. The reaction center complex contains unique pairs of chlorophyll *a* molecules and a **primary electron acceptor** molecule. The electron acceptor is reduced since it accepts electrons. When a photon hits a pigment molecule within the light-harvesting complex, energy is passed from one pigment to another until an electron reaches the reaction center complex. An excited electron leaves a chlorophyll *a* molecule and is transferred to a primary electron acceptor.

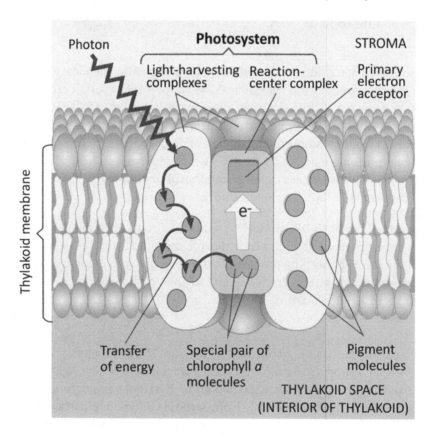

There are two photosystems called PS II and I that are involved in light reactions. *P*680 is a type of chlorophyll *a* pigment found in the reaction center complex of PS II. The number associated with *P*680 means that chlorophyll *a* absorbs light having a wavelength of 680 nm. *P*700 is a type of chlorophyll *a* pigment found in the reaction center complex of PS I and absorbs light with a wavelength of 700 nm.

In a linear electron flow process, electrons move through photosystems and other molecular components within the thylakoid membrane via the following eight steps:

1. A photon strikes a pigment molecule in PS II.

2. An electron is transferred from an excited $P680$ to the primary electron acceptor.

3. An enzyme catalyzes the splitting of the water molecule.

4. A photoexcited electron moves from the primary electron acceptor of PS II to PS I through the ETC.

5. Chemiosmosis: ATP is produced from stored potential energy in a proton gradient.

6. The electron of $P700$ is excited and transferred to PS I primary electron acceptor.

7. Photoelectrons are passed via a series of redox reactions to a second ETC through ferredoxin (Fd).

8. $NADP^+$ reductase catalyzes the electron transfer from Fd to $NADP^+$ to form NADPH.

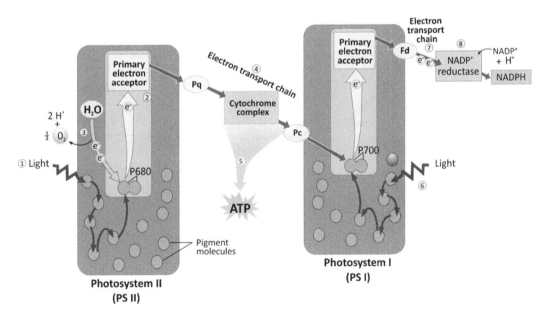

The Calvin (Dark) Cycle

The Calvin cycle synthesizes a three-carbon sugar called glyceraldehyde 3-phosphate (G3P). To produce one net G3P, nine ATPs and six NADPH molecules are required. Three cycles, with one carbon dioxide per cycle, must be completed to make one G3P. The three main stages of the Calvin (Dark) cycle are carbon fixation, reduction, and regeneration of the carbon dioxide acceptor called RuBP.

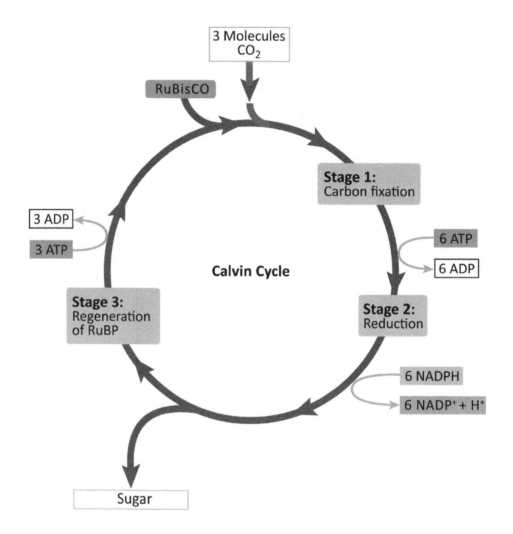

In **carbon fixation**, ribulose bisphosphate (RuBP) is attached to one carbon dioxide molecule. Rubisco catalyzes the first step and produces a short-lived six-carbon intermediate that breaks down to two molecules of 3-phosphoglycerate. In **reduction**, 3-phosphoglycerate combines with ATP to form 1,3-bisphosphoglycerate. NADPH reduces the carboxyl group on 1,3-bisphosphoglycerate (two electrons are added) to yield G3P (glyceraldehyde 3-phosphate). For every three molecules of carbon dioxide that go into the cycle, six G3P molecules are created. Only one three-carbon sugar is counted since the remaining G3Ps are needed to complete the cycle. Therefore, the cycle starts with fifteen carbons worth of carbohydrates (three molecules of the five-carbon RuBP). There are eighteen carbohydrate-derived carbons or six molecules of G3P. One G3P molecule exits the cycle, and the net G3P is used to synthesize molecules such as glucose. The remaining five molecules are recycled to create three molecules of RuBP. In **regeneration**, through a complex set of reactions, the five molecules of G3P have their carbon skeletons rearranged, to form three molecules of RuBP. Three ATP molecules are required. RuBP is then able to receive carbon dioxide, thereby restarting the cycle.

Chemistry

Matter

States of Matter

Matter is a physical substance that has a mass and occupies space. Common examples of matter include trees, water, and living organisms. The elements found in the periodic table are matter or substances that consist of the same atom. Matter may be composed of several types of elements. An **atom** is made up of subatomic particles such as protons, neutrons, and electrons. **Protons** are positively-charged particles, whereas **neutrons** are neutrally charged; these two subatomic particles comprise the **nucleus**, or center, of an atom. **Electrons** are negatively-charged particles. They orbit the nucleus in shells, or what is termed an electron cloud. The properties of each subatomic particle are shown in the table below. Each element has a specific or unique number of protons. **Molecules** are composed of a group of atoms that are bonded to each other.

Properties of Protons, Neutron, and Electrons				
Particle	Mass (kg)	Charge (C)	Mass (amu)	Charge (e)
Proton	1.67262×10^{-27}	$+1.60218 \times 10^{-19}$	1.00728	$+1$
Neutron	1.67494×10^{-27}	0	1.00866	0
Electron	9.10939×10^{-31}	-1.60218×10^{-19}	0.00055	-1

amu = atomic mass unit

Matter can exist in three distinct states: solid, liquid, and gas. The physical state of a substance will mainly be dependent on the forces that are holding the atoms together. The **Kinetic Theory of Matter** states that matter is composed of molecules or atoms that are always in motion. The distance between each atom or molecule in a given state of matter will vary. For example, a **solid** contains particles such as molecules (e.g., H_2O in ice) or collections of the same atoms (e.g., the carbon in graphite) that are closely packed together. The distance or separation between particles is negligible. A solid has a definite shape and volume.

The atoms or molecules in a solid are held by relatively strong forces that keep the particles connected, thereby limiting any freedom of movement. The thermal energy associated with these particles results in a molecular or atomic vibration and allows the transfer of heat. However, the movement of these atoms or molecules is relatively negligible, and the shape/volume of the solid remains unchanged. Some important properties of solids include density, melting point, solubility, and thermal/electrical conductivity.

Solids are typically categorized as amorphous or crystalline. An **amorphous solid**, such as glass, consists of molecules or atoms that are randomly arranged. A **crystalline solid** contains atoms or molecules with fixed positions on a lattice. Crystalline solids can be ionic, metallic, molecular, or composed of a network. **Ionic solids** such as sodium chloride (NaCl) are made up of cations and anions that are held together by **ionic bonds**, a type of chemical bond that involves a relatively strong electrostatic force between two oppositely charged ions. **Metallic solids** are made of up metals that are covalently bonded to each other (e.g., Al in aluminum). **Molecular solids**, such as H_2O in water, are held together by relatively weaker forces (e.g., intermolecular forces such as hydrogen bonding). **Network solids** contain atoms that are covalently bonded. Diamond is an example because the carbon molecules have covalent molecules between them.

A **liquid** consists of particles that have some attractive forces between them. The particles are moderately separated and will take on a loose shape that is dependent on the container that holds the liquid. Liquids will have a definite volume but can flow and change in shape. Some common properties of liquids include viscosity and surface tension. **Viscosity** refers to the internal resistance that inhibits liquid flow. At the surface of the liquid, particles are pulled inward due to attractive forces. Consequently, the surface area is reduced. **Surface tension** refers to the energy needed to increase the surface area of a liquid.

A **gas** is a state of matter in which the forces of attraction between each particle are relatively weaker or nonexistent. Gas particles have a greater degree of separation compared to liquids and solids. As a result, gases do not have a definite volume or shape and will expand such that they take on the shape of a closed container. Some properties of gases include volume, pressure, and temperature.

Plasma is a special state of matter that consists of ionized gas. Specific electrons are separated from the atoms or molecules such that positive ions and free electrons are allowed to coexist. Plasma may be partially or fully ionized; for example, the sun's heat results in the removal of electrons from hydrogen and helium to form a plasma. Plasma can be artificially created (e.g., plasma TVs) and is responsible for the aurora, or southern/northern lights.

Classification of Matter

Two types of matter that exist on the macroscopic scale are pure substances and mixtures. **Pure substances** can be categorized as elements or compounds. **Mixtures** may be homogeneous or heterogeneous.

If matter has a constant composition or consists of a substance that cannot be physically separated, it is called a **pure substance**. A pure substance has a fixed chemical composition and fixed physical properties. Pure substances can be decomposed into a compound or an element. Liquid water and neon gas are examples of pure substances. A **compound** is a type of pure substance that is made up of two or more separate elements (e.g., pure water [H_2O] or sodium chloride [NaCl]). Each element in the compound is combined in a fixed proportion and may be broken down chemically to simpler elements (e.g., water splitting to hydrogen gas and oxygen). Not all molecules are compounds, but all compounds are molecules. For example, the hydrogen gas (H_2) molecule is not a compound, but compounds such as water are molecules.

Elements are pure substances that are made up of one type of atom and cannot be chemically broken down to a simpler substance. Some examples of elements are copper (Cu) and gold (Au).

If matter can be separated physically, the substance is a **mixture**, or a combination of two or more pure substances that are mixed in any ratio. For example, sugar (sucrose) can be added to pure water to form a mixture. Each component (sugar and water) will keep its original identity; the sugar and water molecules will not break apart. The components within each mixture can be separated by distillation or evaporation, chromatography, and filtration. The combination of sugar and water is an example of a food mixture. Lemonade is produced by mixing lemon juice, sugar, and water. Other examples of mixtures include brass (copper and zinc). Smog is another type of mixture that is composed of air (N_2, O_2), nitrogen oxides, and sulfur oxides.

If the mixture is uniform (whereby the components are evenly spread throughout), it is called a **homogenous mixture**. Solids, liquids, and gases can be homogenous mixtures. A homogenous mixture may be referred to as a **solution**. For example, air is a homogenous mixture or gaseous solution. Brass (copper and zinc) is a homogenous mixture or solid solution. Adding salt to pure water and dissolving it forms a liquid solution. Therefore, solutions are homogenous mixtures that have a uniform distribution of components or particles.

A **heterogeneous mixture** contains a nonuniform composition in which various components within the mixture are separated into specific regions. The different regions of a heterogeneous mixture are typically visible and can be separated. Potato soup is an example of a heterogeneous mixture because the potato chunks and other vegetables are visible. The potato pieces, for example, can be isolated and removed from the soup with a spoon. Vegetable oil and water initially form a liquid-liquid **emulsion** (a heterogenous mixture of multiple immiscible liquids) when shaken vigorously but will separate after some time. If the heterogeneous mixture includes both solid and liquid components, it is called a **suspension**. If the components are part liquid (or solid) and part gas, the mixture is an **aerosol**. When a soda can is opened, bubbles of gas (carbon dioxide) are released at the top, forming an aerosol.

Physical and Chemical Properties of Matter

Melting and Boiling Points

Physical properties of substances can be measured without any change to their chemical composition. Melting, freezing, and boiling points are examples of physical properties. Other examples include color, density, and odor. The temperature range where a solid crystalline substance transitions to a liquid is called the **melting point**. The freezing point of a substance is the temperature at which the substance changes from liquid form into a solid. The **boiling point** is the temperature at which the vapor pressure of the substance is equivalent to the surrounding atmospheric pressure (typically 760 mm Hg or 1 atm at sea level).

Phase Transitions

Changes in the state of matter can take place when the pressure, temperature, or volume changes. A solid to liquid phase transition is called **melting**, a liquid to gas transition is called **evaporation**, and a solid to gas transition is called **sublimation**. If the reverse phase transition is considered, a liquid to solid transition is called **freezing**, a gas to liquid transition is called **condensation**, and a gas to solid transition is called **deposition**.

$$H_2O(s) \rightarrow H_2O(l); \; melting \; \; H_2O(l) \rightarrow H_2O(s); \; freezing$$

$$H_2O(l) \rightarrow H_2O(g); \; evaporation \; \; H_2O(g) \rightarrow H_2O(l); \; condensation$$

$$H_2O(s) \rightarrow H_2O(g); \; sublimation \; \; H_2O(g) \rightarrow H_2O(s); \; deposition$$

Vapor Pressure

Phase transitions constantly occur and can interconvert with one another.

$$H_2O(l) \rightleftarrows H_2O(g)$$

The chemical system is at a **dynamic equilibrium** when the rates of vaporization and condensation are equal. Within a closed container, some of the gaseous particles may exert a **vapor pressure**, or a force that results from the collision of gaseous water molecules against the container wall and water surface. The vapor pressure is the partial pressure that is measured at dynamic equilibrium.

Gas Laws

Charles's law describes the relationship between volume and temperature. If the temperature is increased (pressure is constant), the volume of the gas will increase. The following equation describes Charles's law:

$$\frac{V_1}{T_1} = \frac{V_2}{T_2}$$

V_1 and T_1 are the initial volume and temperature. V_2 and T_2 are the final volume and temperature.

Boyle's law explains the relationship between gas pressure (P) and the volume of the gas. If the volume of a gas is decreased (temperature is constant), the gas particles will be compressed and result in more collisions. This means the pressure of the gas increases.

$$P_1 V_1 = P_2 V_2$$

P_1 and P_2 are the initial and final pressure.

Avogadro's law describes the relationship between the moles of gas and its volume at a fixed temperature. As the number of moles increases, so does the volume.

$$\frac{V_1}{n_1} = \frac{V_2}{n_2}, P \text{ and } T \text{ constant}$$

The combination of Charles's, Boyle's, and Avogadro's laws give the ideal gas law:

$$PV = nRT$$

P is the pressure, V is the volume, n is the number of gaseous moles, R is a gas constant, and T is the temperature. A common unit of R is 8.206×10^{-2} with units of $L \times atm \times mol^{-1} \times K^{-1}$.

Chemical Equations and Reactions

Chemical Equations

A **chemical reaction** involves the transformation of reactants into products and is described by a **chemical equation**. Chemical bonds in the reactants break, and atoms rearrange to form new chemical bonds, thereby creating products. A chemical reaction is represented symbolically using a chemical equation. The equation describes the chemical formulas (e.g., CO_2), the phase labels (e.g., gas), the direction of the reaction using arrows ($\rightarrow$), and a coefficient (e.g., **2** CO_2). Consider the following water-splitting reaction of water (H_2O) to hydrogen gas (H_2) and oxygen gas (O_2). The chemical bonds between H and O are broken and then rearranged to form new reaction products.

$$2H_2O(g) \rightarrow 2H_2(g) + O_2(g)$$

The chemical formula, H_2O, on the left-hand side of the chemical equation (before $\rightarrow$) is called a **reactant** and is present at the beginning of the reaction. The right side of the reaction equation (after $\rightarrow$) shows the **products**. The reaction starts with a compound and then produces two pure molecular elements. The plus sign (+) indicates that two products are formed. The chemical reaction equation could also be written as the following:

$$H_2O(g) + H_2O(g) \rightarrow H_2(g) + H_2(g) + O_2(g)$$

The + indicates that multiple reactants are combining. The arrow symbol ($\rightarrow$) shows the direction of the reaction and means the reaction will form products in the forward direction. Coefficients are placed in front of a chemical formula and indicate the number of molecular or formula units. Coefficients simplify the equation and ensure a balanced equation such that the masses on each side are equal. Chemical reactions must follow the **law of conservation of mass**, which states that matter cannot be created or destroyed. Therefore, the mass of the reactants must be equivalent to the mass of the products.

Coefficients are not the same as superscripts or subscripts. For example, the coefficient of 2 in H_2O indicates two water molecules. The subscript of 2 in H_2O means two hydrogen atoms. The physical state of each reactant and product is shown in parentheses: (s) = solid, (l) = liquid, (g) = gas, (aq) = aqueous solution (in water). If the reaction is carried out under heat, a Δ is placed over the reaction arrow: $\xrightarrow{\Delta}$. If the reaction is carried out with a catalyst (e.g., platinum, Pt), the chemical symbol is placed over the arrow: $\xrightarrow{Pt}$.

Types of Chemical Reactions

The water-splitting reaction is an example of a **decomposition reaction** because two products, H_2 and O_2, are produced from one reactant. The general reaction is described as $A \rightarrow B + C$. If the reverse reaction is considered, $B + C \rightarrow A$, it would be an example of a **combination reaction** because two substances combine to form a single product (e.g., H_2O). A **combustion reaction** is a common type of chemical reaction that occurs when a compound or element is burned in air or with oxygen. For example, the gasoline that is injected into an automobile motor is mixed with air and ignited to power a vehicle. The reaction is exothermic and produces heat. If pure or molecular elements are burned, the product is typically a common oxide for that element. For instance, if iron is burned in oxygen, it produces iron oxide. If an organic compound composed of C, H, and O is combusted in oxygen gas (O_2), the products of the reaction will always be carbon dioxide (CO_2) and water (H_2O). The general combustion reaction for a hydrocarbon (C and H) is as follows:

$$C_xH_y + ZO_2 \rightarrow X\,CO_2 + \frac{Y}{2}H_2O$$

For example, the combustion of cyclohexane (C_6H_{12}) gives the following:

$$C_6H_{12} + 9O_2 \rightarrow 6\,CO_2 + \frac{12}{2}H_2O$$

A **double** or **exchange displacement (replacement) reaction** can be described by the following reaction equation:

$$AB + CD \rightarrow AD + CB$$

Species A and C act as a **cation**, or the positively-charged ion, and species B and D are the **anions**, or negatively-charged ions. The reaction of potassium hydroxide and hydrobromic acid is a double-replacement reaction that produces water and potassium bromide.

$$KOH\ (aq) + HBr(aq) \rightarrow H_2O(l) + KBr(aq)$$

In the acid-base reaction, OH exchanges with Br from the acid and K exchanges with H from the acid. **Acid-base reactions** are also called **neutralization reactions** because water and salt are produced, thereby neutralizing the acid and base. There is no excess of hydrogen or hydroxide ions if the acid and base react with the same molar amount. The pH of a strong acid and strong base reaction is equal to 7. Other types of double-displacement reactions that occur in aqueous solutions are **precipitate** or **precipitation reactions**. The cation and an anion combine to form a solid or insoluble ionic substance. A cloudy or colored solution typically indicates the formation of a precipitate. The **exchange reaction** of potassium iodide (LiI, solution 1) and lead (II) nitrate ($Pb(NO_3)_2$, solution 2) create a precipitate called lead (II) iodide (PbI_2).

$$2\ LiI(aq) + Pb(NO_3)_2\ (aq) \rightarrow 2\ LiNO_3(aq) + PbI_2(s)$$

The reactants are strong electrolytes and will initially dissolve completely to create cation and anions. In the exchange reaction, the lead (II) ion (Pb^{2+}) combines with the iodide ion (I^-) to form an insoluble ionic compound or precipitate. The table below is useful for predicting if a double-displacement reaction, formed by mixing two electrolyte solutions, will result in a precipitate.

Solubility Rules	
Soluble Cation Salts	**Exceptions**
Group 1A: Li^+, Na^+, K^+, NH_4^+	No exceptions
NO_3^- (nitrates) and $C_2H_3O_2^-$ (acetates)	No exceptions
Cl^-, Br^-, I^-	Insoluble with $Ag^+,\ Pb^{2+},$ Hg_2^{2+} (mercury (I) ion)
SO_4^{2-}	Insoluble with group IIA ions: $Ca^{2+}, Sr^{2+}, Ba^{2+}, Pb^{2+}, Ag^+$
Insoluble anion salts	
OH^- (hydroxide) and S^{2-} (sulfide)	Soluble with group IA and IIA ions: $Li^+, Na^+, K^+, NH_4^+,$ $Ca^{2+}, Sr^{2+}, Ba^{2+}$
CO_3^{2-} (carbonate) and PO_4^{3-} (phosphate)	Soluble with group IA ions: Li^+, Na^+, K^+, NH_4^+

Single-displacement (replacement) reactions will result in the exchange of one pair of species. For example, in the oxidation-reduction reaction of copper (Cu) with silver nitrate ($AgNO_3$), Cu and Ag exchange places to produce solid silver (Ag) and copper (II) nitrate, $Cu(NO_3)_2$.

$$Cu\ (s) + 2AgNO_3(aq) \rightarrow 2Ag(s) + Cu(NO_3)_2(aq)$$

Single- and double-replacement reactions can be oxidation-reduction (redox) reactions. **Redox reactions** involve the exchange of electrons from one reactant to the other. In the reaction equation above, Cu is oxidized and loses two electrons ($Cu \rightarrow Cu^{2+} +2e^-$). Thus, this half-reaction corresponds to **oxidation** because copper loses electrons. In contrast, the silver ion gains two electrons: $Ag^{2+} + 2e^-$. Thus, this half-reaction corresponds to **reduction** because silver is gaining electrons. Therefore, copper loses electrons to silver, and silver precipitates out of the solution.

Oxidation Numbers in Redox Reactions

An **oxidation number** or **oxidation state** is a hypothetical charge that is given to an atom that is used to track electron flow. The actual charge for that atom determines its oxidation number. An oxidation number is written with a sign (+ or −) followed by a number (e.g., −5). An atomic or ionic charge is designated by a superscript with a number followed by the sign. For example, the magnesium ion (Mg^{2+}) has a charge of 2+ and an oxidation number of +2. For monatomic ions, the oxidation number is equal to the charge. The following table shows rules for determining the oxidation numbers of elements, ions, and compounds:

Rules for Finding the Oxidation State/Number		
	Oxidation Number	**Exceptions**
Elements	0	None
Monatomic ions	Group 1A: +1 for Li^+, Na^+ Group 2A: +2 for Mg^{2+} +3 for Al^{3+}	None
Hydrogen	+1 in most compounds (nonmetals)	−1 in hydrides (compounds with metals, CaH_2)
Halogens (e.g., F^-)	−1 for halogen ions F^-, Br^-, I^-	If the halogen is bonded to oxygen or another halogen, the values may change.
Oxygen	−2 in most compounds	−1 in H_2O_2 If bonded to F, the value will change.
Compounds or ions	The sum of the oxidation number is 0 (e.g., Al_2O_3).	The oxidation number is equal to the charge on the polyatomic anion: $C_2H_3O_2^- = -1$, $SO_4^{2-} = -2$, $CO_3^{2-} = -2$, $PO_4^{3-} = -3$, $OH^- = -1$

The table above can be used to find the oxidation numbers of copper and silver. The reaction of Al and Cu is shown by the following equation:

$$\overset{0}{Cu}\ (s) + 2\ \overset{+1}{Ag}\ NO_3(aq) \rightarrow 2\ \overset{0}{Ag}\ (s) + \overset{+2}{Cu}\ (NO_3)_2(aq)$$

The solid copper in the reactant side is a pure element, so its oxidation number will be equal to 0. Silver nitrate ($AgNO_3$) is an ionic compound with an oxidation number of 0. However, the oxidation numbers for the cation (Ag^+) and the anion (NO_3^-) will not be zero. The oxidation number of the nitrate anion is −1. There is only one nitrate ion, so the oxidation number of the silver ion is +1. On the product side, a pure element of silver is produced and will have an oxidation number of 0. Therefore, the oxidation number of silver changes from −1 to 0, which indicates that silver was reduced. Copper (II) nitrate is the other product that is formed and will have an oxidation number of 0. The ionic compound contains two nitrate ions and one copper ion. The oxidation number of a nitrate ion is −1 because its charge is typically 1−. Therefore, the oxidation number of copper must be +2 because:

$$[2 \times -1\ (NO_3^-)] + [1 \times +2\ (Cu)] = 0$$

The oxidation number of copper changes from 0 to +2, which indicates that copper was oxidized. Silver acts as the oxidizing agent because it oxidizes, or removes, electrons from another species (Cu). Copper is the reducing agent because it reduces, or gives, electrons to another species (Ag). A total of two electrons are removed from solid copper (oxidation) and transferred to two silver ions (reduction).

Acid-Base Reactions

Brønsted-Lowry acid-base reactions involve proton transfers between an acid and base species. **Brønsted-Lowry acids** are proton donors (H^+), and **Brønsted-Lowry bases** are proton acceptors. The general reaction takes the following form:

$$\underset{\substack{Br\o nsted-\\Lowry\\Acid}}{HA} + \underset{\substack{Br\o nsted-\\Lowry\\Base}}{H_2O(l)} \rightleftarrows \underset{\substack{conjugate\\acid}}{H_3O^+(aq)} + \underset{\substack{conjugate\\base}}{A^-}$$

The term A is the **conjugate base** or anion of the acid that is created when the Brønsted-Lowry acid loses a proton. The **conjugate acid** or cation is created when the Brønsted-Lowry base accepts a proton. Consider the following weak acid-base reaction between nitrous acid and water:

$$\underset{\substack{Br\o nsted-\\Lowry\\Acid}}{HNO_2} + \underset{\substack{Br\o onsted-\\Lowry\\Base}}{H_2O(l)} \rightleftarrows \underset{\substack{conjugate\\acid}}{H_3O^+(aq)} + \underset{\substack{conjugate\\base}}{NO_2^-}$$

There are two conjugate acid-base pairs: HNO_2: NO_2^- and H_2O: H_3O^+.

An **Arrhenius acid-base reaction** involves the formation of a proton or hydroxide ions in an aqueous solution. A species that increases the hydrogen ion (or hydronium) concentration is called an **Arrhenius acid**. Phosphoric acid is an example of an Arrhenius acid.

$$H_2SO_4(aq) \rightarrow 2\,H^+(aq) + SO_4^{2-}(aq); \text{ sulfuric acid is a strong acid or electrolyte}$$

or

$$H_2SO_4(aq) + 2H_2O(l) \rightarrow 2H_3O^+(aq) + SO_4^{2-}(aq)$$

A species is called an **Arrhenius base** if it increases the concentration of hydroxide ions when added to water. For example, the addition of calcium hydroxide to water produces two equivalents of hydroxide anion.

$$Ca(OH)_2(aq) \rightarrow Ca^{2+}(aq) + 2\,OH^-(aq)$$

Strong bases and acids are strong electrolytes that completely ionize in water or proceed completely to the right in the reaction. A forward arrow is used to indicate complete ionization. The table below lists examples of strong acids and bases.

Strong Acids	Strong Bases (Groups IA and IIA)
HI Hydroiodic acid	LiOH Lithium hydroxide
HBr Hydrobromic acid	NaOH Sodium hydroxide
HCl Hydrochloric acid	KOH Potassium hydroxide
HNO_3 Nitric acid	$Ca(OH)_2$ Calcium hydroxide
$HClO_4$ Perchloric acid	$Sr(OH)_2$ Strontium hydroxide
H_2SO_4 Sulfuric acid	$Ba(OH)_2$ Barium hydroxide

Weak acids and bases are weak electrolytes and will not dissociate completely. Acetic acid ($HC_2H_3O_2$) is a weak acid/electrolyte that is found in vinegar. The acid partially dissociates in an aqueous solution. A reverse and forward arrow ($\rightleftarrows$) is used to show that reaction can proceed in either direction with one reaction side slightly favored; for example, the longer reverse arrow indicates that the reactant side of the equation is favored.

$$\overset{\displaystyle H^+}{\overbrace{HC_2H_3O_2 \; (aq) + H_2O \; (l)}} \; \rightleftarrows \; C_2H_3O_2^- \, (aq) + H_3O^+ \, (aq)$$

$$\quad\;\; \text{acid} \qquad\qquad \text{base}$$

Arrhenius acids or bases are Brønsted-Lowry acids/bases; however, not every Brønsted-Lowry acid/base is an Arrhenius acid/base. Water acts as the Arrhenius base and accepts a proton from the acetic acid molecule ($HC_2H_3O_2$). Water is a Brønsted-Lowry acid and base.

Neutralization reactions are another type of acid-base reaction that yields an ionic compound (salt) and water. Consider the reaction of hydrochloric acid (HCl) and potassium hydroxide (KOH), which produces potassium chloride (salt, KCl) and water (H_2O). The reaction is an exchange or double-replacement reaction whereby the cation of one species combines with the anion of another species (e.g., H^+ + ^-OH).

$$\overset{\displaystyle H^+}{\overbrace{HCl \; (aq) + KOH \; (aq)}} \; \longrightarrow \; KCl \; (aq) + H_2O \; (l)$$

$$\quad\; \text{acid} \qquad\quad \text{base} \qquad\qquad \text{salt} \qquad \text{water}$$

Lewis acid-base reactions involve the transfer of an electron pair (two electrons) from a Lewis base to a Lewis acid. A **Lewis base** is a species that donates an electron pair to another species, thereby forming a covalent bond in the reaction process. A Lewis acid will accept an electron from the other species (Lewis base) and create a covalent bond. Ammonia (NH_3) is an example of a weak base that partially ionizes in water. The reaction of ammonia (NH_3) and an acid (e.g., HBr) is another example of a Lewis acid-base reaction. The proton from the strong acid reacts with the weak base, NH_3, to produce ammonium

(NH_4^+). Lewis dot structures are typically shown to illustrate the transfer of electrons from one species to another, as demonstrated below.

$$H^+ \quad + \quad :\underset{\cdot\cdot}{\overset{\cdot\cdot}{N}}:H \quad \longrightarrow \quad \left[H:\underset{\cdot\cdot}{\overset{\cdot\cdot}{N}}:H \right]^+$$

Electron-pair acceptor   Electron-pair donor

Periodic Table

Periods and Groups

The **periodic table** contains various elements that are arranged by increasing atomic number (Z) and organized by properties. The **atomic number (Z)** of an atom is the total number of protons inside the nucleus, and this number stays fixed for a particular element. Therefore, an **element** is a substance that contains atoms of the same type that have the same atomic number. Each row on the table is called a **period**, and each column is referred to as a **group**. From left to right, the groups are labeled from 1 to 18. The **main group elements** are labeled from IA to VIIIA. **Transition metal elements** are labeled from IB to VIIIB.

The **inner transition elements** refer to the two rows of elements that are located at the bottom. The first row of inner transition elements is called the **lanthanides**, and the second row is known as the **actinides**. Elements within group IA are called **alkali metals** and are soft metals (except hydrogen, H) that will readily react with water. These metals can quickly form 1+ charges during a chemical reaction. The **alkaline earth metals** are found in group IIA and readily form 2+ charges.

The **halogens** are located in group VIIA. Halogens are reactive and can readily react with some group IA elements and form a 1– charge. For example, chlorine can vigorously react with sodium to form sodium chloride (NaCl). The **noble gases** are found in group VIIIA and exist at moderate temperatures/pressures (e.g., 25°C and 1 atm) with no charge. Noble gases have little reactivity at standard conditions.

An image of the periodic table is below.

Group →	1	2	3	4	5	6	7	8	9	10	11	12	13	14	15	16	17	18
Period ↓																		
1	1 H																	2 He
2	3 Li	4 Be											5 B	6 C	7 N	8 O	9 F	10 Ne
3	11 Na	12 Mg											13 Al	14 Si	15 P	16 S	17 Cl	18 Ar
4	19 K	20 Ca	21 Sc	22 Ti	23 V	24 Cr	25 Mn	26 Fe	27 Co	28 Ni	29 Cu	30 Zn	31 Ga	32 Ge	33 As	34 Se	35 Br	36 Kr
5	37 Rb	38 Sr	39 Y	40 Zr	41 Nb	42 Mo	43 Tc	44 Ru	45 Rh	46 Pd	47 Ag	48 Cd	49 In	50 Sn	51 Sb	52 Te	53 I	54 Xe
6	55 Cs	56 Ba	* 71 Lu	72 Hf	73 Ta	74 W	75 Re	76 Os	77 Ir	78 Pt	79 Au	80 Hg	81 Tl	82 Pb	83 Bi	84 Po	85 At	86 Rn
7	87 Fr	88 Ra	* 103 Lr	104 Rf	105 Db	106 Sg	107 Bh	108 Hs	109 Mt	110 Ds	111 Rg	112 Cn	113 Nh	114 Fl	115 Mc	116 Lv	117 Ts	118 Og

		*	57 La	58 Ce	59 Pr	60 Nd	61 Pm	62 Sm	63 Eu	64 Gd	65 Tb	66 Dy	67 Ho	68 Er	69 Tm	70 Yb
		**	89 Ac	90 Th	91 Pa	92 U	93 Np	94 Pu	95 Am	96 Cm	97 Bk	98 Cf	99 Es	100 Fm	101 Md	102 No

By Offnfopt: Own work, Public Domain, https://commons.wikimedia.org/w/index.php?curid=62296883

Metals, Nonmetals, and Metalloids

Metals are substances or mixtures that are primary solids (except mercury, Hg) and make up most of the periodic table (the left-hand side). Metals can be electrically and thermally conductive, malleable (hammered to make a sheet), and ductile (drawn to produce a wire). They can have a specific luster and may be hard/opaque/shiny. Metals can form an alloy when mixed with other metals and tend to have high densities because the atoms are tightly packed.

Nonmetals are found on the right-hand side of the periodic table (e.g., nitrogen, sulfur, and bromine). Sixteen nonmetals (e.g., C, P, I) are found between groups III and VIIIA. Some of these nonmetals have negligible electrical conductivity. However, there are some exceptions. For example, diamond (sp^3, hybridized carbon) is not electrically conductive, but allotropes of carbon, such as graphene and carbon fiber (sp^2, hybridized carbon), have relatively high electrical conductivity although less than metals. Nonmetals tend to be hard or brittle solids (sulfur and carbon), liquids (only bromine), and gases (chlorine and oxygen gas).

Metalloids have both metal and nonmetal characteristics. They are found between metals and nonmetals and are organized diagonally within the periodic table. Boron (B), arsenic (As), and silicon (Si) are examples of metalloids. Some metalloids are poor electrical conductors but are shiny like metals. At higher temperatures, metalloids may become good electrical conductors. Most metalloids are semiconductors.

Element Symbols

Each element block contains an atomic number and one or two letters that represent the chemical symbol for that element. The element symbol is typically defined from the element name. The element block also includes an average mass number that is generally equal to the mass of the protons and neutrons for one atom of that element. Specifically, the number given below the element symbol is the **atomic mass**, a weighted average for several unique atoms that occur naturally. One **atomic mass unit (1 amu)** is one-twelfth of the mass of a carbon atom that contains six protons and six neutrons (12 amu). Consider the sulfur element block shown below.

16
S
32.06

The chemical symbol *S* signifies sulfur, and 16 corresponds to the atomic number of sulfur (Z = 16). If one sulfur atom contains a neutral charge, the number of protons (Z = 16) must also equal the number of electrons. Therefore, there are 16 electrons. The number below the chemical symbol (e.g., 32.06) is the element's atomic mass or average mass number. The average mass number is a weighted average of several types of sulfur atoms that each differ in total mass due to the different number of neutrons. For example, if the **mass number (A)** of sulfur is 32, the number of protons is 16, and the number of neutrons is also 16. For another type of sulfur atom, the number of protons is still 16, but the number of neutrons is 17, giving it a mass number of 33. The average mass number shown in the sulfur element block must contain a larger fraction of atoms that have 16 neutrons (the naturally occurring element) because the average is closer to 32.

Trends in the Periodic Table

The **periodic law** describes how elements, arranged by atomic number, will vary periodically with respect to their physical and chemical properties.

In other words, the arrangement of each element in the periodic table shows a specific trend and allows for the prediction of that property. Some physical and chemical properties include metal reactivity, atomic radius, electron affinity, ionization energy, and electronegativity.

Metal reactivity decreases across a row (left to right) and decreases up a column (bottom to top) on the periodic table. For nonmetals, the reactivity increases across a row (left to right) and increases up a column (bottom to top). Noble gases are exceptions because they have little reactivity. The metallic character of the elements decreases diagonally (e.g., from francium to fluorine).

The atomic radius may have several definitions, such as the covalent, or ionic, radius. The **covalent radius** is half the distance of a covalent bond, from one nucleus to the other, that forms between two nonmetallic atoms. Along a period or row, the atomic radius decreases as the atomic number increases. The decrease is due to the **effective nuclear charge**, or the positive charge an electron feels from the protons. Because the effective nuclear charge increases from left to right, the added protons pull the valence electrons inward, thereby decreasing the size of the atomic radius. Within a row, alkali metals are larger than noble gas atoms. Within a vertical column or group, the atomic radius of the atom increases with respect to the period number. For example, the atomic radius of cesium is larger than sodium. The atomic radius increases top to bottom or as the period increases because more electrons are added to the valence electron shells (the principal quantum number increases).

Electron affinity (EA) is the amount of energy required to place an electron onto the orbital of a neutrally-charged atom to form a negative ion. The periodic trend for electron affinities is less straightforward. For example, the EA for group IA elements will increase down a column. The stability of a negatively charged atom, due to the addition of an electron, will decrease (e.g., from Li^- to Cs^-). When lithium accepts an electron to form lithium anion, energy will be released. Group IIA elements have a filled s shell; adding an electron would mean that energy would have to be added for an electron to be placed into a p orbital. Therefore, these elements will not form stable ions. Moving left to right across a row, the EA decreases (more negative) with an exception given to group VA. The fluoride anion has greater stability than the lithium anion, so it's expected that the halogens are likely to bear a negative charge.

The minimum amount of energy that is needed to remove an electron from a gaseous atom or ion from the outermost shell is called the **first ionization energy**. For example, the first ionization energy, or energy needed to remove an electron from carbon, is 1086 kJ/mol.

$$C(1s^2 2p^4) \rightarrow C(1s^2 2p^3) + e^-$$

Within a period, ionization energies typically increase with respect to the atomic number. Alkali metals, group IA elements, tend to have the lowest ionization energies, which explains why these metals lose electrons readily. Noble gases, group VIIIA, will have the largest ionization energies for any row. The stability and nonreactivity of noble gases make the removal of an electron difficult. Because the square of the effective nuclear charge increases across a row, the ionization energy increases, thereby making electron removal more difficult. For main group elements, when moving down a column, the ionization energy decreases because the atomic size/radius increases. It requires less energy to remove an electron that is farther away from the nucleus because the effective nuclear charge is smaller (e.g., the force of attraction is weaker at longer distances).

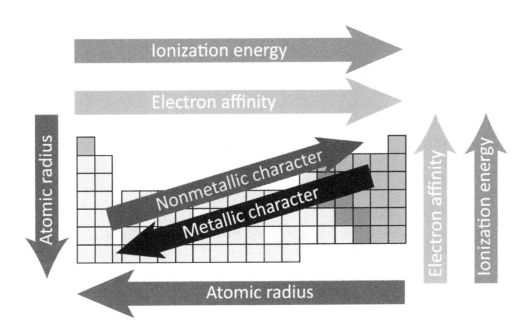

Atoms have a specific measure of readiness to form a chemical bond that is called **electronegativity**. Elements that are found near the bottom on the far-left side (e.g., francium) tend to have a limited ability to attract electrons and are the least electronegative. Elements with relatively low electronegativity tend to give up one or more electrons to form a chemical bond. In contrast, elements located toward the top and right sides (e.g., fluorine) are the most electronegative and have the greatest ability to attract electrons. These elements tend to acquire a negative charge. In general, the electronegativity increases across a row, from left to right, but decreases down a column, from top to bottom. Therefore, metals tend to form cations, whereas nonmetals will form anions. Each element has an associated electronegativity value.

Atomic Structure

Atomic Models

The modern view of the atom is based on observations of alpha particle-scattering experiments that were performed in 1911 by Hans Geiger, Ernest Marsden, and Ernest Rutherford. When alpha particles (helium nuclei) were directed toward a gold metal foil, some of the particles were deflected in several directions. The observation puzzled the scientists because they expected most of the alpha particles to pass through the atoms found within the metal foil. Before 1911, it was widely believed that the atom consisted of negatively-charged electrons dispersed within a positively-charged sphere. The atomic model was equated to a plum-pudding or blueberry muffin model in which electrons were dispersed within a sphere. The model was analogous to how blueberries (electrons) were spread out within the muffin. The muffin acted as the positively charged sphere. Rutherford thought that the alpha particles would show a slight deflection because the subatomic particles (electrons) were evenly dispersed. The existence of subatomic particles such as the proton had not been discovered or fully understood. The results of Rutherford's experiment didn't support the plum-pudding model because some alpha particles were deflected instead of passing through the atom. As a result, Rutherford proposed a new atomic model that supported the findings. The results indicated the following:

1. The space of the atom is mostly empty, and 99.95% of an atom's mass is found at the nucleus. The nucleus is the space at the center of an atom that contains the positively-charged protons and neutrally charged neutrons.

2. The atom is electrically neutral because the number of protons is equal to the number of electrons.

3. The negatively-charged electrons, on the other hand, move about the unoccupied space and around the nucleus. For comparison, the nucleus would occupy a sphere that has a diameter of 1.5 inches (e.g., a ping-pong ball), and the electrons would occupy a space that is approximately 3 miles in diameter.

Electron Motion in the Atom

Since Rutherford's experiments, the current view of the atom has remained mostly unchanged. In 1913, the **Bohr model** introduced and proposed a simplified atomic model that showed electrons moving in a fixed orbit around a nucleus, similar to how planets move around the sun. The Bohr model was successful in predicting the emission spectra of simple atoms, such as the hydrogen atom. For example, the Bohr model correctly predicted the wavelength of emitted light (red and blue light) from a hydrogen atom and was consistent with the experimental line spectra of the hydrogen atom. However, it was less accurate when applied to multi-electron atoms (e.g., carbon). Furthermore, the Bohr model was not an accurate representation of how electrons moved within an atom.

The **quantum mechanical view** of the atom describes electrons as having wave-like properties and occupying regions around the nuclei with a specific probability. The **Heisenberg uncertainty principle** states that the position and momentum of an electron cannot be determined simultaneously. Only the probability of finding an electron at some point can be determined within some region. These regions of spaces, occupied by electrons, are described as **atomic orbitals**, or mathematical functions or spaces occupied by an electron or electron pair. Electrons can be divided into different shells that gradually span away from the nucleus. These **atomic shells** may contain a subset of orbitals that vary in size and shape. Atomic shells and orbitals are often thought of as the electron clouds that surround the nucleus. The hydrogen atom contains two electrons that are found in the K shell. There is only one spherical orbital (called $1s$) in the K shell. Regardless of the orbital's size and shape, one atomic orbital can hold at most two electrons, which is a rule known as the **Pauli exclusion principle**. Each electron per orbital has an opposite spin. The L shell is located farther away from the nucleus and contains four orbitals: one spherical orbital (s or $2s$) and three dumbbell-shaped orbitals ($2p_x$, $2p_y$, $2p_z$). The K shell can only hold up to two electrons because there is only one orbital; however, the L shell can hold up to a maximum of eight electrons because there are four orbitals (each orbital holds two electrons). The M shell is the third atomic shell that lies farther out compared to the L and K shells, and houses one spherical orbital (s orbital or $3s$), three dumbbell-shaped orbitals (three p orbitals or $3p_x$, $3p_y$, $3p_z$), and five leaf clover–like orbitals called d orbitals (five $3d$ orbitals). The total number of electrons within the M shell is 1. The image below shows a simple atomic model and the electron cloud (quantum mechanical view) of the L and K shells.

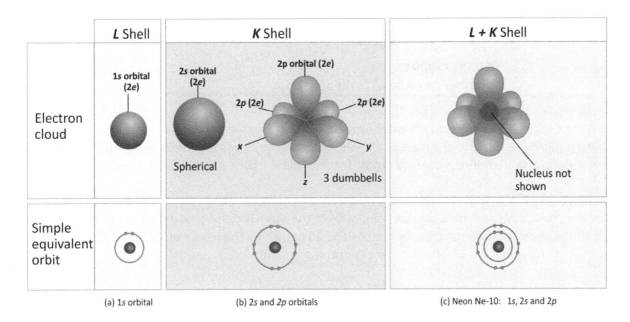

The first row shows the electron cloud picture, and the second row shows a simple orbit model of the L and K and combined shells. The last column combines the L and K shells. The positively-charged protons found within the nucleus attract the negatively-charged electrons. An atom that has an equal number of protons and electrons has a neutral charge. As the atomic number of an atom increases, so does the number of electrons. The orbitals and shells are gradually filled or occupied as the atomic number increases. For example, a neutral carbon atom contains six protons and six electrons. Two electrons will occupy the s orbital within the L shell. Within the K shell, two electrons will occupy another s orbital, and another two electrons will occupy two electrons within the p orbitals. The electron configuration is $1s^2 2s^2 2p^2$.

Isotopes

Most atoms will have a total charge that is 0, and therefore, they contain the same number of protons and electrons within the atom. For a neutrally-charged atom, the atomic number is equal to the number of electrons. An **ion** refers to an atom that does not have an equal number of electrons and protons. If an atom has fewer electrons than protons, it is positively charged and is referred to as a **cation**. If an atom has more electrons than protons, it is negatively charged and is called an **anion**. For a given element that has a fixed number of protons, some atoms will have a varying mass number due to the different number of neutrons. An **isotope** is an atom of the same element that has a varying number of neutrons but the same number of protons. The image below shows an alternate notation of a chemical symbol when discussing isotopes.

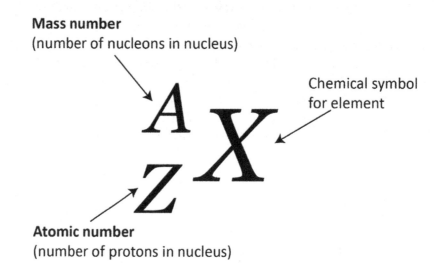

Mass number
(number of nucleons in nucleus)

Chemical symbol
for element

$$_Z^A X$$

Atomic number
(number of protons in nucleus)

The term X refers to the one- or two-letter element symbol. The superscript A is the **mass number (A)**. The mass number is equal to the mass of all protons (Z) and neutrons (N) within an atom. The subscript Z is the atomic number or number of protons. The formula $A - Z = N$ gives the number of neutrons (N).

Average Atomic Mass

If the atomic number and mass number remain fixed, the atom is called a **nuclide**. For example, sulfur-32 is a type of nuclide that contains 16 protons and 16 neutrons. The mass number is 32 because A = 32 and its atomic number Z = 16. The number of neutrons is:

$$A - Z = 32 - 16 = 16$$

If given the number of neutrons for a particular element of sulfur, the mass number can be calculated. For example, if the number of neutrons for one isotope of sulfur is equal to 17, the mass number is:

$$A = N + Z = 17 + 16 = 33$$

Note that the number of protons remains fixed for an isotope of sulfur and that the mass of a neutron and proton are approximately 1 amu. For the different isotopes of sulfur, the chemical symbol may be written in the form $_Z^A S$ or with the name of the element followed by the mass number (e.g., sulfur-**A**).

The three most abundant isotopes of sulfur are sulfur-32 (95.02%), sulfur-34 (4.21%), and sulfur-33 (0.75%) and can be written as follows:

$$^{32}_{16}S, ^{34}_{16}S, ^{33}_{16}S$$

Although the atomic number remains the same, the mass number changes for each isotope. The most abundant isotope of sulfur has a mass number of A = 32. There are 16 protons, 16 neutrons, and 16 electrons in the naturally occurring form of a neutral sulfur atom. Recall that the atomic mass number of sulfur is 32.06 amu. The atomic mass of an element is not necessarily the same as the atomic number due to the number of sulfur isotopes. Sulfur-32 has 16 neutrons, sulfur-33 contains 17 neutrons, and sulfur-34 has 18 neutrons. The average of all atomic masses of sulfur is equal to 32.06 amu. The table below shows the atomic mass and abundance of each isotope.

Isotopes of Sulfur (S)		
Sulfur Isotope	Atomic Mass (amu)	Fractional Abundance
S-32, $^{32}_{16}S$	31.9721	0.9499
S-34, $^{34}_{16}S$	33.9679	0.0425
S-33, $^{33}_{16}S$	32.9715	0.0075
S-36, $^{36}_{16}S$	35.9671	0.0001

Sulfur's average atomic mass is 32.06 amu because sulfur-32 is the most abundant isotope and contains a mass close to 32.0 amu. The average atomic mass depends on the atomic mass for each isotope and its fractional abundance. A **mass spectrometer** is an instrument that can experimentally measure the atomic mass and fractional abundance of different isotopes for a given element. Atoms of a given element are converted to positively charged cations corresponding to specific isotopes, and the mass-to-charge (m/z) ratio and fractional abundance are measured. The spectrometer outputs a graph with the respective fractional abundance versus the m/z ratio. The mass spectrum of sulfur is shown below.

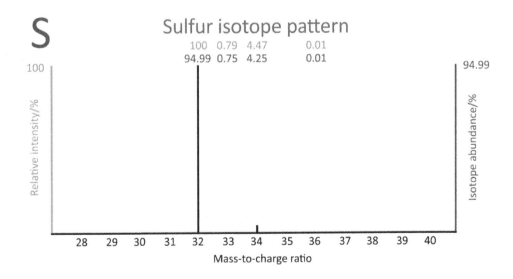

The mass spectrum shows the main peak at 32 m/z (32 amu) and corresponds to sulfur-32. The fractional abundance of sulfur-32 is 0.9499, and its percent abundance is 94.99%. The second most abundant isotope, sulfur-34, is shown at 34 m/z (34 amu) and has a percent abundance of 4.25%. The signals for the remaining isotopes are too small to be seen but are quantified at the top of the spectrum.

The **average atomic mass** of sulfur, as shown in the periodic table, can be determined by averaging over the first three isotopes.

$$Average\ atomic\ mass\ (amu) = \sum (atomic\ mass) \times (fractional\ abundance)$$

$$[(31.9721) \times (0.9499)] + [(33.9679) \times (0.0425)] + [(32.9715) \times (0.0075)]$$

$$32.06\ \text{amu}$$

Sulfur-36 was not accounted for because its fractional abundance is negligible.

Nuclear Chemistry

Nuclear chemistry involves the study of how a nuclear transformation changes the identities of elements within the nuclei of atoms. The transformation typically occurs for unstable nuclei that spontaneously decompose, causing specific subatomic particles to be emitted. The emission of subatomic particles (e.g., electrons, protons, neutrons, or nuclei) by specific elements is called **radioactivity** or **radioactive decay**. A nuclide with an atomic number (Z) greater than 83 tends to be unstable and typically undergoes radioactive decay. The unstable nuclei for that particular element will emit subatomic particles until it becomes more stable.

The nuclear reaction results in the formation of new elements and subatomic particles. The energy changes in a nuclear reaction are much greater than the breakage of a chemical bond (e.g., approximately a million times greater than chemical reactions). The amount of energy that is released can be harnessed for the creation of electricity. The Nobel Prize winner (1903 and 1911), Marie Curie, discovered that elements such as polonium and radium emitted **uranic rays**, a term which is now known as **radiation** or **radioactivity**.

Types of Radioactivity

Radioisotopes are radioactive or unstable isotopes of a specific element that constantly emit subatomic particles from the nucleus of an atom. Some specific isotopes of an element or a nuclide, which have a fixed mass number and atomic number, are more likely to undergo radioactive decay. However, some nuclides are relatively stable and don't readily undergo radioactive decay (e.g., nuclides of argon-36, argon-38, and argon-40). The subatomic particles that are typically emitted by radioisotopes include the proton, neutron, and electron.

$$_{1}^{1}p\ (proton),\ _{0}^{1}n\ (neutron),\ _{-1}^{0}e\ (electron)$$

The subscript and superscripts located to the left of the one-letter symbol have a similar interpretation as the notation of an isotope. For example, the superscript designates the mass number (A). Both the proton and neutron have a mass number of 1 because their atomic mass is each 1 amu. In contrast, the electron has a superscript value of 0 because it's relatively lighter than the neutron and proton. The subscript values take on a slightly different meaning. For a proton, the subscript will be equal to 1 (e.g., there is only one positively-charged proton). The subscript for the neutron is 0 because neutrons are not positively-charged particles. For the electron, a value of −1 is assigned and reflects the electron's charge; it is opposite to that of the proton.

The alpha (α) particle is another type of particle that is released during a nuclear reaction or radioactive decay process. An **alpha (α) particle** is a helium-4 nucleus without any electrons and has the notation $^4_2He^{2+}$. The charge is not usually shown in a nuclear equation, so the notation for an alpha particle is commonly written as ^4_2He. There are two protons and two neutrons because the mass number is 4. If a nucleus is emitting alpha particles, it is emitting **alpha radiation**. The penetrating power of an alpha particle is relatively low (e.g., an alpha particle will not penetrate a piece of paper).

A **nuclear equation** shows the radioactive decay process or nuclear reaction of specific radioisotopes that break down from a parent nuclide to a daughter nuclide along with other subatomic particles. One example, shown below, is the alpha decay (or alpha emission) of uranium-238.

$$\overbrace{^{238}_{92}U}^{\substack{parent \\ nuclide}} \rightarrow \overbrace{^{234}_{90}Th}^{\substack{daughter \\ nuclide}} + \overbrace{^{4}_{2}He}^{\substack{alpha \\ particle}}$$

Uranium-238 is the parent nuclide that initially has 92 protons. During the nuclear reaction, uranium-238 spontaneously decomposes to a lighter daughter nuclide, thorium-234, in addition to an alpha particle, helium-4. The nuclear reaction is an example of alpha decay because an alpha particle is emitted or found on the product side of the equation. The alpha decay of uranium-238 results in a chemical identity change. The number of protons for the daughter nuclide will not necessarily be equal to the parent nuclide. Like a chemical reaction, a nuclear reaction must follow the law of conservation of mass and be balanced on both sides. The mass number (A) must be conserved. The sum of the mass numbers for all reactants must be equal to the sum of the mass numbers for all products.

The mass number of uranium-238 is A_p = 238 (p for product), so the sum of the mass number for thorium-234 (A_{r1} = 234, r1 for reactant 1), and helium-4 (A_{r2} = 4, r2 for reactant 2) must be equal to 238: $A_p = A_{r1} + A_{r2}$ or 238 = 234 + 4. Similarly, the atomic number (Z) must be conserved on both sides of the equation. The atomic number of uranium-238 is Z_p = 92 (p for product), so the sum of the atomic number for thorium-234 (Z_{r1} = 90, r1 for reactant 1) and helium-4 (Z = 2, r2 for reactant 2) must be equal to 92: $Z_p = Z_{r1} + Z_{r2}$ or 92 = 90 + 2.

Beta (β) decay or **beta radiation** is a radioactive decay process in which an unstable nucleus emits a stream of electrons, denoted as β^-, at a relatively high speed. Beta particles have greater penetrating power because they are lighter and smaller than alpha particles; however, they have less ionizing power. Beta particles may penetrate a piece a paper but not a sheet of metal. Importantly, beta decay involves the transformation of a neutron into a proton.

$$neutron \; (^1_0n) \rightarrow proton \; (^1_1p) + \overbrace{electron \; (^{\;\;0}_{-1}e)}^{beta \; particle}$$

Because a neutron is converted to a proton, the new element that is produced will still have the same mass number but a higher number of protons. For example, berkelium (Bk) will decompose to californium (Cf) and emit a beta particle in the process. Note that mass is conserved.

$$\overbrace{^{249}_{97}Bk}^{\substack{parent \\ nuclide}} \rightarrow \overbrace{^{249}_{98}Cf}^{\substack{daughter \\ nuclide}} + \overbrace{^{\;\;0}_{-1}e}^{\substack{beta \\ particle}}$$

A nucleus can emit short-wavelength or high-energy photons, a form of electromagnetic radiation called **gamma (γ) ray radiation**.

$$^0_0\gamma \; gamma \; (\gamma) \; ray \; or \; photon$$

A value of 0 is assigned to the superscripts and subscripts because photons don't have a mass or charge. Therefore, in gamma ray emission, the mass number (A) and atomic number (Z) for the parent nuclide remain unchanged. Gamma rays have low ionizing power but the greatest penetrating power and are hazardous because they can pass through biological material, such as our body. Technetium-99m is a type of nuclide that can exist in an excited state but will decay to a lower energy state, technetium-99m, thereby releasing gamma rays.

$$^{99m}_{43}Tc \rightarrow {}^{99}_{43}Tc + {}^{0}_{0}\gamma \; ; \text{wavelength of } \sim 10^{-12} \text{ m}$$

The m in the superscript of the reactant stands for *metastable technetium-99m*. Concrete and lead are materials that are often used to block gamma radiation. If an unstable nucleus undergoes **positron (β+) emission**, a proton will transform into a neutron.

$$Proton\ ({}^{1}_{1}p) \rightarrow neutron({}^{1}_{0}n) + positron\ ({}^{0}_{+1}e\ )\ Positron\ emission$$

The positron (${}^{0}_{+1}e$) is an antiparticle or anti-electron (+1) because its charge is opposite to an electron (−1) and equal in magnitude. If a positron and an electron collide with each other, both particles are canceled out, and a gamma ray is produced.

$$^{0}_{+1}e + {}^{0}_{+1}e \rightarrow {}^{0}_{0}\gamma$$

The decay of technetium-95 to molybdenum-95 and carbon-10 to boron-10 will produce a positron.

$$^{95}_{43}Tc \rightarrow {}^{95}_{42}Mo + {}^{0}_{+1}e$$

$$\overbrace{{}^{10}_{6}C}^{\substack{parent \\ nuclide}} \rightarrow \overbrace{{}^{10}_{5}B}^{\substack{daughter \\ nuclide}} + \overbrace{{}^{0}_{+1}e}^{positron}$$

The atomic number (Z) of the daughter nuclide decreases by 1 because a proton is converted to a neutron in the parent nuclide. The penetrating and ionizing power of a positron is similar in magnitude to β^{-} particles. In an **electron capture** process, unstable nuclei will decay to stable nuclei by absorbing an electron from one of its inner orbitals within an electron cloud. Like positron emission, a proton is converted to a neutron.

$$^{1}_{1}p + {}^{0}_{-1}e \rightarrow {}^{1}_{0}n$$

Indium-111 can absorb an electron and decay to cadmium-111. The mass number is conserved.

$$^{111}_{49}In + {}^{0}_{-1}e \rightarrow {}^{111}_{48}Cd$$

A nuclide that contains more than 89 protons (Z > 89) can undergo **spontaneous fission** and break up into lighter nuclei. The radioactive decay process results in the production of a neutron and a large amount of energy. The spontaneous fission of uranium-236 produces yttrium-96, iodine-136, and four neutrons.

$$^{236}_{92}U \rightarrow {}^{96}_{39}Y + {}^{136}_{53}I + 4\ {}^{1}_{0}n$$

Radioactive Decay

The radioactive decay of an element or unstable nucleus can be expressed in terms of time. The **half-life** ($t_{1/2}$) is the amount of time needed for half the radioactive element or nuclide to react. The half-life can be expressed in terms of its rate constant (k).

$$t_{1/2} = \frac{0.693}{k}$$

The half-life is inversely proportional to the rate constant. A relatively short half-life indicates that the rate constant is large, and a long half-life means the rate constant is small. For example, the half-life of krypton-89 is 3.16 minutes, and the half-life of cobalt-60 is 5.27 years. Because krypton-89 has a shorter half-life, its rate constant is much greater than cobalt-60's rate constant. If there is initially 10 g of krypton-89, there would be 5 g left of krypton 90 after 3.16 minutes. Similarly, if there is initially 10 g of cobalt-60, there would be 5 g left of cobalt-60 after 5.27 years. The following equation relates the initial $[B]_0$ and final amount $[B]_t$ of a radioactive nuclide after some time (t):

$$ln[B]_t = -kt + ln[B]_0 \; or$$

$$t = -ln\left(\frac{[B]_t}{[B]_0}\right)\frac{1}{k}$$

The half-life of a nuclide can be determined if the initial and final amounts of the nuclide and final time (t) are given. For example, suppose it took 57.6 days for an unknown element Z to decay from 20 to 10 g. First, find the rate constant by rearranging the previous equation.

The term $[B]_t = 10.0 \; grams$ and $[B]_0 = 20.0 \; grams$. The value of t is 57.6 days. The rate constant is:

$$k = -ln\left(\frac{10.0 \; g}{20.0 \; g}\right)\frac{1}{57.6 \; days} = 0.01203 \; days^{-1}$$

The half-life can now be calculated:

$$t_{1/2} = \frac{0.693}{k} = \frac{0.693}{0.01203 \; days^{-1}} = 57.6 \; days$$

It should be immediately clear that the value of t is the half-life because the final amount is only half the initial amount. However, there will be scenarios where the value of t is not the half-life because the final amount is not half the initial amount (e.g., $[B]_t = 5$ g and $[B]_0 = 20$ g). For example, to determine the time at which a particular nuclide decayed to 25% of its initial amount ($[B]_t = 5$ g and $[B]_0 = 20$ g) given that the half-life is equal to 57.6 days, the value of time t is:

$$t = -ln\left(\frac{[B]_t}{[B]_0}\right)\frac{1}{k} = -ln\left(\frac{0.25([B]_0)}{[B]_0}\right)\frac{1}{0.01203 \; days^{-1}} = 115.2 \; days$$

Note that 25% in decimal form is 0.25. The final time is now longer than the half-life. The final answer should probably be evident without calculation. For example, after 57.6 days, half the initial amount is 10 g, and after another 57.6 days, the final amount should be:

$$5 \; g(57.6 + 57.6 = 115.2 \; days)$$

If asked to determine the amount of substance $[B]_t$ at a later time t given the half-life and the initial amount $[B]_0$, the following rearranged equation can be used:

$$[B]_t = [B]_0 e^{-kt}$$

For instance, how much of the same unknown radioactive nuclide is left after $t = 40.0$ days if it has $t_{1/2} = 57.6$ days and an initial amount equal to 20.0 g? Solving for final amount $[B]_t$ at time t gives:

$$[B]_t = [B]_0 e^{-kt} = (20.0\ g)e^{-0.01203\ days^{-1} \times 40.0\ days} = 12.4\ g$$

As a qualitative check, consider the fact that the final amount of 12.4 g after $t = 40$ days is greater than the half-life amount (20 to 10 g after $t_{1/2} = 57.6$ days).

Fission and Fusion Reactions

Transmutation nuclear reactions are initiated by the bombardment of subatomic particles toward parent nuclides and can change the identity of one element to another. Fission and fusion are examples of transmutation reactions. A **fission reaction** involves the splitting of a large nuclide into two or more lighter but stable nuclides. The reaction begins when a nucleus absorbs neutrons that are moving relatively slow. A larger, unstable nucleus is produced but then undergoes nuclear fission. Uranium-235 can absorb neutrons by bombardment, resulting in the formation of krypton-94, barium-139, and several neutrons. A large amount of energy is produced.

$$^{235}_{92}U + ^{1}_{0}n \rightarrow ^{94}_{36}Kr + ^{139}_{56}Ba + 3^{1}_{0}n + energy$$

The production of neutrons results in a **chain reaction** because the produced neutrons from nuclear fission induce another fission reaction; the neutrons bombard other uranium-235 nuclei. Nuclear power plants often employ fission reactions because they produce large amount of energy or electricity.

The energy produced by the atomic bomb relies on nuclear fission and the subsequent chain reaction that follows. The produced neutrons result in multiple nuclear fissions. One fission reaction produces three neutrons $^{1}_{0}n$, which, in turn, bombard three uranium-235 nuclei. One fission reaction creates three fission reactions. The three fission reactions will then lead to nine fission reactions, and so on.

If two or more lighter nuclei are combined to produce a heavier nucleus, the reaction is called a **fusion reaction**. These reactions are more common under extreme pressure and temperature conditions and do not generally occur on Earth. The sun is composed of hydrogen gas and constantly produces light energy and massive amounts of heat by nuclear fusion. For example, deuterium (hydrogen-2 or $^{2}_{1}H$) and tritium (hydrogen-3 or $^{3}_{1}H$) are nuclides found within the sun that can undergo nuclear fusion to produce a neutron and a helium nucleus.

$$^{2}_{1}H + ^{3}_{1}H \rightarrow ^{4}_{2}He + ^{1}_{0}n$$

The Sun's extreme conditions create a plasma state composed of positively charged ions and electrons. These conditions allow for the combination reaction of tritium and deuterium to occur. The extreme temperature and pressure conditions can be replicated on earth by using a particle accelerator. The Torus fusion reactor at the Princeton Plasma Physics Laboratory can create plasma conditions needed for a fusion reaction. Two steps are involved in the detonation of a hydrogen bomb. In the first step, a fission reaction is initiated. Then, the energy provided by the fission reaction creates the extreme conditions required for nuclear fusion to take place. In contrast, an atomic bomb only relies on nuclear fission. Hydrogen bombs are up to a thousand times more destructive compared to atomic bombs because fission and fusion are involved.

Chemical Bonding

A **compound** is a substance consisting of two or more elements that are chemically bonded together. Electrons in the outermost atomic shell are called **valence electrons**. These outer electrons form a chemical bond. For example, consider the bonding of two hydrogen atoms to form hydrogen gas:

$$H + H \rightarrow H_2$$

Each hydrogen atom contains one valence electron. A **chemical bond** forms when the two atoms are joined together. The competition of repulsive and attractive forces between the electrons and protons of each atom creates a chemical bond. The two electrons between each hydrogen atom are distributed or shared equally. The distribution of the electron pair within the chemical bond will determine the bond type. There are generally three bond types. A **covalent bond** results when two atoms share electrons equally. The atoms are typically nonmetallic elements that have a similar electronegativity value. For example, hydrogen gas contains one covalent bond. A **nonpolar covalent bond** results if both atoms are the same element (e.g., H_2).

The electron distribution in the hydrogen molecule is symmetrical because both atoms have the same electronegativity value. A **polar covalent bond** results when both atoms are each a different element. Hydrogen chloride, HCl, is an example of a molecule that has a polar covalent bond. Although the electrons are shared equally, the electrons are attracted more toward the chlorine atom because its electronegativity value is greater. The bonding electrons will move closer to the more electronegative atom. Other examples of molecules that contain polar covalent bonds are H_2O and HBr. The bonding electrons in water will generally lean toward the oxygen atom because it's more electronegative. Similarly, the bonding electrons in hydrogen bromide will move toward bromine because it has a greater electronegativity value. The electron distribution (electron cloud) between the two atoms (e.g., H and Br) is unsymmetrical because each atom has different electronegativity values. The difference in polarity creates a bond dipole where one side of the molecule is electron-deficient or electron-rich.

If two electrons are shared between two atoms, the chemical bond is referred to as a **single bond**. If the two atoms share four electrons, two pairs of electrons are shared, and the chemical bond is called a **double bond**. The sharing of six electrons forms three pairs of shared electrons and results in a chemical bond known as a **triple bond**. When the number of electrons increases within a chemical bond, the bond becomes stronger, and the distance between each atom decreases (shorter bond). Therefore, a triple covalent bond is the strongest and shortest type of covalent bond.

An **ionic bond** is a type of chemical bond that forms as the result of electrostatic attractions between two atoms that are oppositely charged. These types of bonds generally form between a metal and nonmetal. Because metals have low ionization energies, they tend to lose an electron. Nonmetals have a relatively high electron affinity and are more likely to gain an electron. Therefore, when metal and nonmetal atoms are close together, the metal loses an electron to the nonmetal. Consequently, the metal is positively charged (cation), and the nonmetal is negatively charged (anion). Potassium chloride is an example of a compound that contains an ionic bond. Potassium loses an electron to the chlorine atom and creates a strong electrostatic force of attraction.

Ionic bonds are relatively strong due to the strong electrostatic forces of attraction. Ionic compounds tend to have high boiling and melting points. Ionic compounds exist as crystalline solids that are brittle.

The molecular structure of an ionic compound is well defined because the atoms are arranged within a crystal lattice (e.g., sodium chloride has a face-centered cubic crystal lattice). The classification of a chemical bond can be determined by the difference in electronegativity between the two atoms in the bond. A bond is classified as nonpolar covalent if the electronegativity difference between each atom lies between 0 and 0.4.

A bond is polar covalent if the electronegativity difference falls from 0.4 to 2.0. If the electronegativity difference is greater than 2.0, the bond is considered ionic. The electronegativity difference between potassium and chlorine is $\Delta EN = 3.0 - 0.8 = 2.2$, so the bond is ionic. For the H-Br bond, bromine has an EN value equal to 3.0, and hydrogen has an EN value equal to 2.1: $\Delta EN = 3.0 - 2.1 = 0.9$. The H-Br bond is polar covalent. The hydrogen molecule (H_2) will be nonpolar because the electronegativity values are the same. The difference between each EN value is given for each bond in the table below.

Bond Types Based on Electronegativity Difference (ΔEN)		
Molecule or Ionic Compound	Bond Type (ΔEN range)	Electronegativity Difference (ΔEN)
H_2	Nonpolar covalent (0-0.4)	$\Delta EN = |2.1\text{-}2.1| = 0.0$
HBr	Polar covalent (0.4-2.0)	$\Delta EN = |2.8\text{-}2.1| = 0.7$
KCl	Ionic (2.0+)	$\Delta EN = |3.0\text{-}0.8| = 2.2$

Metals such as pure aluminum can form a **metallic bond** with another metal. Like ionic substances, which have atoms that are oppositely charged, metallic bonds are the result of attractive forces between metal ions and electrons. These attractive forces act like glue and keep the metallic substance intact. Metals contain a "sea of electrons," and these electrons can move freely through a metal. As a result, metals tend to conduct heat and electricity with relative ease and have high strength and malleability. As electrons move across the metal, energy moves freely across the metal, and a current is created, thereby making the metal electrically conductive.

Structural formulas may be written as **Lewis structures** in a chemical equation to help visualize how valence electrons move between an atom or a molecule. Lewis structures are not typically expressed for metallic substances due to the free-roaming nature of the electrons.

For covalent compounds, the element is written as a **Lewis symbol**, which is surrounded by dots that represent the number of valence electrons. A Lewis dot can be placed on the left, top, right, or bottom of an element symbol. Only two dots at most are allowed per side. Therefore, only a maximum of eight dots can surround the element. Most elements follow the octet rule; however, there are some exceptions. For instance, hydrogen shares two electrons (duet), whereas boron only shares six valence electrons (sextet).

Lewis symbols are generally written for main group elements (e.g., groups IA–VIIIA). The group number for that element determines the number of dots around a specific element. For example, because sodium belongs to group IA, one dot will be assigned to sodium. Carbon belongs to group 4A, so there will be four dots around that element. During a chemical reaction, atoms will react to obtain a total of eight valence electrons.

In other words, atoms may lose, gain, or share electrons to complete an octet (octet rule). Sodium tends to lose one electron because the sodium ion obtains an octet or an electron configuration like neon. Chlorine belongs to group VIIA and should have seven dots or valence electrons. Chlorine tends to gain an electron or dot, which gives the element a complete octet. Consider the reaction of two chlorine atoms to form chlorine gas.

The Lewis symbols for the chlorine atoms and the Lewis electron dot formula of the product are shown in below.

Lewis symbol

Lewis electron dot formula

$$:\overset{..}{\underset{..}{Cl}} \cdot \; + \; \cdot \overset{..}{\underset{..}{Cl}}: \quad \longrightarrow \quad :\overset{..}{\underset{..}{Cl}} : \overset{..}{\underset{..}{Cl}} :$$

Lewis electron dot formulas are useful for depicting specific types of electron pairs. For example, chlorine gas contains a bonding pair or an electron pair that is shared between each atom. Chlorine gas contains six lone or nonbonding pairs that are not involved in bonding (e.g., the electrons are not shared). The figure below provides an example of the Lewis electron dot formula for ammonia (NH_3) and ammonium (NH_4^+).

Lewis structures for reactants	Lewis structure for product	Structural formula	Molecular model

Bonding pair

Lone pair

Trigonal pyramidal geometry

Lone pair

Tetrahedral molecular geometry

Hydrogen contains one dot because it belongs to group IA. Nitrogen belongs to group VA and will be surrounded by five dots. The five dots are spread out around all four sides. One side will contain two dots (nonbonding electron pair), and three sides will each contain one dot. For ammonia, three bonding pairs can form between hydrogen and nitrogen. Each atom contributes one electron. The nitrogen atom in ammonia will contain one lone pair of electrons that will act as a nonbonding pair.

Only three bonding pairs or covalent bonds can form when the Lewis symbols for hydrogen and nitrogen are combined. Each atom contributes one electron to form one bonding pair. Nitrogen will have one lone pair of electrons that does not participate in chemical bonding with the other hydrogen atoms. Hydrogen contains a duet of electrons, and nitrogen contains an octet. In the structural formula, a dash will replace the Lewis dots. An ammonium ion can form a coordinate covalent bond by donating its lone electron pair to a hydrogen proton. The curved arrow indicates the transfer of two electrons.

The Lewis electron dot formula contains a set of brackets with a 1+ superscript. The positive charge is centralized at the nitrogen atom because the donation of the electron pair makes the nitrogen atom electron-deficient. For atoms that contain double bonds and nonbonding pairs, the bonding electron pairs in a Lewis structure typically can move around. **Delocalized bonding** (or **delocalization**) refers to how electron pairs move from one atom to another within a compound. For example, in sulfur dioxide, lone electron pairs can delocalize from the oxygen atom to the sulfur atom, as shown in the figure below.

Lewis electron dot formula

Structural formula

Each curved arrow indicates the movement of one pair of electrons. Each structure is a **resonance structure** or a possible Lewis dot structure that is involved in delocalization. A bonding electron pair from a double bond moves to the oxygen atom and becomes a nonbonding pair. Simultaneously, the nonbonding pair from the second oxygen atom delocalizes between the oxygen and sulfur atom to form one bonding pair.

Anatomy and Physiology

General Terminology

Anatomy is the study of the body's shape and structure, as well as the interrelationship of body parts. **Gross anatomy** is the study of large, easily observable body structures, such as the bones or the heart. In contrast, **microscopic anatomy** is the study of small body structures that are not visible to the naked eye. Small body structures, such as cells and tissues, can be seen with the aid of a microscope.

The study of how body parts function is called **physiology**, and the study of how the heart works is called **cardiac physiology**. Anatomy and physiology are intertwined. Parts of the body are categorized together as forming an organized unit, within which each part performs a specific function. In general, the structure of a body part dictates its function. For example, the lungs and heart work together to provide oxygen to the body. The lungs contain air sacs, called alveoli, that have thin walls that enable the exchange of oxygen and carbon dioxide. The heart contains muscular chambers that pump oxygen-rich blood through the body.

Levels of Organization in the Body

Organisms contain organs; an **organ** is a structure that performs a specific function and is made up of two or more types of tissues. Some groups of organs, called **organ systems**, work together to perform one or more functions. The blood vessels and heart are an example of an organ system. The heart pumps blood through the blood vessels, and the blood laden with oxygen and nutrients is carried to all cells of the body; these components comprise the cardiovascular system. Human organisms are made up of eleven different organ systems: the integumentary, skeletal, muscular, cardiovascular, nervous, lymphatic, endocrine, respiratory, digestive, urinary, and reproductive systems. In the figure below, the cardiovascular system is used to demonstrate levels of structural organization.

At the smaller end of the scale are tissues and cells. Complex organisms such as humans and trees contain **cells**, the smallest organizational units of a living thing. Different parts of the body (for example, the heart muscle) contain groups of similar cells (in this case, cardiac muscle cells), called **tissues**, that work together to carry out a specific function or set of functions.

There are four basic types of tissues in the human body (connective, epithelial, nervous, and muscle) and they each play a specific role.

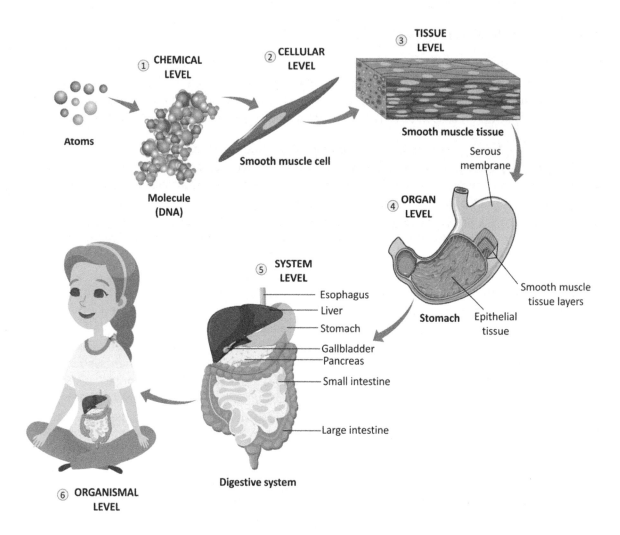

Organ Systems

The **cardiovascular system** includes primary organs such as the blood vessels and the heart. The heart moves blood from its chambers into blood vessels that are found throughout the body's tissues. Blood carries and delivers nutrients, substances, hormones, and oxygen, and it collects waste such as carbon dioxide. White blood cells are found in the blood and help protect the body from bacteria, tumor cells, and viruses.

The **lymphatic system** consists of the lymph nodes, lymphatic vessels, and the lymphoid organs such as the tonsils and the spleen. The cardiovascular and lymphatic systems are complements of one another. For example, if fluid from the blood is leaked into the tissues, then the lymphatic vessels move it back to the bloodstream to ensure that enough blood is circulated in the body. The lymphoid organs keep the blood clean and hold the cells (white blood cells) that are responsible for immunity. The **respiratory system** is responsible for providing oxygen to the body and removing carbon dioxide. This organ system includes the lungs, trachea, bronchi, pharynx, and nasal passages. The **digestive system** can be described as a tube extending from the mouth to the anus. This organ system consists of the mouth (oral cavity), the esophagus, stomach, the small and large intestines, and the rectum. Organs such as the liver, pancreas, and salivary glands act as accessory organs to the digestive system. For instance, the small intestine receives digestive enzymes from the pancreas, and the liver produces bile that helps break down fats. The digestive system breaks down ingested food and absorbs and delivers the nutrients (from the food) to the blood. The blood delivers these nutrients to all cells in the body. The breakdown of food takes place between the oral cavity and the small intestine. Water reabsorption takes place in the large intestine. Undigested and digested food move through the anus as feces.

The **urinary** or **excretory system** removes waste byproducts, for example, nitrogen compounds such as uric acid and urea, from the blood and flushes them outside the body as urine. The urinary system is made up of the bladder, urethra, kidneys, and ureters. An important function of the urinary system is to regulate the body's blood pressure, electrolyte (salt and water) concentration, and pH or acid-base balance of blood.

The primary function of the **reproductive system** is to create offspring. The female ovaries produce the ova or egg, and the male testes create the sperm. The female duct system is composed of the uterus, uterine tubes, and the vagina. The male reproductive structures consist of the penis, scrotum, accessory glands, and the duct system that transfers the sperm outside the body.

Anatomical Terminology

The **anatomical position** refers to the body in its standard position whereby the body is erect with the feet in a parallel position. The arms hang at the sides. The palms face forward instead of hanging in a cup position and facing toward the thighs. Since the palms face forward, the thumbs point away from the body.

Directional and orientational terms are used to indicate where one body structure is located with respect to another structure. For instance, the ears are found on each side of the head, left and right. In anatomical terms, the phrase would be that the ears are "lateral with respect to the nose." The following table shows several orientational and directional terms.

Term	Meaning	Example
Anterior (ventral)	In front of or toward the body	The breastbone is ventral (anterior) to the spine.
Distal	Farther from the body's origin, a point of attachment of a limb to the trunk of a body.	The elbow is distal to the bicep; the knee is distal with respect to the thigh
Deep (internal)	Away from the surface of the body or more internal	The heart is deep to the rib cage
Inferior (caudal)	Away from the head or below	The knee is inferior to the navel
Intermediate	Between a medial or later structure	The heart is intermediate to the right and left lungs.
Lateral	On the outer side or away from the body's midline	The elbows are lateral to the navel
Medial	At or toward the body's midline or on the inner side	The sternum (or heart) is medial to the arm
Posterior (dorsal)	At or toward the backside of the body; behind	The lungs (or heart) are posterior to the breastbone.

129

Term	Meaning	Example
Proximal	Near the origin of the body part; the point of attachment of a limb to the trunk of a body	The wrist is proximal to the fingers.
Superior (cephalic or cranial)	Toward the upper part of a structure	The cranium is superior to the sternum.
Superficial (external)	At or toward the surface of the body	The skin is superficial to the muscles.

Regional terms refer to the visible landmarks on the body's surface. The anterior view includes the cephalic, cervical, thoracic, abdominal, pelvic, and pubic regions. The table that follows the graphic lists the labels associated with each region.

Anterior or ventral view	Anterior and/or posterior	Posterior or dorsal view
Cephalic: The head	Upper limb	Cephalic: The head
Frontal: The forehead	Acromial: shoulder point	Occipital: The back of the head or base of skull
Orbital- The eye area	Deltoid (anterior)	Cervical: neck region
Nasal: The nose area	Brachial: The arm	Back (dorsal)
Buccal: The cheek area	Antecubital (anterior)	Scapular: shoulder blade area
Oral: The mouth	Olecranal: The posterior surface of elbow	Vertebral: The spinal column area
Mental: The chin	Antebrachial: The forearm	Lumbar: Back area between hips and ribs (the loin)
Cervical: The neck region	Carpal (anterior): The wrist	Sacral: The area between hips located at the base of the spine
Thoracic: The area between the neck and abdomen; chest	Manus: The hand	Gluteal: The buttock
Sternal: The breastbone area	Digital: fingers	
Axillary: The armpit	Lower limb	Lower limb
Pectoral: Relating to in or on the chest	Coxal (anterior): The hip	Sural (posterior): The calf
Abdominal: The anterior body trunk that is inferior to the ribs	Femoral: The thigh (anterior and posterior)	Popliteal: The posterior knee area
Umbilical: The navel	Patellar (anterior): knee	
Pelvic: An area overlying the pelvis in an anterior manner	Crural (anterior): The leg or shin	
Inguinal: The area where the thigh meets the trunk of the body; the groin	Fibular: lateral parts of the leg (anterior and posterior)	
Pubic-The genital area.		
Pedal (foot)		Pedal (foot)
Tarsal: The ankle		Calcaneal: the foot or heal
Digital: toes		Plantar: sole of the foot

Body Planes and Sections

Three types of sections and planes can be found in the body. A **plane** is the body divided into sections, and a **section** is an imaginary cut along the body. The planes of the body are the median (midsagittal), frontal (coronal), and transverse. The **midsagittal** or **median section** is the cut down the median plane of the body, whereby the left and right parts of the body are equal in size. A **sagittal section** is a cut or slice along the longitudinal (lengthwise) plane of the body. The sagittal section cuts the body into the left and right parts. The term "parasagittal" refers to a plane adjacent or parallel to the plane which divides the body into halves. The **coronal** or **frontal section** is cut along a lengthwise plane; it divides the organ or body into a posterior and an anterior part. The **transverse section** refers to a cut along a horizontal plane (like a cross-section) and divides the organ or body into its inferior and superior parts. The image below shows the planes of the body. Note that the model is standing in anatomic position.

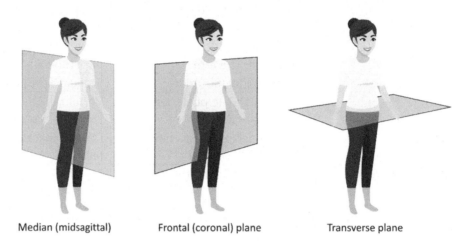

| Median (midsagittal) | Frontal (coronal) plane | Transverse plane |

Body Cavities

The ventral and dorsal body cavities provide a varying degree of protection to the organs. The **ventral body cavity** is larger than the dorsal body cavity and contains structures inside the abdomen and chest.

The ventral cavity can be divided into several parts: the thoracic, mediastinum, abdominopelvic, and pelvic cavity.

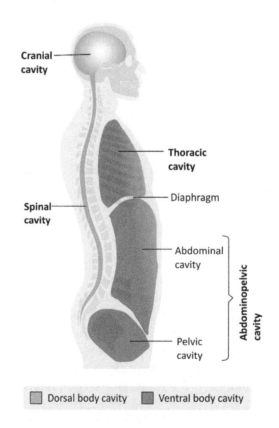

The **dorsal body cavity** contains two cavities, the cranial and the spinal cavity. The two cavities are continuous with each other. The **cranial cavity**, inside the skull, contains the brain. The

spinal cavity stretches from the cranial cavity to the end of the spinal cord; the spinal cavity is posterior to the abdominal cavity.

The **ventral body cavity** is divided into two other cavities: the **thoracic cavity** and the **abdominopelvic cavity**. These two cavities are separated by the **diaphragm**, a dome-shaped muscle underneath the lungs. The **thoracic cavity**, which is protected by the rib cage, contains the heart and lungs. In the thoracic cavity, the **mediastinum** (central region) separates the lungs into the left and right cavities. The **mediastinum cavity** contains the visceral organs, the heart, and the trachea. The **abdominopelvic cavity** is inferior to the diaphragm and can be divided into the abdominal cavity and pelvic cavity. The intestines, liver, and stomach are found in the superior abdominal cavity.

The **orbital cavities** in the skull house the eyes. The **middle ear cavities** in the skull are medial to the eardrums. The mouth or **oral cavity** contains the tongue and teeth. The oral cavity and the **digestive cavity** are continuous with each other. The **nasal cavity** is posterior to the nose or inside the nose and is part of the respiratory system.

The **pelvic cavity**, posterior to the abdominal cavity, houses the rectum, bladder, and reproductive organs. The abdominopelvic cavity can be divided into four approximately quadrants, as shown in the image below.

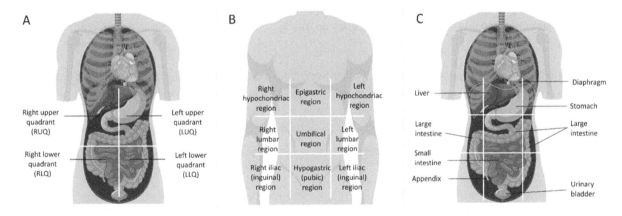

Anatomists typically divide the abdominopelvic cavity into nine individual regions using four planes, as shown in part B in the image above. The centermost region, which surrounds the navel (umbilicus), is the **umbilical region**. Superior to the umbilical region is the **epigastric region**, and inferior to the umbilical region is the **hypogastric region**. The **right and left inguinal (iliac) regions** are lateral to the hypogastric region. The right and left **hypochondriac regions** house the lower ribs and flank the epigastric region. The right and left **lumbar regions** are lateral to the spinal column and are located between the hip bones and bottom ribs.

Histology

Histology, or microanatomy, is the study of tissues at the microscopic level. The study of organs, **organology**, and the study of cells, **cytology**, are general topics in the area of histology. Groups of cells that have structural similarities and similar functions are called **tissues**. The four main types of tissues are the muscle, connective, epithelial, and nervous tissues. These tissues form the fabric of the body. Muscle tissue allows for movement. Connective tissue supports other tissues in the body and connects them together. Epithelial tissues cover other tissues and lines some organs and passages in the body.

Finally, nervous tissues allow for the control of the body through conveying impulses to and from the brain and receptors and effectors (e.g., muscles) throughout the body.

Muscle Tissue

Muscle tissues can generate a force that is needed to create movement. These muscles are designed to shorten or contract to create movement. The three main types of muscles are smooth, skeletal, and cardiac muscles. The **visceral** or **smooth muscle** has no visible striations. Each cell has one nucleus and is tapered at each end. Smooth muscle lines the walls of hollow organs such as the blood vessels, the uterus, and the stomach. As the wall of the smooth muscle shortens, the organ cavity shrinks. When the smooth muscle relaxes, the organ cavity dilates, or enlarges. The contraction and relaxation process allows substances to be mixed or moved through the organ towards a specific path.

Smooth muscle contracts more slowly than skeletal and cardiac muscle. The contractions of smooth muscle may last longer, and they have an important function in the stomach. For example, the small intestine is made up of two layers of smooth muscle. These muscles undergo **peristalsis**, a wavelike motion that keeps food moving in the small intestine.

Skeletal muscles are voluntary (under conscious control). Contraction of these muscles causes the skin or bones to be pulled on, resulting in body movements or changes in facial expression. Skeletal muscles are relatively long, multinucleate, cylindrical, and characterized by striations or stripes. Skeletal muscle cells are also called **muscle fibers** since the cells can elongate, thereby providing a long axis for contraction.

Cardiac muscle is located only in the heart wall where it forms the myocardium. The myocardium acts as a pump by contracting, thereby propelling blood through the blood vessels throughout the body. Cardiac muscle also has striations, like skeletal muscle, but cardiac cells are shorter and contain a single nucleus. These cells are branched and fit closely together, similar to clasped fingers, and are connected by gap junctions.

The intercalated discs have gap junctions, which allow the free passage of ions from one cell to another. Because the cells are held together by the discs, a **functional syncytium** is created. The syncytium, a single cell that contains several nuclei, allows the rapid conduction of an electrical signal causing the heart to contract. Humans cannot consciously control the contraction of the heart; the cardiac muscle contracts involuntarily.

Connective Tissue

The most common tissue in the body is **connective tissue**. It connects the different parts of the body; it binds, supports, and protects other tissues. Connective tissues are distinguished by blood supply variations and the extracellular matrix. Connective tissues typically have a good blood supply with the exception of the tendons, ligaments, and cartilage. These structures with low blood supply tend to heal slowly when an injury occurs. The **extracellular matrix** is a nonliving substance found on the outside of cells. Connective tissues have varying amounts of the extracellular matrix.

The extracellular matrix has two components: the fibers and a structureless ground substance. The **ground substance** is mostly made up of water in addition to cell adhesion proteins and charged polysaccharide molecules. In the ground substance, connective tissue cells are glued to matrix fibers with the aid of adhesion proteins. The polysaccharide molecules trap water molecules when intertwined. The consistency of the matrix depends upon the number of polysaccharide molecules. The greater the number of polysaccharide molecules, the firmer the matrix becomes. If there is a low number of polysaccharide molecules, then the matrix becomes more fluid.

If the number of molecules is somewhere in the middle, then the matrix is gel-like. The fibers inside the matrix include white collagen fibers, elastic yellow fibers, and reticular fibers. The collagen fibers have high tensile strength, and the yellow fibers can stretch and recoil. The reticular fibers are fine collagen fibers (type III) that make up the internal skeleton of the soft organs. The spleen is a soft organ that is supported by a skeleton of reticular fibers (as shown below). Connective tissue cells produce these collagen fibers and secrete them in the extracellular space, forming unique fibers.

Types of Connective Tissue

The major classes of connective tissue, listed in order from the softest (most fluid) to the most rigid, are blood, loose connective tissue, dense connective tissue, cartilage, and bone. Blood carries the nutrients, respiratory gases, white blood cells, and wastes for the cardiovascular system. Vascular or blood tissue is a connective tissue since it contains blood cells that are surrounded by a fluid matrix called blood plasma. The blood fibers are soluble proteins that are visible only during clotting.

Areolar, adipose, and reticular are three types of loose connective tissue. **Areolar connective tissue** is a soft and pliable tissue that protects and cushions the body organs. It is the most widely distributed tissue throughout the body. Areolar connective tissue holds or glues internal organs together to keep organs from shifting inside the body. The lamina propria is a type of areolar tissue that underlies all mucous membranes. In general, areolar connective tissue acts as a water and salt reservoir. All body cells release wastes and obtain nutrients from this tissue fluid. Phagocytes typically move through this tissue and pick up or destroy bacteria and dead cells. During inflammation of the body, the areolar tissue soaks up excess fluid, causing that area to swell, a process called **edema**.

Adipose connective tissue is a type of areolar tissue that predominantly contains fat cells. Oil makes up most of the cell's volume and displaces the nucleus to one side. Adipose makes up the subcutaneous tissue under the skin and insulates the body. Adipose protects the body from bumps and from extremes of heat and cold. Adipose cushions the eyeballs and is also found in the kidneys. The hips, the belly, and breasts are fat "depots" since they store fat, which provides fuel.

Reticular connective tissue is a network of interwoven reticular fibers that have reticular cells. The cells resemble fibroblasts. This tissue makes up the internal framework, or **stroma**, of the organs, and can support **lymphocytes**, which are white blood cells. The lymph nodes, spleen, and bone marrow contain stroma.

Dense fibrous connective tissue makes up the dermis or lower layer of the skin and is arranged in sheets. Dense fibrous tissue contains collagen fibers that compose the main matrix. This tissue is surrounded by fiber-forming cells called **fibroblasts**. These cells create the building blocks of the collagen fibers. Dense fibrous tissue forms ropelike and strong structures such as the ligaments and tendons. **Tendons** connect the skeletal muscles to the bones. The **ligaments** connect bones to each other; they stretch more than tendons since they contain more elastic fibers.

Compared to bone, **cartilage** is a soft and flexible tissue. It contains cartilage cells called **chondrocytes**. Only a few parts of the body contain cartilage. The most common type of cartilage is called **hyaline cartilage**, which contains an abundance of collagen fibers hidden in a rubber-like matrix. The hyaline cartilage is bluish-white and glassy in appearance. It forms the windpipe and the trachea, and it is attached to the ribs of the breastbone. Hyaline cartilage covers the bone ends of joints. Less hard than bone, hyaline cartilage is sometimes eventually replaced by bone in the course of the body's development. For example, the skeleton of a fetus is made mostly of hyaline cartilage, but after the baby is born, the cartilage becomes replaced by bone. Cartilage in long bones do not undergo the cartilage-to-bone transition since these long bones grow in length. **Fibrocartilage** is highly compressible and comprises the cushion-like disks between the vertebrae of a spinal column. **Elastic cartilage** exists in structures that have elasticity; for example, the external ear contains elastic cartilage.

Bone is also known as **osseous tissue** and is made up of bone cells called **osteocytes**. These cells sit in pits or cavities called **lacunae**. The cavities are surrounded by layers of a hard matrix that includes calcium salts along with a high number of collagen fibers. Due to one of its physical attributes—rock-like hardness—bone tissue can protect many body organs (for example, the skull protects the brain).

Epithelial Tissue

The **epithelium** or **epithelial tissue** is a glandular tissue that covers the body's surfaces both inside and out. The functions of the epithelial tissue are protection, filtration, secretion, and absorption. Any substance that the body receives or gives off must go through the epithelium. Epithelial tissue protects against chemical damage and bacteria. This tissue absorbs food nutrients from the stomach and the small intestine. Glandular epithelial tissue produces mucus, oil, sweat, and digestive enzymes. Characteristics of the epithelium are as follows:

- Epithelial cells fit close together, bound by specialized cell junctions (for example, desmosomes) to form continuous sheets (except glandular epithelium).

- The surfaces are **apical**, meaning that the membranes have a free edge. The surfaces are exposed to the cavity of an internal organ or to body's exterior. Some epithelia have cilia or microvilli, and other epithelia are smooth and slick.

- The anchored surface of the epithelium sits on a **basement membrane**, a structureless material that acts like a glue that holds the epithelium in place.

- Epithelial tissues are **avascular**, meaning they have no blood supply; they depend on diffusion from the capillaries to obtain food and oxygen. Well-nourished epithelial cells can regenerate easily.

Simple epithelial tissue forms a single layer of cells. The functions are absorption, secretion, and filtration. Stratified epithelial tissue is two or more layers of cells; it is found at the free surface of epithelial membrane. Its function is protection.

The table below shows the classification and functions of epithelia:

Cell Shape	Layers	
	Simple	Stratified
Squamous (flat)	It rests on a basement membrane; cells are tightly packed; filtration and exchange occur by diffusion. It is found in air sacs of lungs (alveoli) and the walls of capillaries where gases or nutrients are exchanged. It forms a serous membrane (serosae) that covers organs in cavities and lines the ventral body cavity.	The most common type of stratified epithelium in the body. It is found on the surface of the skin, mouth, and esophagus where friction occurs.
Cuboidal (cube-shaped)	Found in glands and associated ducts such as the pancreas and salivary glands. Forms walls of the kidney tubules and covers the surface of the ovaries.	It usually has two cell layers and is found near the basement membrane. Rare in the body but found in ducts of large glands.
Columnar (column shape)	Contain tall cells that are packed together. Contain goblet cells that produce a lubricating mucus. It lines the digestive tract from the stomach to the anus. Forms the mucous membranes that line body cavities. The cells are open the organ body's exterior. They line the stomach wall where acids are secreted to break down food. Forms a pseudostratified epithelium that rests on a basement membrane. The nuclei are located above the basement membrane at different heights. Ciliated pseudostratified version lines the respiratory tract and the mucus produced by goblets cells act to capture dust and debris; for example, the cilia push the mucus upward from the lungs.	The surface is columnar, but the basal cells vary in shape and size. Rare in the body but found in ducts of large glands.
Transitional	Transitional epithelium is only stratified.	Forms the lining of the ureters, urinary bladder, and part of the urethra. The cells can slide past one another and allow the ureter wall to stretch. Cells of the basal layer are cuboidal or columnar. The epithelium can undergo considerable stretching (cells become squamous like) and are domelike when relaxed.

The **glandular epithelium** contains one or more cells that produce and secrete a specific product. The secretion product contains protein molecules in an aqueous fluid. The glandular cells obtain specific substances from the blood to make these products. Endocrine and exocrine are two types of glands. The endocrine contains ductless glands (for example, glands in thyroid, pituitary, and adrenals) that secrete hormones that diffuse into the blood vessels and weave through the glands. The **exocrine glands** have ducts and secrete their products through the ducts of the epithelial surface. These glands are found in the pancreas (internal and external), in the liver, and in sweat glands and oil glands.

Nervous Tissue

The nervous tissues contain cells called **neurons**. The neurons conduct electrochemical impulses from one part of the body to another, and it can receive electrochemical impulses from parts of the body. The main characteristics of nervous tissues are conductivity and irritability.

The cytoplasm for each neuron cell is drawn out or extended so that it can conduct an impulse to distant locations in the body. **Neuroglia** are supporting cells that insulate, protect, and support the neurons. The nerves, spinal cord, and brain contain these supporting cells.

Integumentary System

The **integumentary system** makes up the external covering of the body and protects deep tissue from injury. The word integumentary means "covering," but the integumentary system has many functions besides protection. Hair, fingernails, and skin are examples of organ systems that cover the body. The integumentary system cushions and insulates the deeper body organs and protects the body from cuts and bumps. The skin can waterproof the body and can act as a cushion against injury. Keratin toughens cells and acts as a physical barrier, and fat cells act as a cushion against blows. The organ system also protects against chemical damage from acids and bases.

The skin acts as a chemical plant and produces proteins that are important for immunity. The skin produces vitamin D; under sunlight, cholesterol molecules in the skin are converted to vitamin D under sunlight. It also regulates the temperature of the body; the skin acts as a mini-excretory system when a person is exerting themselves. Salts, water, and urea are excreted when a person sweats.

The integumentary system protects us from microbes and harsh sunlight such as ultraviolet (UV) radiation. The skin secretes an acidic substance, called the acid mantle, that inhibits the invasion of bacteria. The melanin that is created by melanocytes, located at the bottom layer of the skin's epidermis, provides protection from UV damage. The integumentary system also protects against thermal damage from hot or cold substances; for example, the system contains heat-cold pain receptors. The skin keeps molecules such as water in the body and keeps excess water, along with other substances, from entering the body. The skin prevents the body from drying out (desiccation) since it contains water-resistant glycolipids and keratin.

Structure of the Skin

The outer **epidermis** is composed of a stratified squamous epithelium that can harden and become tough. The underlying layer, the **dermis**, is generally tear-resistant and is composed of dense connective tissue. Both structures, the dermis and epidermis, are connected firmly. Burns or friction can cause the two layers to separate; interstitial fluid then builds up in a cavity between the layers. The fluid-filled cavity is called a blister.

The **hypodermis** or subcutaneous tissue is basically fat or adipose tissue that is deep to the dermis. It's not part of the skin but anchors the skin to underlying organs and provides a place to store nutrients. The hypodermis functions as a shock absorber and insulates deeper tissues from severe temperature changes in the environment. It is the deepest layer of the skin, and its thickness can vary from person to person. For instance, a woman's rounded body curves are due to the presence of fat or adipose tissue. The characteristic is specific to women because their hypodermis layer is thicker than men's.

Epidermis

The epidermis mostly contains cells called **keratinocytes**. Through a process called keratinization, these cells produce keratin, a fibrous protein that acts as a tough protective layer. **Desmosomes** connect keratinocytes throughout the epidermis. The image below shows the different layers of the epidermis.

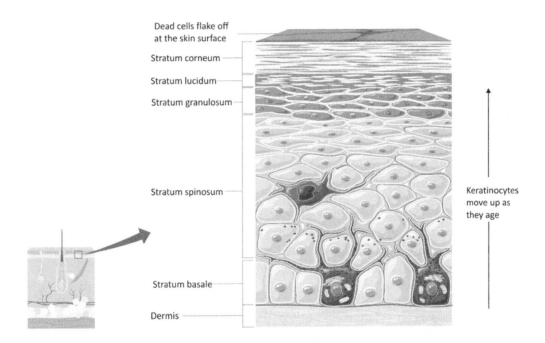

A close look at the epidermis indicates that there is no supply of blood flowing through each structural layer, showing that the epidermis is avascular. When someone nicks themselves when they shave, they are cutting off several layers of the cell. The epidermis is made up of five layers called **strata**. The order of the layers, from outermost to innermost, is stratum corneum, stratum lucidum, stratum granulosum, stratum spinosum, and stratum basale. The **stratum corneum** is roughly twenty to thirty cell layers thick and makes up three quarters of the epidermal thickness. The shingle-like dead cells of the stratum corneum, called **cornified cells**, are filled with keratin.

The stratum corneum provides the body with a durable overcoat that protects deeper cells from extreme temperatures as well as biological, physical, and chemical damage. Water retention is an important function of the stratum corneum. However, these cells can flake off slowly under friction such as rubbing, and they can manifest as dandruff, a food source for dust mites. Given that an average person acquires a new epidermis every thirty-five days, a person can shed up to forty pounds of these flakes over a lifetime.

The **stratum lucidum** lies underneath the corneum and makes up the clear, dead cells that leave the granulosum. The **stratum granulosum** is a superficial layer that contains flat cells with deteriorating organelles and a cell cytoplasm filled with granules. Cells that leave the granulosum die and form the lucidum. The **stratum spinosum** is another superficial layer that contains thick bundles of filaments composed of pre-keratin. This layer contains dendritic cells, keratinocytes, and desmosomes. Both the granulosum and spinosum flatten as they are pushed upward and away from the dermis.

The **stratum basale** or **stratum germinativum** is found closest to the dermis and contains adequately nourished epidermal cells. These nutrients diffuse from the dermis. Stem cells continually undergo division and produce millions of cells daily. The germinating layer also produces epidermal cells while maintaining the stem cell population through division. Daughter cells from the epidermal cells are pushed upward, away from the dermis, and become part of the superficial layers such as the stratum spinosum followed by the stratum granulosum.

Dermis

The **dermis** is a strong and stretchy envelope or hide that keeps the body together. Elastic fibers and collagen are found throughout the dermis. Collagen provides the dermis with toughness and binds or attracts water to keep the skin hydrated. Elastic fibers provide the skin with elasticity. The dermis is made up of areolar and dense irregular connective tissue. There are two major regions in the dermis called the papillary and reticular areas. The superficial dermal region near the epidermis is called the **papillary layer**. The **dermal papillae** make up the papillary layer and cause indentation of the epidermis. The layer is uneven with peg-like projections from the superior surface. Several capillary loops in the papillary layer provide nutrients to the epidermis.

Papillae have definite patterns that result in loops and whorled ridges at the surface of the epidermis. These result in enhanced gripping and friction on the fingers and feet. The papillary patterns are genetically determined. The created ridges on the fingers contain sweat pores and leave sweat films, called **fingerprints**, on surfaces that have been touched.

The thickness of the dermis varies; for example, the dermis is thin on the eyelids but thick on soles of the feet. The dermis has an abundant supply of blood vessels, and it functions to maintain body temperature homeostasis. For instance, if the body temperature is high, the capillaries swell with heated blood. The skin begins to warm up and redden, resulting in the radiation of heat from the skin's surface. If the external environment is cold, blood bypasses the dermis capillaries so that the internal body temperature remains elevated and body heat is conserved.

The deepest layer of the skin is called the **reticular layer**, and it contains dense irregular tissue, oil/sweat glands, blood vessels, and pressure receptors (for example, lamellar corpuscles). Phagocytes are found in the dermis; they keep microbes from penetrating deeper into the body.

Skeletal System

The **skeletal system** is made up of cartilage, joints, ligaments, and bones. **Ligaments** are the fibrous cords that keep the bones together at the joints. The bones can come together, or **articulate**, at the joints to enable movement. For example, the skeleton anchors the skeletal muscles such that muscle contractions result in body movements. The skeletal system also supports and protects body organs and produces blood cells within the marrow of bones. There are two main divisions in the skeletal system: the axial skeleton and the appendicular skeleton. The **axial skeleton** consists of bones that make up the longitudinal axis of the body. The **appendicular skeleton** contains the bones of the girdles and limbs that attach to the axial skeleton.

Functions of Bones

Bones provide support, protection, and storage, and they enable movement. They make up the internal framework that supports the body and envelopes the soft organs. For example, the skull is part of the skeletal system that encloses the brain and provides support and protection. The vertebrae surround the spinal cord. Bones enable body movement. Skeletal muscles are connected to the bones by tendons. These muscles use bones as levers to move the body and its parts, thereby allowing us to walk, throw a ball, and complete the compendium of movements and activities we can do. Bones store essential minerals such as calcium and phosphorous.

The internal cavity (marrow) of a bone also stores fat. Bones contain most of the body's calcium in the form of calcium salts. Based on the body's needs, calcium can be deposited in and withdrawn from the bones and blood. The flow of calcium into the blood and bones is dynamic and controlled by hormones. Within the marrow cavities of specific bones, **hematopoiesis**, or blood cell formation, takes place.

The adult skeleton contains about 206 bones. The two types of bone tissue are called compact and spongy. **Compact bone**, also called **cortical bone**, is dense with a homogeneous and smooth appearance. **Spongy bone**, also called **cancellous bone**, is spiky and sponge-like in appearance. Bones come in many sizes and shapes. For instance, the pisiform bone (wrist bone) is pea-sized, and the femur (thigh bone) is two feet long with a ball-shaped head.

Bones are classified based on their shape, as shown below.

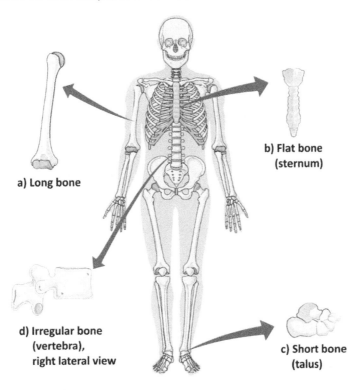

a) Long bone

b) Flat bone (sternum)

c) Short bone (talus)

d) Irregular bone (vertebra), right lateral view

Long bones are usually greater in length than in width, and they have a shaft with enlarged or bulging ends. With the exception of the wrist, ankle, and kneecap (the patella), all bones of the limbs are long bones. **Flat bones** are thin, curved, and flat and consist of two thin layers of compact bone. A layer of spongy bone is sandwiched between the thin layers of flat bone. The ribs, breastbone (sternum), and most of the skull bones are flat bones.

Short bones are typically cube-shaped and consist mostly of spongy bone and an outer layer of compact bone. The ankle and wrist are examples of short bones. **Sesamoid bones**, such as the patella, are a special type of short bone. **Irregular bones** are similar to short bones and are mostly spongy bone with an outer layer of compact bone. The vertebrae, which make are the spinal column, are irregular bones.

Structure of Bone

In a long bone, the shaft, or **diaphysis**, is what makes up the bone's length. The diaphysis is made of compact bone, and it is covered with the **periosteum**, a fibrous connective tissue membrane that protects it. The perforating fibers, or Sharpey's fibers, which are hundreds of connective tissue fibers, secure the periosteum to an underlying bone. The ends of the long bones are called the **epiphyses** and consist of a thin layer of compact bone. The epiphysis encloses an area that is filled with spongy bone. The epiphysis is covered with **articular cartilage**, which is a glassy hyaline cartilage that reduces friction at the joint. This cartilage is covered with a lubricating fluid. The articular cartilage is somewhat thicker than the periosteum.

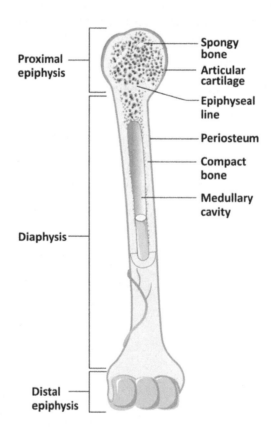

The **epiphyseal line** is a thin line of bony tissue that spans the epiphysis; this region is not made of spongy bone. The line is a remainder of the **epiphyseal plate**, the flat plate of hyaline cartilage that is evident in young, growing bones. These plates allow the long bone to grow lengthwise. After puberty is over, when hormones inhibit the growth of long bones, the plates are mostly replaced by bone. As a result, epiphyseal lines mark the previous location of the epiphyseal plates. The **endosteum** is a delicate connective tissue that covers the inner bony surface of the shaft. In infants, the shaft cavity is called a **medullary cavity**. The cavity contains red marrow, which produces blood cells. By the age of seven, the red marrow is replaced with yellow marrow. Adipose, or fat tissue, is stored in yellow marrow. Adult skeletons contain red marrow in the cavities of spongy bone in the axial skeleton, the epiphyses of long bones, and the hip bones.

Bone markings are characterized by bumps, ridges, and holes. These markings identify where tendons, muscles, and ligaments attach and where nerves and blood vessels pass through. Two categories of bone markings are processes or projections and cavities or depressions, which manifest as bone indentations. Generally, bone terms that begin with "F" are depressions, and names starting with "T" are projections.

Bone Markings	
Name of bone mark	**Description**
Projections that are Sites of Ligament/Muscle Attachment (1)	
Crest	A narrow ridge of prominent bone
Epicondyle	A raised area above a condyle
Line	A narrow ridge of bone less prominent than the crest
Process	Any type of bony prominence
Spine	A sharp and slender pointed projection
Trochanter	A large irregular shaped prominence (e.g., femur)
Tubercle	A small, rounded projection
Tuberosity	A large round or rough projection
Projections that Form Joints (2)	
Condyle	A rounded articular projection
Facet	A smooth and almost flat articular surface
Head	A bony expansion on a narrow neck
Ramus	An arm-like bar
Openings and Depressions (3)	
For Passage of the Nerves and Blood Vessels	
Fissure	A narrow slit-like opening
Foramen	A round opening through a bone
Groove	A furrow
Notch	An indentation found at the edge of a structure
Other Types	
Fossa	A shallow depression in a bone
Meatus	A tunnel-like passageway
Sinus	Contains a cavity within a bone that is filled with air. The cavity is lined with a mucous membrane.

Microscopic Anatomy

Spongy bone is made up of small needle-like pieces of bone called **trabeculae**. Much of the spongy bone is "open space" that is filled by nerves, marrow, and blood vessels. **Osteocytes** are mature bone cells in compact bone that are located in **lacunae** or tiny cavities in the bone matrix. The lacunae are organized into concentric circles, known as **lamellae**, that are found around Haversian or central canals. The **Haversian system**, or **osteon**, contains a complex of lamellae containing a central canal and matrix rings.

The osteon is the functional and structural unit of compact bone. The Haversian canals run lengthwise through the bony matrix and carry nerves and blood vessels to all regions of the bones.

The **canaliculi** or tiny canals radiate outward from the Haversian canals to the lacunae. These tiny canals form a transportation system that links bone cells to a nutrient supply and waste removal system in the hard bone matrix. As a result, bone cells are well-nourished and can heal quickly when a bone injury occurs.

Muscular System

The muscular system's main function is to contract so that movement can occur. Skeletal muscles are large, fleshy muscles that are attached to the bone. These muscles form the muscular system, and when these muscles shorten, the body can walk, jump, smile, and carry out other such movements and actions. The three major types of muscle tissue are smooth, cardiac, and skeletal muscle. Skeletal and smooth muscle cells are elongated and are called **muscle fibers**. The contraction of these muscles depends on myofilaments.

Skeletal Muscle (Striated and Voluntary)

The skeletal muscles are organs that are packaged with skeletal muscle fibers and are attached to the skeleton. These muscles cover the cartilage and bone and provide the body with a smooth contour. The muscle fibers can be described as cigar-shaped and are usually relatively large, with a range of up to one foot. Skeletal muscle fibers are multinucleated cells with stripes, or striations, along the fibers. Even though these fibers are voluntarily controlled, they can be activated unwillingly by our reflexes. Skeletal muscle fibers can contract rapidly with a large amount of force, but they require rest after a certain amount of activity. Skeletal muscles can exert force without tearing since the muscle fibers are held together by connective tissue.

Each muscle fiber is covered with a delicate tissue sheath called an **endomysium**. These sheathed fibers collectively form a bundle of fibers called a **fascicle**. The fascicle is wrapped with a **perimysium**, a coarse fibrous membrane. The **epimysium**, a tough overcoat of connective tissues, binds many fascicles and covers all the muscle.

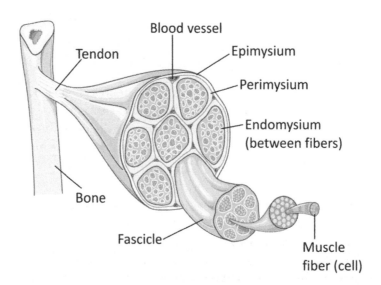

The ends of the epimysium blend into a sheet-like **aponeurosis**, or strong, cordlike tendon, as shown above. Tendons are made up of tough collagen fibers and, thus, provide durability. The tendon conserves space and indirectly connects to the cartilage, bone, or some other connective tissue covering. The tendon is durable enough to pass through rough bony projections and over a joint. Skeletal muscles vary in the arrangement of fibers. Although these fibers are often depicted as having a spindle shape, some fibers are arranged in circles, and other fibers are shaped like a fan.

Microscopic Anatomy of Skeletal Muscles

The **sarcolemma**, a plasma membrane, wraps the multinucleate skeletal muscle fibers cells and myofibrils. The **myofibrils** are long, ribbonlike organelles that fill the cytoplasm and push aside the nuclei. Every myofibril is surrounded by a **sarcoplasmic reticulum.** The reticulum contains interconnecting tubules and sacs that act to store and release calcium on demand. For instance, when a muscle fiber is stimulated to contract, calcium is released. Alternating dark (A) and light (I) bands span the length of the myofibrils and give a banded or striated appearance on the muscle fiber. These banding patterns provide insight into the working structure of myofibrils.

Myofibrils are complex organelles that are made up of bundles of thick and thin threadlike protein myofilaments. **Sarcomeres** are small contractile units that link together in chains to make up the myofibrils. These functional and structural units are aligned end to end along the length of the myofibrils. The arrangement of the **myofilaments**, found in the sarcomeres, is what produce the striations that are seen in skeletal muscles. Each sarcomere is marked and visually distinguishable by light and dark bands. The **light I band** contains a darker area called the **Z disc**, and the **dark A band** has a light central region known as the **H zone**. At the center of the H zone, there are tiny protein rods that hold and bind adjacent thick filaments. The center is referred to as the **M line**.

There are two sorts of threadlike protein myofilaments: thick filaments and thin filaments. The thick filaments contain bundled molecules of myosin, a protein, and enzymes. The enzyme ATPase breaks ATP down to produce the energy needed for muscle contraction. Thick myosin filaments span the entire length of the A band (the darker region). The midpart of the thick filaments (within the H zone) is smooth, but the ends that span the remainder of the A band are studded with small heads. During contraction, these myosin heads form cross bridges and link the thick and thin filaments together. The thick myosin filaments are attached to the Z discs or lines through the elastic filaments called **titin**. The giant protein titin, also called **connectin**, can span one micrometer in length and acts as a molecular spring. Since titin runs through the core of the thick filament, it keeps myosin in place.

The thin filaments are made up of **actin**, a contractile protein, as well as some regulatory proteins that allow the binding of actin to myosin heads. These thin filaments connect to the Z disc or line. The I band includes the thin filaments and parts of two adjacent sarcomeres. For a relaxed sarcomere, the thin filaments are not in the H zone or central region. Consequently, the H zone looks lighter. The A band, excluding the H zone, is darker since it contains both the thin and thick filaments. During contraction, the thin filaments slide against the thick filaments, and they completely overlap one another. As a result, the H zone disappears.

Smooth Muscle (No Striations, Involuntary)

Smooth muscles cannot be voluntarily controlled and do not have striations. These muscles are found in tube-like visceral organs such as the respiratory passages, the stomach, and the urinary bladder. The muscles are spindle-shaped and encased by a scant endomysium. The uninucleate fibers are often arranged in two layers; one layer runs longitudinally and the other runs circularly. As each layer contracts and relaxes in an alternating position, the size and shape of the organ changes. Smooth muscles allow food to pass along through the digestive tract, thereby allowing the bowels to be emptied.

Cardiac Muscle (Striated, Involuntary)

Cardiac muscle is found only in the heart and makes up the bulk of the heart walls. It pumps and propels blood through the blood vessels to the body's tissues. Cardiac muscle is striated, uninucleate, and involuntarily controlled. Small portions of endomysium are arranged in eight shaped bundles and cushion the cardiac cells. The contraction of the heart causes its internal chambers to become smaller. As a result, blood leaves the heart and is forced into the large arteries. Cardiac muscle fibers are joined by intercalated discs.

Nervous System

The **nervous system** includes the brain, spinal cord, sensory receptors, and nerves. It is the master control system and the body's communication system. The nervous system allows the body to respond to external stimuli (for example, sound, light, and temperature changes) and internal stimuli (such as a decrease in the supply of oxygen). The nervous system is a fast-acting control system. The skin contains cutaneous sensory receptors located in the dermis. These tiny receptors are the part of the nervous system that indicates pressure, touch, temperature, and pain. Each receptor provides information regarding the external environment and sends signals to the spinal cord or brain about any changes or potential threats.

The nervous system works with other organs to maintain hemostasis. The **endocrine system**, like the nervous system, controls and monitors activities occurring in the body, but to a lesser extent than the nervous system. The endocrine system is composed of glands such as the thyroid and adrenal glands, in addition to the pancreas. Endocrine glands create molecules and secrete hormones. These hormones regulate other structures. For example, some hormones that are released into the blood travel to a target organ. Some hormones even control reproductive growth.

The nervous system has three main functions: sensory input, integration, and motor output. **Sensory input** involves the monitoring of changes that take place inside and outside the body. Sensory receptors monitor changes in cues called **stimuli**. Information that is gathered is called **sensory input**. **Integration**

involves the processing and interpretation of sensory input, followed by decision making. The decision results in a response that leads to the activation of muscles or glands by **motor output**.

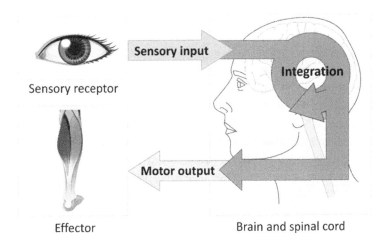

Sensory receptor

Effector

Brain and spinal cord

Structure of the Nervous System

The nervous system is divided into the central and peripheral nervous systems. The **central nervous system (CNS)** is made up of the spinal cord and brain. The CNS functions as the integrating and command center for the nervous system. Once the CNS interprets incoming sensory information, instructions are given to the muscles or motor division. These instructions are based on past occurrences and current circumstances. The **peripheral nervous system (PNS)** consists of components of the nervous system that are found outside the CNS. The PNS is mostly nerves that extend from the brain and spinal cord. For example, cranial nerves carry impulses back and forth from the brain. Spinal nerves carry impulses back and forth from the spinal cord. Both nerve systems act as communication lines and connect to other parts of the body by carrying impulses. For example, impulses can travel from the sensory receptors to the CNS or from the CNS to the muscles or glands.

Functional Classification of PNS Structures

PNS structures can be separated into two divisions: the sensory division and the motor division. The **sensory division** allows the CNS to perceive external and internal sensations. The afferent or sensory division is made up of nerves that send impulses to the CNS from sensory receptors found in many parts of the body. **Somatic afferent fibers** are types of sensory fibers that deliver impulses from the joints, skin, and skeletal muscles. **Visceral afferent fibers** transmit impulses from the visceral or internal organs such as the heart, lungs, liver, intestines, or pancreas.

The **efferent**, or **motor division**, relays pulses from the CNS to effector organs such as the glands and muscles. Therefore, efferent pulses cause a motor response. Efferent division can be divided into the somatic and autonomic nervous systems. The **somatic**, or **voluntary nervous system**, allows a person to control most of their skeletal muscles. The **autonomic**, or **involuntary nervous system**, controls involuntary events and includes activities related to the cardiac muscles, smooth muscles, and glands. The involuntary nervous system can be further divided into the parasympathetic and sympathetic systems. The **parasympathetic nervous system** can conserve energy by slowing the heart rate, increasing gland and intestinal activity, and relaxing sphincter muscles in the gastrointestinal tract. Therefore, the parasympathetic system keeps the body from being overworked and restores the body to a calm state. The **sympathetic nervous system** prepares the body for a "flight or fight" response in the event of a dangerous situation. An example of a response from the sympathetic system would be the flash flood of hormones such as epinephrine or adrenaline to increase the body's heart rate and alertness in response to hearing a huge crash. Extra blood is then sent to the muscles so that the body can prepare for facing potential danger.

Structure and Function of the Nervous Tissue

The neuroglia cells (glial or glia cells) are the supporting cells in the CNS that make up the nerve glue. There are different types of neuroglia cells that protect, support, or insulate the neurons. Each type of neuroglia has a special function. **Astrocytes** are star-shaped cells that make up almost half the neural tissue. These cells have many projections, which have swollen ends that stick to the neurons. Astrocytes allow the neurons to be anchored to the blood capillaries to obtain nutrients. In addition, they determine the capillary permeability and have a role in allowing exchanges between the neurons and blood capillaries. Astrocytes help control the chemical environment in the brain and protect the neurons from harmful substances that might be found in the blood. In the brain, they even sweep up leaked potassium ions that are needed to generate nerve impulses or for communication purposes.

Microglia are another type of glia cells; they act as scavengers in the CNS. These spiderlike phagocytes mediate immune response and monitor the health of nearby neurons. Microglia remove dead brain cells, bacteria, and debris. **Ependymal cells**, or **ependymocytes**, are a type of glial cell that lines the central cavities of the spinal cord and brain. The beating of their cilia helps circulate the cerebrospinal fluid and creates a protective, watery cushion that envelopes the CNS. **Oligodendrocytes** are similar to astrocytes and are involved in the production of **myelin**, a fatty insulating sheath located on the axons of nerve fibers. These neuroglia use their flat extensions to cover the nerve fibers tightly. Both neurons and neuroglia are structurally similar and have cell extensions. However, only nerves can transmit nerve impulses. Unlike most neurons, neuroglia do not lose their ability to divide. Brain tumors, such as gliomas, are the result of uncontrolled cell growth formed by neuroglia.

Satellite cells and Schwann cells are two major types of supporting cells in the PNS. The **satellite cells** are protective and cushioning cells in the peripheral neuron cell bodies. The **Schwann cells** make up the myelin sheaths that cover the nerve fibers.

Endocrine System

The second major controlling system within the body is called the endocrine system. The **endocrine system** regulates processes such as growth, development, reproduction, and metabolism. The body's cells are coordinated and directed with the help of the endocrine and nervous system. For instance, the endocrine system can release special types of signaling molecules called **hormones**, which are chemicals that control complex processes in the body and carry instructions for more than a dozen endocrine glands.

The endocrine system is slower-acting compared to the nervous system and uses hormones that act as chemical messengers rather than nerve impulses. **Endocrinology** is the study of the endocrine organs, its diseases, and the secretion of hormones. There are more than fifty different hormones in the human body that vary in function. These hormones may be released into the fluid around the cells or into the blood and then transported throughout the body's cardiovascular system. These signaling molecules, released by the endocrine glands, move through the blood and change the target cells' activity. Insulin molecules can bind to protein receptors on nearby cells, causing bloodborne glucose molecules to enter the cells. As a result, cellular activity increases dramatically. Other processes that are controlled by hormones include mobilizing body defenses against stressors, regulating cellular metabolism, controlling growth and maturation, and balancing the use of cellular energy. Hormones also maintain the body's electrolytes, nutrient levels in the blood, and water balance.

Hormone Chemistry and Function

Organs within the endocrine system are generally small, and parts of the endocrine tissue are stored away in separate regions in the body. The major glands include the pituitary, pineal, thyroid, parathyroid, hypothalamus, and adrenal glands. The ovaries, testes, and pancreas are also endocrine glands. Functionally, these glands are essential when it comes to maintaining body homeostasis. Endocrine cells secrete hormones into the extracellular fluid. These chemical messengers "arouse" and change cellular activity at the target tissues. Hormones regulate the metabolic activity of cells found throughout the body by either increasing or decreasing the rate of normal metabolic processes.

Most hormones can be classified as either steroids or amino acid–based molecules. **Steroids** are hormones that are produced from cholesterol. The ovaries and testes, or **gonads**, produce sex hormones that can be classified as **steroid hormones**. These sex hormones include testosterone, progesterone, and estradiol. The adrenal cortex can also produce hormones that can be classified as steroids. Steroids made by the adrenal cortex include androgens, estrogens, progestin, mineralocorticoids, and glucocorticoids. **Amino acid–based molecules** can consist of amines, proteins, and peptides. Other types of hormones are amino acid derivatives that are nonsteroidal. **Prostaglandins**, the third class of hormones that act on a local level, are produced from highly active lipids and released from most cell membranes.

Hormone Action

Hormones target specific tissue cells and organs. Organs that are targeted by hormones are called **target organs**, and tissue cells that are targeted by hormones are called **target cells**. Each target cell contains a unique protein receptor that is specific to a hormone. Therefore, a cell will only respond to a hormone that properly attaches to its receptor on its plasma membrane or in the cell interior. Proper binding allows the hormones to influence the cell. Hormones can alter the cell membrane's electrical state (its potential) or change the permeability of the plasma membrane by closing or opening ion channels. Hormones can render enzymes inactive or active, inhibit or promote the secretion of a product, turn gene transcription off or on, and inhibit or stimulate the division of cells.

Hormones trigger changes in cells by direct gene activation or by a second-messenger system. The thyroid and steroid hormones use the direct gene activation mechanism. Because steroids are lipid-soluble molecules, they can diffuse through the target cell's plasma membrane.

In **direct gene activation**, the steroid may bind to receptors in the cytoplasm or a steroid inside the nucleus. Steroids that bind to the cytoplasm receptors create a complex that moves into the nucleus to activate specific genes. Steroids that enter the nucleus (1 in the figure below) bind to a specific receptor (2) and initiate a transcription/translation process. For example, the hormone-receptor complex (3) will then stick to a specific site found on the cell's DNA (4). As a result, specific genes will be activated, thereby allowing the transcription of messenger RNA (mRNA) (5), followed by mRNA translation in the cytoplasm (6). New proteins are then produced in the cytoplasm of the cell.

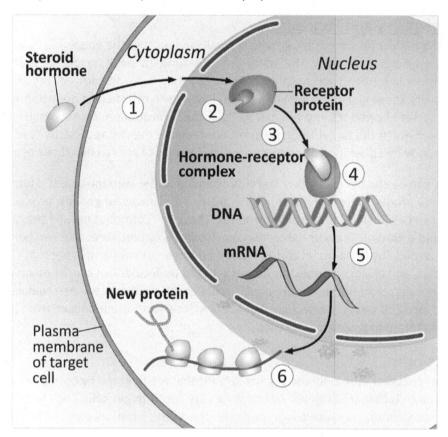

In the **second-messenger system**, steroid hormones influence cell activity indirectly by activating second-messenger molecules. Peptide and protein hormones tend to act through second-messenger systems because they are not water-soluble and cannot enter the target cell directly. In the first step (1 in the figure below), hormones bind to receptors located on the plasma membrane of a target cell. In the second step (2), the hormones act as the first messenger by activating the receptor protein, thereby setting off a series of reactions called a **cascade** that turns on an enzyme. In the third step (3), the activated enzyme catalyzes several reactions that result in the production of second-messenger molecules called **cyclic adenosine monophosphate (cAMP)**. In the last step (4), the cAMP molecules provide oversight to additional intracellular changes that include processes such as glycogen breakdown and the regulation of lipid production.

Steroid, peptide, and protein hormones may have other second messengers, such as cyclic guanosine monophosphate (cGMP) and calcium ions. For example, **epinephrine** is a hormone, a derivative of an amino acid (peptide molecule) that acts as a primary messenger. Epinephrine acts through the second-messenger system and causes calcium ion, a secondary messenger, to build up in the cell's cytoplasm.

Calcium ions can then enter many smooth muscle cells and cause contraction. Epinephrine, also called adrenaline, can even increase heart rate, blood pressure, and muscle strength.

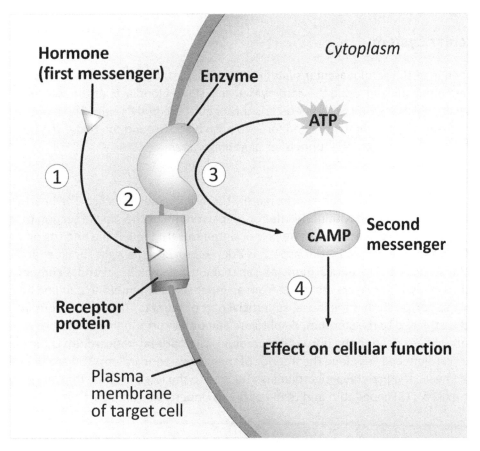

Stimuli

Most hormones are controlled via negative feedback mechanisms and are released based on some external or internal stimuli. For example, the hypothalamus will release hormones in response to signals from the internal and external environment, such as body temperature and hunger. As the hormone level rises, the hypothalamus inhibits the release of that hormone, and the response of the target organ remains unaffected. The blood levels of many hormones can fall within a very narrow concentration range. Although many endocrine organs respond to a variety of stimuli, there are three modes in which the stimuli can activate the endocrine glands. The hormonal, humoral, and neural mechanisms are the most common systems that regulate the release of hormones. The **hormonal stimulus** is the most common, whereby endocrine glands are prompted into action by other types of hormones. For example, the hypothalamus can stimulate the anterior pituitary gland to release its hormones.

The pituitary hormones then stimulate other endocrine organs, such as the thyroid glands. Hormone release is rhythmic. For instance, hormones created by the target (thyroid) glands will increase in the blood and then serve as feedback to prevent the release of the anterior pituitary and hypothalamus hormones. **Humoral stimuli** involve a process in which the changing blood levels of nutrients and ions stimulate the release of hormones. For instance, as the calcium ion concentration decreases in the blood within the capillaries connecting to the parathyroid glands, it prompts the release of parathyroid hormone (PTH). This hormone reverses the declining concentration level of calcium ion, allowing the calcium ion level to increase again, thereby preventing the release of PTH. Endocrine cells can respond to **neural stimuli** when the nerve fibers stimulate hormone release. For example, during times of stress, the sympathetic nervous system stimulates the adrenal medulla. Specifically, the sympathetic fibers signal the medulla to secrete the catecholamines called epinephrine and norepinephrine.

Cardiovascular System

The major function of the **cardiovascular system** is the transportation of nutrients, oxygen, hormones, cell wastes, and other substances. In the cardiovascular system, blood acts as the transport vehicle for these substances, which are vital for homeostasis throughout the body's cells. The blood pressure and the beating of the heart provide the needed force to push blood around the body. The heart is the pump, and the blood vessels are the tunnels, or plumbing system.

Heart Anatomy

The heart is cone-shaped, hollow, and approximately the size of a person's fist. The heart weighs less than one pound and is enclosed within the inferior **mediastinum**, or the medial section of the thoracic cavity. The lungs border the heart, and its **apex** is oriented toward the left hip and sits on the diaphragm. The **base**, or posterosuperior aspect, is oriented toward the right shoulder and is found underneath the second rib. The **pericardium** is a sac that encloses the heart and is composed of three layers (as shown below). The layers are made from an inner serous membrane pair and an outer fibrous layer. The **fibrous pericardium** is the loose, superficial part of the sac. The outer fibrous layer protects the heart and is attached to the sternum, diaphragm, and other surrounding structures. The two-layered **serous pericardium** lies deep to the fibrous pericardium. The **parietal pericardium** is the parietal layer of the serous pericardium and lies along the interior of the fibrous pericardium. Toward the upper part, or superior to the heart, the parietal pericardium is attached to the large arteries that leave the heart. The parietal layer makes a U-shaped turn and then continues underneath the heart's surface.

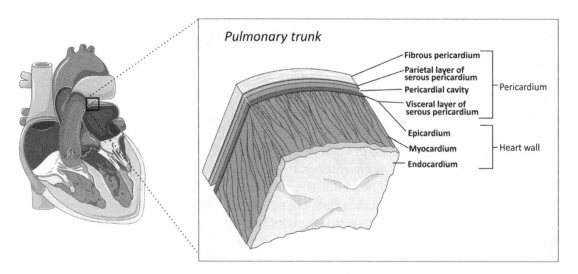

The **epicardium**, or **visceral pericardium**, makes up part of the heart's wall and is the visceral layer of the serous pericardium. The epicardium and visceral layer of the pericardium are the same structure. The epicardium is the outermost layer of the heart wall and the innermost layer of the pericardium. The pericardial cavity is found between the serous pericardium and the visceral layer. The serous pericardial membranes produce a lubricating serous fluid that collects in the pericardial cavity. The fluid provides a frictionless environment and allows the serous pericardial layers to move across one another smoothly. Without the fluid, the heart would not beat so easily.

The heart wall is composed of three main layers called the epicardium, myocardium, and endocardium. As stated previously, the **epicardium**, or visceral pericardium, is the outermost layer. The **myocardium** is a muscle layer that contracts and is made up of thick twisted bundles of cardiac muscle that are whorled into ring-like arrangements. Each myocardial cell is connected by intercalated discs that contain gap junctions and desmosomes. Ions flow from cell to cell via the gap junctions at the intercalated discs. A network of dense fibrous connective tissue, called the **skeleton of the heart**, reinforces the myocardium. The heart chambers are lined with a thin, gleaming sheet of endothelium called the **endocardium**. The endocardium is the innermost layer and is continuous with the linings of the blood vessels that enter and leave the heart. Two **ventricles** and two **atria** make up the four hollow chambers, or cavities, of the heart.

Each cavity is lined with an endocardium and keeps blood flowing smoothly throughout the heart. The main receiving chambers that assist with filling of the ventricles are found in the superior atria. However, these atria are not as vital in terms of the bulk of the heart's pumping activity. Under low pressure, the blood flows from the veins of the body into the atria and then to the ventricles. The discharging chambers refer to the inferior thick-walled ventricles and are the true pumps of the heart. As the ventricles contract, blood is pushed out of the heart and into circulation throughout the body. The heart's anterior surface consists primarily of the right ventricle, and the apex of the heart contains the left ventricle. The **interatrial septum** divides the heart longitudinally and divides the atria. The **interventricular septum** divides the left and right ventricles.

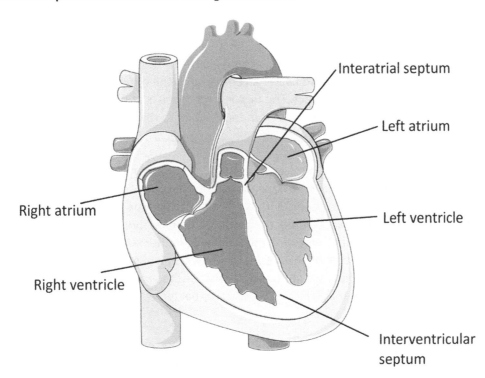

The heart contains two ventricles and functions as a double pump whereby veins carry blood toward the heart and arteries carry blood away from it. The right side of the heart works as a pulmonary circuit pump and receives oxygen-poor blood from the veins. These veins come from the capillary beds of the body tissues and run through the large inferior vena cava and the large superior vena cava. Blood is then pumped out through the pulmonary trunk, which splits into the left and right pulmonary arteries. Blood is then carried to the capillary beds of the lungs where oxygen is loaded and carbon dioxide is released.

The oxygen-rich blood then leaves the capillary beds where gas exchange occurred and is returned to the left portion of the heart through four pulmonary veins.

The **pulmonary circulation** is a circuit whereby blood moves from the right pump/ventricle to the lungs and back to the left receiving chamber, or atrium. The main purpose of this circuit is to transfer blood to the lungs so that carbon dioxide exits into the lungs and oxygen enters the blood. The oxygen-rich blood is then returned to the left atrium and flows into the left ventricle where it is pumped out into the aorta. The **systemic circulation** is the second circuit where blood moves from the left ventricle to all the body tissues and back into the right atrium. The circuit supplies oxygen and nutrients to the body's organs. The aorta and systemic arteries branch to all capillary beds of all body tissues whereby oxygen is delivered to these tissues. Oxygen-poor and carbon dioxide-rich blood then circulates back to the right atrium through the systemic veins. Blood then enters the inferior or superior vena. Because the left ventricle pumps blood over a longer pathway (the systemic circuit), the left ventricle is thicker and is a more powerful pump than the right ventricle.

Respiratory System

The respiratory and cardiovascular systems work together to supply the body oxygen gas and remove carbon dioxide. The organs of the respiratory system are responsible for managing the gas exchange (oxygen and carbon dioxide) between the external environment and the blood. These organs include the bronchi and their smaller branches, larynx, lungs, nose, pharynx, and trachea. The lungs contain terminal air sacs called **alveoli**. Gas exchange in the blood takes place only in the alveoli. The remaining respiratory organs are conducting passageways that carry air into the lungs. These conducting passageways can humidify, purify, and warm the incoming air. Therefore, as air reaches the lungs, it is damp and warm, and there is less dust and bacteria compared to the outside air. The respiratory tract can be divided into an upper and lower tract. The **upper tract** consists of the passageways that run from the nose to the larynx. The **lower tract** extends from the trachea to the alveoli.

Nose
The only external and visible part of the respiratory system is the **nose**. As a person breathes, air enters the nose and passes the **nares**, or **nostrils**. Toward the interior of the nose, there is a **nasal cavity** that is divided by a midline called the **nasal septum**. Within the slit-like superior part of the nasal cavity is a mucous membrane called the **mucosa**. The mucosa contains the olfactory receptors that sense smell. The **respiratory mucosa** makes up the remaining mucosa lining in the nasal cavity. This mucosa sits on an abundant network of thin-walled veins that keeps the air warm when inhaled. The respiratory mucosa's glands produce a sticky mucus that not only moistens the air and traps bacteria/debris but also contains lysozyme enzymes that chemically break down bacteria.

Pharynx
In between the nasal cavity and the larynx is a muscular passageway called the **pharynx**. Commonly known as the **throat**, this structure is approximately 5 inches long and functions as the passageway for air and food. The pharynx is continuous and located anteriorly to the nasal cavity and connected through the **posterior nasal aperture**. The three primary regions of the pharynx are the **nasopharynx**, **oropharynx**, and **laryngopharynx**. From the nasal cavity, air enters through the superior part of the nasopharynx, and then travels down through the oropharynx and laryngopharynx, and then the larynx. On the other hand, food moves through the mouth, along with air, and goes through the oropharynx and laryngopharynx. However, food enters the esophagus posteriorly through the **epiglottis** (a flap).

Larynx

The **larynx** is inferior to the pharynx and functions by routing food and air through specific channels. The larynx is known as the **voice box** and has a role in speech. Eight rigid hyaline cartilages and an epiglottis make up the larynx. The Adam's apple, the largest of these cartilages, is a shield-shaped piece of hyaline cartilage that protrudes anteriorly and is part of the larynx. The **epiglottis** is a spoon-shaped flap made of elastic cartilage. The epiglottis is referred to as "the guardian of the airway" because it protects the superior larynx opening. It allows the passage of air to the lower respiratory passages. However, when fluids or food are swallowed, the larynx pulls upward, causing the epiglottis to tip and form a lid over the larynx opening. This process allows food to enter the esophagus and the stomach in a posterior manner. If food or fluids enter the larynx, a cough reflex is initiated to prevent those substances from moving into the lungs. However, the cough reflex is not triggered when a person is unconscious.

Trachea

Once air passes down through the larynx, it enters the windpipe, or **trachea**, which is approximately four inches in length, and reaches the mid-chest at approximately the level of the fifth thoracic vertebra. The trachea is reinforced with C-shaped hyaline cartilage rings, which make the trachea walls fairly rigid. The rings have two functions. The open portions of the rings near the esophagus allow it to expand toward the anterior end as a person swallows food. The solid parts of the wall keep the trachea patent and provide support, regardless of the pressure changes that take place during breathing. The **trachealis** is a muscle that makes up the trachea wall and is posterior to the esophagus. Ciliated mucosa lines the wall of the trachea and beats continuously in the superior (upper) direction. The cilia are surrounded by goblet cells. As these cells produce mucus, the cilia propel the mucus (which traps debris and dust particles) away from the lungs and to the throat where it can be spat or swallowed.

Main Bronchi

The trachea is divided into the left and right main bronchi. Each bronchus runs in a slanted fashion (approximately 100-120 from the trachea) before heading into the **hilum**, or medial depression, of each lung. The right bronchus is generally shorter, wider, and straighter compared to the left. Therefore, it's common for an inhaled foreign substance or object to get stuck in the right bronchus. As air reaches the bronchi, it becomes warm and humid and cleansed of most of the impurities. Inside the lungs, the main bronchi branch into smaller divisions and route directly to the air sacs.

Lungs

The **lungs** occupy all of the thoracic cavity except for the mediastinum, the most central area of the cavity. The lungs envelop the blood vessels, heart, esophagus, and bronchi. Fissures separate the lungs into lobes. The left lung contains two lobes, and the right contains three lobes. The pulmonary, or visceral pleura, covers the surface of each lung. The parietal pleura covers the walls of the thoracic cavity. Pleural fluid, a serous fluid, is produced by the pleural membranes and allows the lungs to glide over the thorax easily during breathing. The main bronchi are subdivided into secondary and tertiary bronchi, or smaller branches, that end at the **bronchioles**, the smallest air-conducting passageways. This branched network within the lungs is called the respiratory, or bronchial, tree. The terminal bronchioles lead to and terminate in smaller conduits or respiratory zone structures called the **alveoli**, or air sacs. The respiratory bronchioles, alveolar ducts, alveoli, and alveolar sacs make up the respiratory zone and are the only site of gas exchange. The remaining respiratory passages are conducting zone structures that are gateways to and from the respiratory zone.

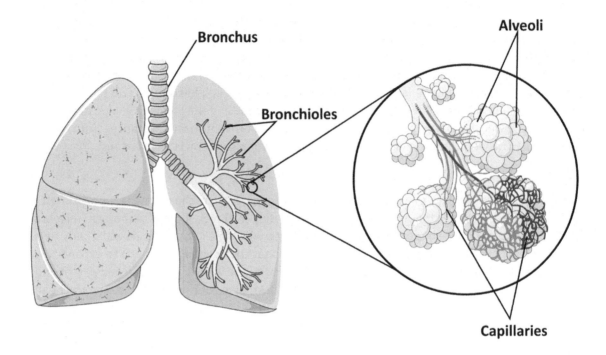

Digestive System

The digestive system breaks down food into essential nutrients that are required for metabolic processes, such as the production of energy, or adenosine triphosphate (ATP). Four main processes of the digestive system include ingestion, digestion, absorption, and defecation. The digestive system is divided into two primary groups that include the alimentary canal and the accessory digestive organs.

The Gut

The organs of the **alimentary canal**, or **gastrointestinal (GI) tract** (gut), consist of a coiled and continuous hollow muscle tube that winds from the mouth to the anus. Organs of the alimentary canal include the mouth, pharynx, and esophagus as well as the stomach and small and large intestines. The walls of the gut from the esophagus to the large intestine are made of the same four tissue layers, or **tunics**, as shown below.

Stomach

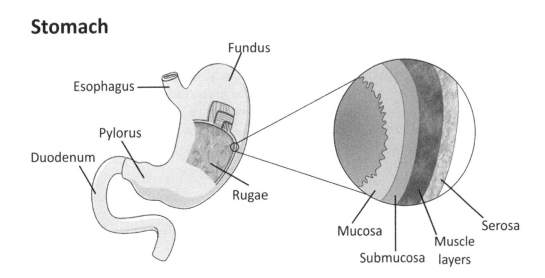

The four tissue layers are called the mucosa, submucosa, muscularis externa, and serosa. The innermost layer of the alimentary canal is a moist mucous membrane called the **mucosa**. The mucosa lines the **lumen**, or hollow cavity, of an organ. It's made mostly from surface epithelium plus a small portion of **lamina propria** (connective tissue) and a scanty layer of smooth muscle. The epithelium is primarily composed of simple columnar tissue that extends past the esophagus. Beneath the mucosa is a soft connective tissue called the **submucosa**. This tissue contains nerve endings, blood and lymphatic vessels, and mucosa-associated lymphoid tissue.

The alimentary canal wall also contains the **muscularis externa**, which wraps around the submucosa. This smooth muscle layer is made up of two layers: an inner circular layer and outer longitudinal layer. The outermost layer of the canal wall is called the **serosa**. There are two layers, and half the serous membrane pair makes up the visceral peritoneum. The **visceral peritoneum**, or serosa, is made up of a single layer of flat cells that produce a serous fluid and is continuous with the **parietal peritoneum**. The abdominopelvic cavity is lined with the slippery parietal peritoneum.

The alimentary canal has two intrinsic nerve plexuses. Part of the autonomic nervous system, the submucosal and myenteric nerve plexus, regulate the mobility and secretory activity of the GI tract organs.

Stomach

The stomach is sandwiched between two types of peritoneum called the lesser and greater omentum. The **lesser omentum** is made up of a double layer of peritoneum, and the **greater omentum** is riddled with fat to help cushion, insulate, and protect the abdominal organs.

The lesser omentum extends from the liver toward the lesser curvature of the stomach. The greater omentum wraps downward and envelops the abdominal organs and greater curvature of the stomach. The **cardial region** of the stomach surrounds the cardioesophageal sphincter. Food enters the cardial or cardia from the esophagus. The **fundus** is an expanded part of the stomach, and the **body** is the midportion of the stomach. The **greater curvature** of the stomach is the convex lateral surface, and the

lesser curvature is the concave medial surface. As the stomach narrows, the body of the stomach becomes the **pyloric antrum**, followed by a terminal part of the stomach called a **pylorus**, a funnel-shaped segment. The pylorus is continuous with the small intestine and goes through the pyloric sphincter, or valve.

The stomach is approximately six to ten inches in length and can hold one gallon of food when full. When the stomach is empty, it shrinks into large folds called **rugae**. The stomach is not only a site for the breakdown of food, but also acts as a temporary storage tank. In addition to the longitudinal and circular muscle, it contains a third oblique layer called the **muscularis externa**. This innermost layer allows the stomach to move, mix, churn, and pummel food while simultaneously moving it along the GI tract. Therefore, food is physically broken down into smaller pieces. Once food is processed in the stomach, it forms a thick cream called **chyme**. The chyme will pass through the pylorus into the small intestine. The **pyloric sphincter** regulates the flow of chyme.

The stomach's other function involves the chemical breakdown of food. The stomach's mucosa contains simple columnar epithelium. The single layer of mucous cells produces a protective layer of bicarbonate-rich alkaline mucus that sticks to the stomach mucosa. The mucus protects the stomach wall from being digested by enzymes and from acidic damage. The stomach's mucosa is dotted with millions of deep gastric pits.

The gastric glands can divide into two channels and contain the mucous neck cells, parietal cells, chief cells, and enteroendocrine cells. The gastric glands contain specific cells that secrete gastric juice that is composed of several components. For example, humans contain cells that produce an intrinsic factor that is responsible for the absorption of vitamin B_{12}. Without the production of the intrinsic factor, absorption of vitamin B_{12} would not occur readily in the **ileum**, a section within the small intestine. The parietal cells also produce **hydrochloric acid (HCl)**, a corrosive acid that makes stomach acid. HCl initiates the activation of the inactive enzyme **pepsinogen** to the active enzyme **pepsin**. At a low pH, a polypeptide portion of pepsinogen cleaves, thereby creating an active site on pepsin.

Pepsinogens are initially inactive protein-digesting enzymes that are produced by the **chief cells** but become active after reacting with HCl. The **mucous neck cells** produce an acidic mucus and are found in the upper region of the fundic glands. Although the function of the neck cells is unknown, they are identifiable by their wedge-shaped nucleus. The **enteroendocrine cells** secrete specific hormones that are vital in the regulation of digestive activities. For example, these cells secrete the hormone **gastrin**, which stimulates stomach emptying and the release of gastric juice. **Stem cells** are unspecialized cells that are found at the top of the glands within the gastric mucosa and are open within the pits. These cells undergo cell division to replace secretory cells of the gastric glands and surface mucosa cells that die. Therefore, stem cells are vital to replenishing the surface epithelium on a continual basis. Within the stomach, much of the digestive activity takes place in the pyloric region.

Urinary System

The urinary system's role is to regulate water and filter nitrogen waste from the blood. The primary organs of the urinary system include the urinary bladder, kidneys, urethra, and paired ureters. Urine can be temporarily stored in the ureters and urinary bladder and then transported to the kidneys before exiting the body. The kidneys have the primary role of eliminating nitrogen-containing wastes, drugs, and toxins from the body. The kidneys maintain the purity of our internal fluids by filtering gallons of fluid from the bloodstream daily.

The filtrate is processed by allowing excess ions and wastes to exit the body as urine. Some substances in the filtrate are returned to the blood. The kidneys also control blood volume while maintaining the right balance between salts and waters and acids and bases. Other functions of the kidneys include blood pressure regulation and the stimulation of red blood production within the bone marrow. Specifically, the kidneys produce an enzyme called **renin** to control the blood pressure and the hormone **erythropoietin** to stimulate red blood cell production. Kidney cells can even transform vitamin D supplements into the active form that is needed by the body.

Kidneys

The kidneys are small, dark red organs that have the shape of a kidney bean. Each kidney is approximately the size of a large bar of soap. These organs lie against the dorsal body wall behind the parietal peritoneum within the superior lumbar area. The kidneys are mostly protected by the lower part of the rib cage. Due to the liver, the right kidney is slightly lower than the left kidney.

The kidney contains a medial indentation called the **renal hilum** and is convex laterally. The image shows the structures of the kidney, which include renal blood vessels, nerves, and ureters. At the top of the kidney is the **adrenal gland**. There are three protective layers in the kidney, from deep to superficial, called the fibrous capsule, perirenal fat capsule, and the renal fascia. The **fibrous capsule** encloses each kidney and gives it a shiny appearance. The **perirenal fat capsule** is a fatty mass that also surrounds each kidney and cushions it against blows.

The most superficial layer is the **renal fascia**, which is made of dense fibrous connective tissue. The renal fascia anchors the adrenal gland and kidney to its surrounding structures. The perirenal fat capsule is vital for holding the kidneys in their respective body position. During massive weight loss, the fatty mass can dwindle, thereby dropping the kidneys to a lower position. The drooping condition is generally called **ptosis** and can cause the ureters to become kinked such that urine is not able to pass through the ureters. Because the ureters are kinked, fluid pressure is exerted on the kidney tissue and causes a condition called **hydronephrosis**.

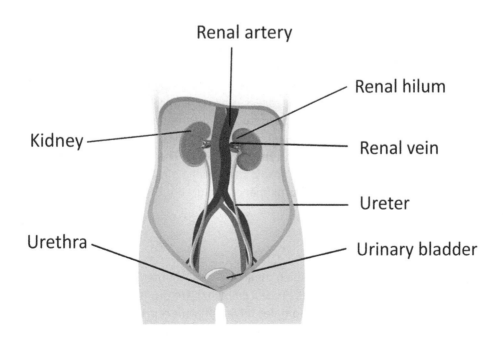

There are three main regions in the kidney. The outer region is called the **renal cortex**. Deeper than the cortex, in the middle of the kidney, is the **renal medulla**. The medulla has several triangular regions called **medullary (renal) pyramids**. The base of the pyramid faces the cortex. The tip of the pyramid is called the **apex** and points to the kidney's inner region. Each pyramid is separated by cortex-like tissue extensions called **renal columns**. The **renal pelvis** is the innermost region and is lateral to the hilum. It is a flat, funnel-shaped tube that is continuous with the ureter when exiting the hilum.

The **calyces** are extensions of the pelvis and form cup-shaped drains that surround the pyramid tips. Urine is collected at the calyces and is continuously drained from the pyramid tips into the renal pelvis. After urine flows from the pelvis to the ureter, it is transported to the bladder where it is temporarily stored before exiting the body.

Blood Supply in the Kidneys

The kidneys have a vital role in blood cleansing and composition adjustment. These processes occur continuously, and nearly one-quarter of the body's blood supply passes through the kidney within a minute. Each kidney is supplied with blood through the **renal artery**. As the artery nears the hilum, it divides into segmental arteries that further form several branches of arteries called **interlobar arteries**. The interlobar arteries move through renal columns into the cortex and branch into **arcuate arteries** at the cortex-medulla junction. The arcuate arteries form an arch over the medullary pyramids but then branch into **cortical radiate arteries**, which supply blood to the renal cortex. The blood then becomes deoxygenated (venous blood) and flows through the veins, along the arterial pathway but in reverse. In other words, the venous blood will flow in the following direction: cortical radiate, arcuate, interlobar, and renal veins. The renal vein emerges from the kidney hilum and is emptied into the inferior vena cava.

Nephrons

Nephrons, the tiny filters responsible for producing urine, make up the structural and functional units within the kidney. There are more than a million nephrons and thousands of ducts that collect fluid from many nephrons.

The renal corpuscle and renal tubule are the two main structures in a nephron. The **renal corpuscle** contains a knot of capillaries called a **glomerulus**. The glomerular, or Bowman's capsule, is a cup-shaped hollow structure that envelops the glomerulus. The podocytes are octopus-like cells within the inner layer of the capsule. These cells contain long branching extensions called **foot processes** that intertwine and stick to the glomerulus. Between the foot processes are openings called **filtration slits** that give podocytes a porous membrane around the glomerulus. The afferent arteriole feeds nutrients to the glomerulus, which runs from the feeder vessel, which is called the cortical radiate artery. The efferent arteriole receives blood that has passed through the glomerulus. The renal tubule is approximately 1.25 inches long and extends from the glomerular capsule to the collecting duct. The different regions of the tubule, from the glomerular capsule, are the proximal convoluted tubule (PCT), nephron loop (loop of Henle), and distal convoluted tubule (DCT).

Reproductive System

The primary sex organs are called **gonads**, which means "seeds". In men, the sex organs are **testes**, and for women, they are called **ovaries**. **Gametes** are sex cells that are produced by the gonads. Hormones are also secreted by the gonads. Males and females have different reproductive systems that serve to produce offspring. Males produce male gametes called **sperm**, which are delivered to the woman's reproductive tract. The paired testes in men contain a sperm-producing (exocrine) and testosterone-producing (endocrine) function. Women create female gametes called **ova** (eggs). During suitable conditions, the sperm and egg combine to create a fertilized egg called a **zygote**. The female uterus provides an environment where the fetus can develop until birth.

Male Reproductive System

Testes

The golf ball-sized testis is attached to the trunk via a connective tissue sheath called the **spermatic cord**. This tissue wraps around nerves, blood vessels, and the ductus deferens. The tunica albuginea is a white fibrous connective tissue capsule that surrounds each testis. These capsules (septa) have extensions that connect to the testis and divide into several large web-shaped lobules. One to four sperm-producing factories called **seminiferous tubules** are found in each lobule. These tubules empty sperm into the rete testis, another set of tubules found on one side of the testis. From the rete testis, sperm enters the **epididymis**, the first part of the duct system that wraps the external testis surface. The interstitial cells are embedded in soft connected tissue that surrounds the seminiferous tubules. These cells produce androgens, such as testosterone.

Duct System

The accessory organs of the male duct system are responsible for the transportation of sperm within the body. They are the epididymis, ductus (vas) deferens, and urethra. As shown in the image below, the epididymis is highly convoluted and bowl-shaped and wraps the posterior end of the testis.

Immature sperm is temporarily stored in the epididymis. As sperm travels along the convoluted pathway, a process that takes approximately twenty days, it matures and gains the ability to swim. **Ejaculation** occurs when a man becomes sexually stimulated. The process causes the epididymis to contract, thereby forcing sperm to be expelled into the **ductus deferens**, the secondary duct. The vas, or ductus, deferens, runs from the epididymis via the spermatic cord, in an upward fashion, through the inguinal canal. The main function of the vas deferens is to push live sperm from the storage sites into the urethra. The urethra extends from the base of the urinary bladder to the tip of the penis and is the terminal end of the male duct system. The three main regions of the urethra are the prostatic, membranous, and spongy (penile) urethra. The male urethra serves the urinary and reproductive systems and therefore carries both urine and sperm to the body's exterior.

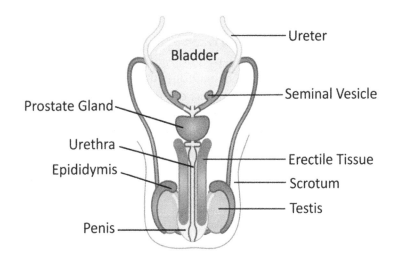

Accessory glands of the male reproductive system include the seminal vesicles, single prostate, and the paired bulbourethral glands. The **seminal vesicles** are large hollow glands that have the shape and size of a small finger and are found at the base of the bladder. These vesicles make approximately 60 percent of the seminal fluid and produce a thick yellow secretion that is rich in vitamin C, fructose, prostaglandins, and other nourishing substances. The seminal fluid contains substances that activate the sperm as it moves through the tract. The **prostate** consists of one doughnut-shaped gland that is approximately the size of a peach pit. The prostate produces a milky fluid and, like the vesicles, plays a role in activating sperm. When ejaculation occurs, fluid enters the urethra through many small ducts. The **bulbourethral glands** are pea-sized glands below the prostate gland that produce a clear, thick mucus that drains into the penile urethra.

During sexual stimulation, the mucous secretion is the first to pass through the urethra. Before ejaculation, the mucus will be secreted and clean out any traces of acidic urine in the urethra. The mucus also acts as a lubricant. **Semen** is a milky white sticky mixture that acts as a transport medium for sperm and other accessory gland secretions. Mature sperm are cellular tadpoles that contain a tail, midsection, and head. Mitochondria are found in the midsection and wrap around special filaments. The sperm head contains the nucleus and compacted DNA.

Female Reproductive System

Ovaries

The ovaries are attached to the sidewalls of the pelvis by the **suspensory ligaments**. These organs are fastened to the uterus medially through the **ovarian ligaments**. The **broad ligament** is a fold of peritoneum that holds the ovaries and encloses the ovarian and suspensory ligaments. The ovaries produce ova (exocrine product), estrogen, and progesterone (endocrine products). The ovaries are the shape of an almond but twice as large and contain sac-like structures called **ovarian follicles**.

An immature egg, called an **oocyte**, is found within each follicle. The oocyte is surrounded by one or more layers of distinct cells called **follicle cells**. The follicle enlarges and produces a fluid-filled central region, called an **antrum**, as the developing egg matures. During follicle enlargement, the follicle matures into a Graafian, or vesicular, follicle, and the developing egg becomes ready for ejection from the ovary in a process called **ovulation**. In women, ovulation generally occurs every twenty-eight days but may occur more or less frequently. Following ovulation, the follicle ruptures and transforms into a yellow body called the **corpus luteum**.

The Duct System

The duct system of the female reproductive tract is composed of the uterus, uterine tubes, and vagina. The **fallopian (uterine) tubes** make up the initial part of the duct system and provide a site where fertilization of the ovulated oocyte can occur. Each uterine tube is approximately four inches long and extends medially from the ovary into the superior part of the uterus. The broad ligaments support the uterine tubes. The female duct system has no contact between the ovaries and uterine tubes. The **uterine tube** is made up of two components called the infundibulum and the fimbriae. The **infundibulum** is a funnel-shaped cavity, and the **fimbriae** are finger-like projections located at the end of the fallopian tube near the ovary. The fimbriae partially cover the ovary. During ovulation, an oocyte is expelled from the ovary, propelled by fluid currents from the waving fimbriae, and moves into the uterine tube toward the uterus.

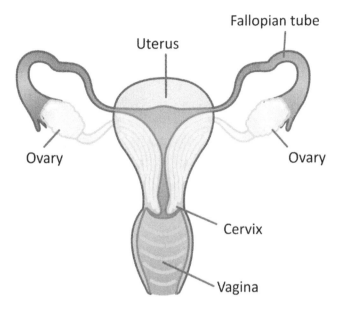

The **uterus** is a womb and a hollow organ that works to receive, retain, and nourish the fertilized egg. Oocytes are carried to the uterus by peristalsis and the rhythmic beating of the cilia, but many are lost in the peritoneal cavity. Initially the size and shape of a pear, the uterus will increase in size during pregnancy. The broad ligament suspends the uterus within the pelvis, and the round, uterosacral ligaments anchor the uterus. The main part of the uterus is called the **body**, and the rounded region, superior to the uterine tube entrances, is called the **fundus**. The **cervix** is a narrow outlet that protrudes inferiorly into the vagina.

Practice Test #1

Mathematics

1. Add $1000 + (-55)$.
   a. 945
   b. 1055
   c. 955
   d. 45

2. Add $-675 + (-246)$.
   a. -429
   b. 921
   c. -921
   d. 429

3. Add $-431 + 99$.
   a. -510
   b. -332
   c. 332
   d. 510

4. Add $0.555 + 0.0235$.
   a. 0.5785
   b. 0.79
   c. 0.079
   d. 0.05785

5. Add $5.41 + 11.9$.
   a. 17.31
   b. 1.731
   c. 16.5
   d. 1.65

6. Add $18 + 0.567$.
   a. 23.67
   b. 18.567
   c. 185.67
   d. 1.8567

7. Add $18{,}765 + 34{,}876$.
   a. 53,639
   b. 53,640
   c. 53,641
   d. 53,642

8. Estimate the sum $86,542 + 91,224$ by first rounding the addends to the nearest ten-thousand place.
    a. 178,000
    b. 179,000
    c. 177,700
    d. 180,000

9. Estimate the sum $2.567 + 4.109$ by first rounding the addends to the nearest ones place.
    a. 8
    b. 7
    c. 6.7
    d. 5

10. Find the perimeter of a square garden with a side length of 16 meters.
    a. 32 meters
    b. 256 meters
    c. 8 meters
    d. 64 meters

11. Find the perimeter of the following rectangle:

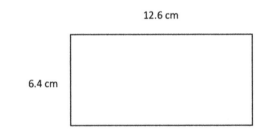

12.6 cm

6.4 cm

    a. 19 cm
    b. 38 cm
    c. 12.6 cm
    d. 25.2 cm

12. If a square has a perimeter of 48 inches, what is the length of each side?
    a. 8 inches
    b. 24 inches
    c. 12 inches
    d. 4 inches

13. Subtract $89,076 - 45,195$.
    a. 43,981
    b. 43,881
    c. 44,981
    d. 33,881

14. Subtract −65 − 4.
   a. −61
   b. 69
   c. −69
   d. 61

15. Subtract 98 − (−45).
   a. 143
   b. 53
   c. −143
   d. −53

16. Subtract −45 − (−17).
   a. −28
   b. 28
   c. −62
   d. 62

17. Subtract 65.814 − 14.87.
   a. 51.727
   b. 50.943
   c. 59.944
   d. 50.944

18. Subtract 4.2 − 0.054.
   a. 3.66
   b. 4.146
   c. 4.1946
   d. 4.156

19. Subtract 65 − 0.9999.
   a. 64.001
   b. 64.01
   c. 64.0001
   d. 65.1

20. Estimate the difference 95,198 − 54,987 by first rounding the numbers to the nearest ten-thousands place.
   a. 55,000
   b. 50,000
   c. 40,000
   d. 45,000

21. Estimate the difference 56,999 − 45,298 by first rounding the numbers to the nearest thousands place.
   a. 22,000
   b. 21,000
   c. 20,000
   d. 10,000

22. Estimate the difference $43.892 - 35.789$ by first rounding the numbers to the nearest ones place.

    a. 7

    b. 8

    c. 9

    d. 8.1

23. A tower in India is 1,543 feet tall. Another tower in China is 1,345 feet tall. How much taller is the tower in India than the tower in China?

    a. -288 feet

    b. 288 feet

    c. -198 feet

    d. 198 feet

24. A building in New York City is 876 feet taller than a building in Spokane, Washington. If the building in Spokane is 456 tall, how tall is the building in New York City?

    a. 400 feet

    b. 420 feet

    c. 1,332 feet

    d. 1,432 feet

25. Multiply 413×34.

    a. 14,402

    b. 14,042

    c. 12,390

    d. 13,940

26. Multiply 7000×9000.

    a. 630,000,000

    b. 6,300,000

    c. 63,000,000

    d. 630,000

27. Find the area of a square that has a side length of 17 feet.

    a. 68 square feet

    b. 34 square feet

    c. 289 square feet

    d. 170 square feet

28. Find the area of the following rectangle:

8 yards

3 yards

a. 22 square yards
b. 24 square yards
c. 64 square yards
d. 11 square yards

29. Multiply $-34(-4)$.
a. -136
b. 68
c. 136
d. -38

30. Multiply $45(-2)$.
a. 90
b. -90
c. 43
d. -43

31. Multiply $(-3)(-5)(-6)(-2)$.
a. -180
b. -90
c. 180
d. 90

32. Multiply $(-6)(190)(0)(-17)$.
a. 0
b. 19,380
c. $-19,380$
d. $-1,140$

33. Multiply 7.5×0.7.
a. 0.525
b. 5.25
c. 52.5
d. 525

34. Multiply 7.567 × 2.41.
   a. 1.823647
   b. 0.1823647
   c. 18.23647
   d. 182.3647

35. Estimate the product 5.879 × 19.203 by first rounding the factors to the nearest ones place.
   a. 120
   b. 114
   c. 100
   d. 95

36. Estimate the product 15,763 × 21,892 by first rounding the factors to the nearest ten-thousands place.
   a. 400,000,000
   b. 40,000,000
   c. 200,000,000
   d. 352,000,000

37. Find the area of a rectangular room that is 8.75 feet wide and 12 feet long.
   a. 105 feet
   b. 10.5 square feet
   c. 105 square feet
   d. 1050 square feet

38. Simplify $\frac{-109}{-109}$.
   a. -1
   b. 0
   c. 1
   d. 109

39. Simplify $\frac{0}{-967}$.
   a. 0
   b. undefined
   c. 1
   d. −967.

40. Multiply and simplify $\frac{25}{2} \times \frac{7}{6}$.
   a. $\frac{32}{12}$
   b. $\frac{32}{8}$
   c. $\frac{175}{8}$
   d. $\frac{175}{12}$

41. Simplify $\frac{16}{10}$.

    a. 4

    b. $\frac{8}{5}$

    c. $\frac{4}{3}$

    d. $\frac{8}{3}$

42. Multiply and simplify $\frac{18}{5} \times \frac{10}{2}$.

    a. 18

    b. $\frac{180}{10}$

    c. $\frac{28}{7}$

    d. $\frac{36}{50}$

43. Multiply and simplify $65 \times \frac{2}{5}$.

    a. $\frac{130}{5}$

    b. 13

    c. 26

    d. $\frac{325}{5}$

44. Find the area of the following triangle:

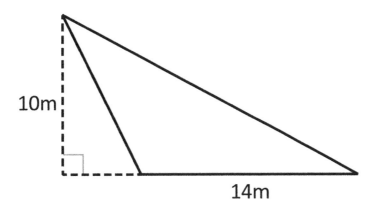

   a. 140 square meters
   b. 70 square meters
   c. 24 square meters
   d. 40 square meters

45. What is the reciprocal of $\frac{14}{5}$?

   a. $\frac{14}{5}$

   b. 14

   c. 5

   d. $\frac{5}{14}$

46. Divide and simplify $\frac{15}{4} \div 5$.

   a. $\frac{75}{4}$

   b. $\frac{3}{4}$

   c. $\frac{15}{20}$

   d. $\frac{15}{5}$

47. Divide and simplify $\frac{5}{8} \div \frac{15}{4}$.

   a. $\frac{1}{6}$

   b. $\frac{10}{60}$

   c. $\frac{75}{32}$

   d. $\frac{20}{120}$

48. Find the least common denominator (LCD) of $\frac{1}{15}$ and $\frac{5}{6}$.

    a. 6

    b. 15

    c. 30

    d. 90

49. Add and simplify $\frac{15}{17} + \frac{2}{17}$.

    a. $\frac{17}{17}$

    b. 1

    c. $\frac{13}{17}$

    d. $\frac{30}{17}$

50. Add and simplify $\frac{1}{8} + \frac{1}{6}$.

    a. $\frac{2}{14}$

    b. $\frac{1}{7}$

    c. $\frac{7}{12}$

    d. $\frac{7}{24}$

51. Subtract and simplify $\frac{18}{25} - \frac{14}{15}$.

    a. $-\frac{16}{75}$

    b. $\frac{16}{75}$

    c. $\frac{4}{10}$

    d. $\frac{2}{5}$

52. Convert $6\frac{1}{7}$ to an improper fraction.

    a. $\frac{6}{7}$

    b. $\frac{13}{7}$

    c. $\frac{43}{7}$

    d. $\frac{44}{7}$

53. Convert $\frac{76}{9}$ to a mixed number.

   a. $\frac{9}{76}$

   b. $4\frac{8}{9}$

   c. $8\frac{9}{4}$

   d. $8\frac{4}{9}$

54. Multiply and simplify $4\frac{1}{3} \times \frac{3}{8}$.

   a. $\frac{7}{24}$

   b. $\frac{39}{24}$

   c. $\frac{24}{39}$

   d. $\frac{1}{2}$

55. Add and simplify $4\frac{1}{2} + 1\frac{1}{12}$.

   a. $\frac{5}{14}$

   b. $\frac{76}{12}$

   c. $\frac{67}{12}$

   d. $\frac{25}{12}$

Reading Comprehension

Questions 1–5 are based on the following passage:

Fluoride use is one of the main factors responsible for the decline in prevalence and severity of dental caries and cavities (tooth decay) in the United States (*1*). Brushing children's teeth is recommended when the first tooth erupts, as early as 6 months, and the first dental visit should occur no later than age 1 year (*2–4*). However, ingestion of too much fluoride while teeth are developing can result in visibly detectable changes in enamel structure such as discoloration and pitting (dental fluorosis) (*1*). Therefore, CDC recommends that children begin using fluoride toothpaste at age 2 years. Children aged 3 years or younger should use a smear the size of a rice grain, and children aged older than 3 years should use no more than a pea-sized amount (0.25 g) until age 6 years, by which time the swallowing reflex has developed sufficiently to prevent inadvertent ingestion. Questions on toothbrushing practices and toothpaste use among children and adolescents were included in the questionnaire component of the National Health and Nutrition Examination Survey (NHANES) for the first time beginning in the 2013–2014 cycle. This study estimates patterns of toothbrushing and toothpaste use among children and adolescents by analyzing parents' or caregivers' responses to questions about when the child started to brush teeth, age the child started to use toothpaste, frequency of toothbrushing each day, and amount of toothpaste currently used or used at time of survey. Analysis of 2013–2016 data found that greater than 38% of children aged 3–6 years used more toothpaste than that recommended by CDC and other professional organizations. In addition, nearly 80% of children aged 3–15 years started brushing later than recommended. Parents and caregivers can play a role in ensuring that children are brushing often enough and using the recommended amount of toothpaste.

Thornton-Evans G, Junger ML, Lin M, Wei L, Espinoza L, Beltran-Aguilar E. Use of Toothpaste and Toothbrushing Patterns Among Children and Adolescents — United States, 2013–2016. MMWR Morb Mortal Wkly Rep 2019;68:87–90. DOI: http://dx.doi.org/10.15585/mmwr.mm6804a3

1. What is responsible for the decline in tooth decay in the United States?
    a. Tooth brushing
    b. Fluoride
    c. Toothpaste
    d. Dentist visits

2. Why should parents/caregivers limit the amount of toothpaste given to children under the age of six?
    a. Young children don't get cavities.
    b. Their baby teeth will fall out, so they need not worry.
    c. They don't need fluoride.
    d. They might swallow the toothpaste, causing dental issues.

3. How did the study gather information?
    a. By talking to caregivers
    b. By asking children
    c. By asking adolescents
    d. By observing children

4. Using the context clues from the passage, what does the word *inadvertent* mean?
    a. Deliberate
    b. Unintentional
    c. Incorrect
    d. Advantageous

5. Which is NOT a detail included in the passage?
    a. More than half of children start brushing their teeth too late.
    b. First dental visits should be no later than one year old.
    c. Regular brushing should begin at eight to ten months of age.
    d. Children should use fluoride starting at two years old.

Questions 6–10 are based on the following passage:

Among many other factors, the risk of adult obesity is greater among adults who were obese as children, with racial and ethnic disparities existing by the age of two. If nothing else is done in the United States beyond what is being done now, simulated growth trajectories that model today's children show that over half (59% of today's toddlers and 57% of children aged two to nineteen) will be obese by age thirty-five. Early feeding patterns, including how babies are fed and how caregivers use food in response to an infant's mood, affect acute growth, future eating patterns, and the risk of obesity. Similarly, family and caregiver modeling of healthy behaviors, food offerings, and active playtime, as well as characteristics of neighborhoods such as walkability and traffic volume, may affect children's nutrition and physical activity habits.

As sectors come together to reduce the obesity epidemic, we are aware how challenging success will be due to factors such as 1) the contributing risk factors of genetic and biological attributes; 2) individual behaviors (parenting styles, dietary patterns, physical activity levels, medication use, sleep, stress management); and 3) community and societal factors that influence individual, family, and collective access to healthy, affordable foods and beverages; access to safe and convenient places for physical activity; and exposure to the marketing of unhealthy products.

By using self-reported data of height and weight from the Behavioral Risk Factor Surveillance System, CDC's Division of Nutrition, Physical Activity, and Obesity (DNPAO) has published state-specific obesity maps since 1999. Obesity is defined as a body mass index (BMI: a person's weight in kilograms divided by the square of height in meters) of 30.0 or higher. These maps have shown the growing epidemic that has affected our nation from coast to coast. Although the data collection methods changed in 2011, which somewhat limits our ability to assess trends, the 2017 data continue to show that obesity prevalence among adults remains high across the country. The state-specific prevalence ranges from a low of 22.6% in Colorado to a high of 38.1% in West Virginia.

Petersen R, Pan L, Blanck HM. Racial and Ethnic Disparities in Adult Obesity in the United States: CDC's Tracking to Inform State and Local Action. *Prev Chronic Dis*. 2019;16:E46. Published 2019 Apr 11. DOI:10.5888/pcd16.180579

6. Which of the following is a true statement if we do not change our tactics to address obesity?
   a. Obesity levels in adults will level out.
   b. As long as they weren't obese as children, adults will be fine.
   c. Over half of American children will be obese by age thirty-five.
   d. Children of obese parents will likely be obese as well.

7. The author writes that there are many challenges to tackling obesity, including individual, community, and societal behaviors. What other factors contribute to the challenge?
   a. Fast food
   b. Biological and genetic attributes
   c. Food industry tactics and food science
   d. Paying to play sports

8. Increasing which of the following features in a neighborhood might have a positive impact on a child's nutrition and physical activity habits?
   a. Single-family homes
   b. Traffic
   c. Convenience stores
   d. Walkability

9. How is obesity defined?

    a. Weight

    b. Size

    c. Appearance

    d. BMI

10. Based on context clues from the passage, what does the word *disparities* mean?

"Among many other factors, the risk of adult obesity is greater among adults who had obesity as children, with racial and ethnic disparities existing by the age of two."

    a. Differences

    b. Experiences

    c. Beliefs

    d. Similarities

Questions 11–15 are based on the following passage:

The approximate two-thirds decline in adult cigarette smoking prevalence that has occurred since 1965 represents a major public health success. In 2018, 13.7% of U.S. adults ages 18 years or older smoked cigarettes, the lowest prevalence recorded since 1965. However, no significant change in cigarette smoking prevalence occurred during 2017–2018. Most cigarette smokers and smokeless tobacco users reported daily use, whereas most e-cigarette and cigar users reported nondaily use. Even nondaily use of cigarettes has been linked to increased mortality risk.

Quitting smoking at any age is beneficial for health. From 2009 to 2018, significant linear increases occurred in quit attempts, recent successful cessation, and quit ratio. Population-based tobacco control interventions, including high-impact tobacco education campaigns like CDC's Tips From Former Smokers campaign and FDA's Every Try Counts campaign, combined with barrier-free access to evidence-based cessation treatments, can both motivate persons who use tobacco products to try to quit and help them succeed in quitting.

The prevalence of adult e-cigarette use increased from 2.8% in 2017 to 3.2% in 2018 but was much lower than the 20.8% of U.S. high school students reporting past thirty-day e-cigarette use in 2018. The prevalence of e-cigarette usage among persons aged 18–24 years is higher than that among other adult age groups, and e-cigarette use in this age group increased from 5.2% in 2017 to 7.6% in 2018. During 2014–2017 there had been a downward trajectory of adult e-cigarette use, but during 2017 and 2018 a significant increase in adult e-cigarette use was detected for the first time. This increase might be related to the emergence of new types of e-cigarettes, especially "pod-mod" devices, which frequently use nicotine salts as opposed to the free-base nicotine used in other e-cigarettes and tobacco products. Sales of JUUL, a pod-mod device, increased by approximately 600% from 2016 to 2017, making it the dominant e-cigarette product in the United States by the end of 2017. Further research is needed to monitor patterns of e-cigarette use and the relationship between use of e-cigarettes and other tobacco products (e.g., cigarette smoking).

The findings in this report are subject to at least three limitations. First, responses were self-reported and were not validated by biochemical testing. However, self-reported smoking status correlates highly with serum cotinine levels. Second, because National Health

Interview Survey (NHIS) is limited to the noninstitutionalized U.S. civilian population, the results are not generalizable to institutionalized populations and persons in the military. Finally, the NHIS sample adult response rate of 53.1% might have resulted in nonresponse bias.

Coordinated efforts at the local, state, and national levels are needed to continue progress toward reducing tobacco-related disease and death in the United States. Proven strategies include implementation of tobacco price increases, comprehensive smoke-free policies, high-impact antitobacco media campaigns, barrier-free cessation coverage, and comprehensive state tobacco control programs, combined with regulation of the manufacturing, marketing, and distribution of all tobacco products.

Creamer MR, Wang TW, Babb S, et al. Tobacco Product Use and Cessation Indicators Among Adults — United States, 2018. MMWR Morb Mortal Wkly Rep 2019;68:1013–1019. DOI: http://dx.doi.org/10.15585/mmwr.mm6845a2external icon

11. According to the text, since 1965, the number of smokers in the U.S. has:
    a. Increased
    b. Decreased
    c. Stayed the same
    d. Been hard to study

12. According to the text, e-cigarette use in adults has _____, and e-cigarette use in adolescents has _____.
    a. Increased; increased
    b. Decreased; decreased
    c. Increased; decreased
    d. Decreased; increased

13. The text refers to evidence-based cessation treatments. Based on context clues, what does *cessation* mean?
    a. Beginning
    b. Ending
    c. Continuing
    d. Assisting

14. Which of these is NOT one of the reported limitations?
    a. Self-reported data
    b. Limited to noninstitutionalized citizens
    c. Adolescents did not report
    d. Non-response bias

15. The study includes multiple ways to reduce smoking, including price increases, tobacco control programs, regulation, and which of the following?
    a. Raising the smoking age
    b. Banning e-cigarettes
    c. Punitive fines
    d. Media campaigns

Questions 16–20 are based on the following passage:

Skipping breakfast and other meals is one behavior studied as a factor influencing weight outcomes and dietary quality. Based on evidence that skipping breakfast reduces total daily caloric intake, some weight-loss recommendations include skipping breakfast (e.g., intermittent fasting) as one strategy to use. United States Department of Agriculture's (USDA) Economic Research Service (ERS) suggests that while skipping meals can cut calories, this may also reduce diet quality.

USDA and other federal agencies engage in nutrition education efforts to improve U.S. diets. ERS researchers investigated how skipping meals—breakfast, lunch, and dinner—affects calorie intake and diet quality among U.S. adults to see if this action conflicts with these education efforts and nutrition advice. Along with dietary effects, if the decision to skip a meal is widespread and sustained, there could be economic implications for agricultural producers, food processors, and others in the food supply chain.

The researchers used two days of food intake data for U.S. adults from the National Health and Nutrition Examination Survey (NHANES) for 2007-2016. These data capture detailed information about the types and amounts of food consumed in two non-consecutive days, as well as when each food was eaten and if it was part of a meal or a snack. The researchers used the Healthy Eating Index (HEI), which is a measure of how well a person's diet conforms with recommendations in the *Dietary Guidelines for Americans*, to gauge diet quality on each day. The HEI is made up of twelve dietary components encompassing food groups (fruit, dairy, whole grains, etc.) and dietary elements (fatty acids, empty calories, sodium, etc.). The HEI sums to a maximum total score of one hundred, with a higher score reflecting better diet quality. The score includes nine adequacy components—eight food groups and fatty acids—where higher consumption raises scores. The other three are moderation components—refined grains, sodium, and empty calories—with higher scores reflecting lower consumption and therefore, better diet quality.

Using the two days of intake for each survey respondent, the researchers used a statistical model that allowed them to control for individual characteristics that do not change between the two days (e.g., demographic variables and unobserved food and eating preferences). What remains are variables that may differ between the two days (e.g., the types and amounts of foods consumed and number of meals eaten), allowing the researchers to estimate how changes in day-to-day eating patterns (skipping a meal) affect the calories consumed and diet quality.

The results show that skipping a meal reduced daily caloric intake between 252 calories (breakfast) and 350 calories (dinner). However, skipping breakfast or lunch decreased diet quality by about 2.2 points (4.3%), while skipping dinner lowered diet quality by 1.4 points (2.6%). The dietary components affected by skipping each meal differed.

Skipping breakfast or lunch reduced the HEI component scores for fruit, whole grains, dairy, and empty calories. Skipping lunch also lowered component scores for vegetables and seafood and plant proteins. Lastly, skipping dinner reduced component scores for vegetables, greens and beans, dairy, protein food, seafood and plant proteins, and empty calories.

Out of all three meals, skipping dinner reduced daily calories the most while lowering diet quality the least.

Zeballos E, Todd JE. The effects of skipping a meal on daily energy intake and diet quality [published online ahead of print, 2020 May 13]. Public Health Nutr. 2020;1-10. DOI:10.1017/S1368980020000683

16. What is the main idea of the passage?
    a. Skipping meals might reduce caloric intake but will also impact dietary quality.
    b. Dieters should find a way to skip a meal to cut calories.
    c. Skipping meals will be bad for the economy.
    d. The advice to never skip breakfast is correct.

17. Which of these factors was NOT included in the data collected?
    a. Type of food
    b. Amount of food
    c. When food was eaten
    d. Where food was eaten

18. If one is looking to reduce calories but limit losses in dietary quality, which is the best option?
    a. Lunch is the best meal to skip.
    b. Dinner is the best meal to skip.
    c. Breakfast is the best meal to skip.
    d. One should never skip meals.

19. Which of the following is NOT a supporting detail from the text?
    a. Skipping a meal reduced caloric intake by about 250-350 calories, depending on the meal skipped.
    b. Skipping a meal reduced diet quality by about 2.5-4.0%, depending on the meal skipped.
    c. Skipping a meal a day resulted in an overall weight loss of one to two pounds per month.
    d. Skipping any meal a day resulted in a reduction of empty calories.

20. The HEI is made up of twelve components including food groups and which of the following?
    a. Fruits and vegetables
    b. Whole grains
    c. Dietary elements
    d. Calorie requirements

Questions 21–25 are based on the following passage:

The majority of studies that have examined the relationship between store access and dietary intake find that better access to a supermarket or large grocery store is associated with healthier food intakes. The relationship between the availability of restaurants (both fast food and full-service) and dietary intake has also been studied. In general, these studies have found that greater availability of fast-food restaurants and lower prices of fast-food restaurant items are related to poorer diet. Access to full-service restaurants shows either no relationship or a positive relationship with healthy dietary intake.

Only a few studies have used longitudinal data to measure how changes in access affect changes in diet. The few that exist focus on changes in shopping behavior and changes in dietary intake, not more distant outcomes such as obesity or other diet-related diseases. Two studies have examined the impact of the opening of a large supermarket in underserved areas in Leeds and Glasgow, UK.

The Leeds study used a pre/post intervention design, with survey interviews of participants about their shopping and food intake five months before and seven months after a Tesco supermarket opened in the area. The Glasgow study used a pre/post study design to assess change in shopping and food intake behaviors surrounding a new store opening, but it also considered a comparison area that had similar neighborhood characteristics but did not have a new store open in the area. The comparison area was added to determine if any changes in shopping or diet could be due to secular changes in diet that were not due to a new store opening.

Results of both studies showed that shopping behavior was affected by the openings of new stores—that is, a significant number of sampled individuals from the neighborhood switched their shopping to the new store. Both studies also show that average fruit and vegetable intake increased among surveyed individuals but that the average increase was small (just over one-third of a serving). The average increase in fruit and vegetable intake among those who switched their main food shopping to the new store was larger, but still under one-half of a full serving size. The increase in fruit and vegetable intake in Leeds was statistically significant, but the increase in Glasgow was not. The Glasgow study, which used a control comparison area, shows that some of the increase in fruit and vegetable intake among sampled individuals could be due to overall increased consumption of these foods in both the control and study area—not due to the better accessibility to the store in the study area. Also noteworthy is that in both studies, respondents who switched to the new store reported better self-reported psychological health.

Access to Affordable and Nutritious Food: Measuring and Understanding Food Deserts and Their Consequences. United States Department of Agriculture. Edited by Michele Ver Ploeg. https://www.ers.usda.gov/webdocs/publications/42711/12703_ap036d_1_.pdf?v=0

21. According to the text, what is related to fast-food access and cheap fast-food prices?
    a. Poorer diet
    b. Healthier diet
    c. Greater vegetable intake
    d. Poorer store access

22. Full-service restaurants show which of the following?
    a. A significant decrease in healthy diets
    b. Greater likelihood of fast-food restaurants in the area
    c. Poor store access in the vicinity
    d. Either no impact or positive impact on diet

23. What did the Glasgow study intend to measure?
   a. Changes in fruit and vegetable consumption
   b. Changes in shopping and food intake
   c. Preferences for Tesco versus other stores
   d. Fast food versus grocery store preferences

24. What other reason is given for the increase in fruit and vegetable consumption?
   a. Seasonal fruit availability
   b. A general increase in availability of fruits and vegetables
   c. A general increase in both areas (control and test) in consumption of fruits and vegetables
   d. A general decrease in availability of other food items

25. Based on the studies, how was shopping behavior impacted most significantly?
   a. In an increase in fruit and vegetable consumption
   b. In a decrease in restaurant business
   c. In an increase in whole grain consumption
   d. In customers switching to the new store

Questions 26–30 are based on the following passage:

Intensive care units worldwide cared for COVID-19 patients with life-threatening multiple organ dysfunction, in other words, sepsis. This trend provides a stark reminder that sepsis is likely to arise as a secondary confounder of any health security threat, whether in the coronavirus pandemic or another public health emergency.

Biomedical Advanced Research and Development Authority (BARDA) focuses on developing safe, effective medical countermeasures, such as vaccines, treatments, and diagnostics, against all potential health security threats the United States faces—chemical, biological, radiological, nuclear, pandemic, and emerging infectious diseases. Being fully prepared for those threats requires real solutions for sepsis.

In 2018, BARDA launched the DRIVe **Solving Sepsis** program to expand the range of tools to reduce the incidence, morbidity, mortality, and cost of treating sepsis, and to prepare for health security threats. Sepsis, a term still unfamiliar to many Americans, is a dysregulated response to infection leading to organ dysfunction.

Any infection can lead to sepsis—a bacterial infection, seasonal influenza, or SARS-CoV-2. Sepsis is far-reaching, affecting individuals of any age from neonates to the elderly, and can be life threatening. The **CDC reports** more than 270,000 lives are lost to sepsis each year in the U.S., among more than 1.7 million cases. In years with major public health events, like **COVID-19** that can lead to viral sepsis, those numbers can climb much higher.

Diagnostics for SARS-CoV-2 infection are critical to the response, but they don't tell the whole story. Roughly twenty percent of those infected become severely ill and require hospitalization. There's a need to identify COVID-19 patients who are on the path to sepsis. BARDA is exploring whether technologies that may predict sepsis can aid healthcare providers and COVID-19 patients in early identification of health deterioration before patients fall victim to sepsis. If providers could identify those patients sooner, both in hospitals and remotely in other care settings, those professionals could make informed, strategic decisions about the critical resources needed and better target early interventions to improve patient outcomes.

Pilot studies launched through the Rapidly Deployable Capabilities team, as part of the BARDA-COVID-19 medical countermeasure response, will evaluate utility of these technologies for COVID-19 patients and potentially against any future public health threat to our nation. Since the sepsis technologies are agnostic to the source of infection, validating their use builds real solutions to any emerging infectious disease outbreak.

Sciarretta, K. Ph.D., Pennini, M. Ph.D. "Why sepsis solutions can help Covid-19 patients." ASPR Blog. https://www.phe.gov/ASPRBlog/pages/BlogArticlePage.aspx?PostID=383

26. What is the relationship between COVID-19 and sepsis?
    a. Sepsis is a variable in any healthcare emergency, especially this one.
    b. Sepsis has been present in every hospitalized COVID-19 patient.
    c. There is no special relationship between the two.
    d. COVID-19 patients are more susceptible to sepsis.

27. According to the article, health security threats include pandemics, infectious diseases, and many other threats such as which of the following?
    a. Natural disasters
    b. Radiological threats
    c. Genetic diseases
    d. Childhood diseases

28. According to the text, what would be beneficial to the treatment of sepsis, especially as it relates to COVID-19?
    a. Better prediction technologies
    b. Better diagnostic technologies
    c. Better treatment technologies
    d. Better public knowledge of the risk

29. Based on contextual clues, what does the word *neonates*, found in the third paragraph, mean?
    a. Teens
    b. Children
    c. Newborns
    d. Adults

30. What are the overall implications of this research?
    a. COVID-19 patients will see immediate relief.
    b. Technologies developed now can help with future health threats.
    c. Companies developing these technologies will get government funding.
    d. Doctors can decrease the number of hospitalizations from sepsis.

Questions 31–35 are based on the following passage:

Approximately 15.5 million cancer survivors (people who received a diagnosis of cancer) were alive in the United States in 2016, and that number is expected to increase to nearly twenty million by 2026 because nearly half of cancer survivors live longer than ten years. Pain is one of the most common symptoms experienced among cancer patients and can be caused by cancer itself (e.g., tumor pressing on nerves, bones, or organs), surgery, treatment and treatment side effects (e.g., peripheral neuropathy, mouth sores, radiation mucositis), or other procedures and tests. Research suggests that pain occurs in approximately 20% to 50% of cancer survivors.

Clinical factors that may be associated with survivor pain are the stage (type and invasiveness) of the tumor, type of anticancer treatment received, time since completing treatment, comorbid conditions, and initial pain management. Effective methods are available to prevent and control pain during and after cancer treatment, including early recognition of pain symptoms, characterization and communication about pain type and severity, pharmacologic and nonpharmacologic pain control options, and patient education to ensure adequate pain and symptom management through all phases of cancer treatment and following treatment. Although pain can be controlled, approximately 30% of cancer survivors do not receive pain medication proportional to their pain intensity. Pain can negatively affect a cancer survivor's daily functional status and quality of life and can persist for years. Cancer survivors may experience psychological distress when pain persists after completion of cancer treatment, and untreated pain can lead to unnecessary hospital admissions. Identification of demographic, physiologic, and behavioral correlates of pain in cancer survivors can provide important information on specific subgroups most in need of pain management.

Cancer survivors can suffer from both short- and long-term pain; however, treatment-related pain typically diminishes over time. Approximately one year after diagnosis, more than 90% of patients observed in the American Cancer Society's Study of Cancer Survivors-I study reported short-term pain symptoms related to their cancer or its treatment; 6% of Australian adult cancer survivors reported pain intensity as "quite a bit/very much" five to six years post-diagnosis, and approximately 20% of childhood cancers survivors (with a mean survival time from diagnosis of 16.5 years) reported recent pain attributed to their previous cancer or cancer treatment. Pain may be more common among certain subpopulations, such as breast and lung cancer survivors, because of the cancer stage or surgery received. The prevalence and severity of chronic pain among cancer survivors has also been shown to vary by racial populations (e.g., pain severity reported among Black people is greater than among whites) and sex (e.g., occurrence of pain reported among females is greater than among males).

Pain can also be associated with other physiologic symptoms. Cancer survivors who report pain also report lack of sleep, fatigue, and mental health issues. Patients with comorbid conditions may have significantly greater physical functional pain and associated limitations and may be less likely to improve with standard pain management.

Despite all the evidence related to the prevalence of pain and comorbidities with pain and the availability of effective pain management strategies, cancer survivors may not be fully aware of the long-term prevalence of cancer-related pain that may persist after treatment completion. Thus, behaviors associated with pain need to be better characterized to help inform clinicians treating cancer survivor populations that could most benefit from additional education, resources, and strategies to manage cancer-related chronic pain. To this end, the purpose of our study was to use the most current national data to describe demographic and physiologic characteristics of cancer survivors who reported physical pain caused by cancer or cancer treatment. Informing patients and providers will aid in promoting collaborative relationships critical to providing optimal pain management.

Gallaway MS, Townsend JS, Shelby D, Puckett MC. Pain Among Cancer Survivors. Prev Chronic Dis 2020;17:190367. DOI: http://dx.doi.org/10.5888/pcd17.190367

31. Based on the text, why is the number of cancer survivors expected to increase in the U.S.?
    a. Because there are more cancer diagnoses
    b. Because we have identified new cancers
    c. Because nearly half of cancer survivors live ten years or more
    d. Because treatments have gotten better

32. Pain among cancer patients has several causes including the cancer itself, surgery, treatment, and which of the following?
    a. Metastasis
    b. Unknown causes
    c. Psychosomatic pain
    d. Treatment side effects

33. What is the subject of this passage?
    a. Cancer
    b. Cancer treatments
    c. Pain in cancer patients
    d. Impact of post-cancer care

34. What is one reason why the authors recommend educating patients and providers regarding physical pain after cancer?
    a. Many providers are unaware of the long-term pain.
    b. Many patients are unaware of the long-term pain.
    c. More research about the causes needs to be done.
    d. They do not recommend education in this passage.

35. Based on context, what does the word *comorbid/comorbidities* (paragraphs three and four) mean?
    a. The patient's cancer has metastasized.
    b. The patient's prognosis is not good.
    c. More than one medical condition is present.
    d. The current condition is related to a previous condition.

Questions 36–40 are based on the following passage:

Frequent mental distress and history of depression are common features among adults with arthritis in all states, with considerable variability across states. These findings are supported by previous studies that estimated anxiety and current depression among adults with and without arthritis. Similar to findings in an earlier report, states with high prevalence of frequent mental distress were geographically clustered, with eight of the ten states in the highest quintile in the Appalachian and southern states. This report also provides further evidence of poorer mental health status among lesbian/gay/bisexual adults with arthritis compared with their heterosexual peers with arthritis.

A meta-analysis of twelve studies reported that persons with chronic conditions (e.g., cancer, end stage renal disease, rheumatoid arthritis, and angina) who reported current depression were three times more likely to have a reduced adherence to medical treatment recommendations (i.e., medication adherence, diet, exercise, and follow-up appointments) than were those who did not report depression. In addition, among persons with rheumatoid arthritis, symptoms of anxiety and current depression are associated with reduced response to treatment and poorer quality of life. Therefore, actively engaging adults with arthritis in evidence-based programs such as the Arthritis Self-Management Program or the more widely available Chronic Disease Self-Management Program can help address the physical and psychological needs in tandem; these programs have shown to reduce depression and improve self-efficacy in adults with arthritis. The higher prevalence of poor mental health outcomes among specific subgroups in this study, including those who are lesbian/gay/bisexual, suggests that organizations serving these persons can be important partners for promoting and increasing access to these evidence-based interventions.

The Community Preventive Services Task Force (Community Guide) recommends active depression screening for all adults, use of trained depression care managers, and educating both patients and providers. Home-based supports, such as the use of community health workers, can support culturally appropriate care and further patient engagement in treatment goal-setting and self-management. Using community health workers can result in greater improvements in participant behavior and health outcomes (e.g., improvement in diabetes control) when compared with usual care.

Because of shortages in mental health care providers, multidisciplinary and population-based strategies that include both clinical and community approaches to addressing mental health service needs are needed for adults with arthritis. For example, allied professionals could use technology such as telemedicine in collaboration with mental health professionals, especially in rural areas and in the delivery of care in community-based settings. The Program to Encourage Active, Rewarding Lives (PEARLS), for example, is a national evidence-based program for late-life depression that brings high quality mental health care into community-based settings that reach vulnerable older adults including those with arthritis.

Price JD, Barbour KE, Liu Y, et al. State-Specific Prevalence and Characteristics of Frequent Mental Distress and History of Depression Diagnosis Among Adults with Arthritis — United States, 2017. MMWR Morb Mortal Wkly Rep 2020;68:1173–1178. DOI: http://dx.doi.org/10.15585/mmwr.mm685152a1

36. What is the main idea of this passage?
    a. More services need to be provided for mental health care for adults with arthritis.
    b. Individuals with medical conditions do not get the care they need.
    c. Telemedicine is an effective way of delivering care.
    d. Depression and anxiety impact a patient's self-management.

37. According to the authors, shortages in mental health care providers mean we need to do which of the following?
    a. Increase the number and type of available medications
    b. Include community and clinical approaches
    c. Teach self-care and management to patients
    d. Increase the number of providers

38. An analysis of twelve studies found that people who reported current depression were more likely to do which of the following?
    a. Not seek initial care
    b. Ignore medical advice and needs
    c. Be very responsible patients
    d. Seek care for all medical needs and concerns

39. Home-based support, such as community health workers, has several advantages including which of the following?
   a. Live-in home health aides
   b. Medication delivery
   c. Culturally appropriate care
   d. Improved patient outlook

40. Which of the following describes states with highest prevalence of mental distress?
   a. Those considered to be Appalachian and southern states
   b. Those that are home to major metropolitan areas
   c. Those with the largest populations
   d. Those that are geographically spread

Questions 41–45 are based on the following passage:

The total annual number of binge drinks consumed per U.S. adult who reported binge drinking increased significantly by 12% from 2011 to 2017, including among non-Hispanic white adults and those aged thirty-five years or older. These increases are consistent with other recent evidence of an approximately 30% increase in high-risk drinking, including binge-level alcohol consumption, particularly among middle-aged and older adults. Because binge drinking contributes a substantial proportion of all alcohol consumption in the United States, these increases also are consistent with an increase in per capita alcohol consumption (derived from sales and shipment data) in the United States, from 2.29 gallons in 2011 to 2.34 gallons in 2017.

The finding that the total number of binge drinks consumed per U.S. adult who reported binge drinking increased significantly among those with lower education and income levels is also consistent with a recent study that found the majority of persons reporting prescription opioid misuse are also adults who reported binge drinking, and that prescription opioid misuse tends to be most common among persons with lower household incomes. Socioeconomic disparities in the total number of binge drinks per adult who reported binge drinking also might have contributed to the lower life expectancies reported among persons with lower socioeconomic status in the United States.

The total annual number of binge drinks per adult who reported binge drinking did not change significantly in most states from 2011 to 2017, although it did increase significantly in nine states. At the state or local levels, examining the total number of binge drinks consumed by adults who reported binge drinking is a relatively new way to assess binge drinking and related harms. However, by combining public health surveillance data on the prevalence, frequency, and intensity of binge drinking, this measure provides a completer and more sensitive indicator of this health risk and facilitates assessment of sociodemographic and geographic disparities in binge drinking. This measure also might be useful for assessing health risks related to binge drinking (e.g., opioid misuse), and for planning and evaluating effective strategies for preventing binge drinking at the state and local levels.

Reducing binge drinking is essential to reducing excessive drinking. These findings highlight the need to reduce the total number of binge drinks per adult who reported binge drinking by reducing the prevalence, frequency, and intensity of binge drinking. Moreover, monitoring binge drinking prevalence alone, the most commonly used measure of binge drinking, portrays an incomplete picture of the problem of binge drinking, and might mask important sociodemographic and socioeconomic disparities in binge drinking behavior. Binge drinking is also strongly affected by the social context within which persons make their drinking decisions. For example, persons living in states with more restrictive alcohol policies are also less likely to binge drink and experience alcohol-attributable harms, including motor vehicle crash deaths, alcoholic liver cirrhosis, and alcohol-involved homicides and suicides than are persons living in states with less restrictive alcohol policies. Evidence-based prevention strategies to decrease excessive drinking that the Community Preventive Services Task Force recommends include increasing alcohol taxes, regulating the number and concentration of alcohol outlets in communities, and enforcing minimum legal drinking age laws.

Kanny D, Naimi TS, Liu Y, Brewer RD. Trends in Total Binge Drinks per Adult Who Reported Binge Drinking — United States, 2011–2017. MMWR Morb Mortal Wkly Rep 2020;69:30–34. https://www.cdc.gov/mmwr/volumes/69/wr/mm6902a2.htm

41. According to the text, which of the following is true of binge drinking?
    a. It has decreased in the last five years.
    b. The prevalence of it is lowest among non-Hispanic white adults.
    c. It is more frequent in states with restrictive policies.
    d. It contributes significantly to alcohol consumption in the U.S.

42. Which of the following is one of the factors that increased binge drinking behaviors?
    a. Easy access to alcohol
    b. A family history of alcoholism
    c. Lower education and income levels
    d. Adults who started drinking at a young age

43. In addition to prevalence, frequency, and intensity of binge drinking, what new measurement was used?
    a. Where the alcohol was consumed
    b. Type of alcohol consumed
    c. Age when binge drinking began
    d. Total number of drinks consumed

44. According to the research, individuals in states with more restrictive alcohol polices are less likely to:
    a. Suffer alcohol-induced homicides
    b. Be arrested for alcohol-induced crimes
    c. Start drinking at a young age
    d. Consume alcohol in general

45. What is the main idea of this passage?
    a. Binge drinking is a dangerous activity that more and more adults participate in.
    b. The reduction of binge drinking is vital to the decrease of excessive drinking in general.
    c. Binge drinking is responsible for a majority of alcohol consumption in the U.S.
    d. Socioeconomic factors are the biggest contributor to binge drinking.

Questions 46–50 are based on the following passage:

Mental health conditions are common complications in pregnancy and an underlying cause for approximately 9% of pregnancy-related deaths. Postpartum depression is associated with lower rates of breastfeeding initiation, poorer maternal and infant bonding, and increased likelihood of infants showing developmental delays. Left untreated, postpartum depression can adversely affect the mother's health and might cause sleeping, eating, and behavioral problems for the infant; when effectively treated and managed, both mother and child benefit.

Professional and clinical organizations have issued recommendations to address perinatal (e.g., during and after pregnancy) depression. The United States Preventive Services Task Force (USPSTF) recommends that all adults be screened for depression, including pregnant and postpartum women, and that clinicians provide or refer pregnant and postpartum women who are at increased risk for perinatal depression to counseling interventions. The American College of Obstetricians and Gynecologists (ACOG) recommends that obstetric care providers screen patients for depression and anxiety symptoms at least once during the perinatal period and also conduct a full assessment of mood and emotional well-being during the comprehensive postpartum visit. If a patient is screened for depression and anxiety during pregnancy, additional screening should also occur during the comprehensive postpartum visit. The American Academy of Pediatrics also recommends that routine screening for maternal postpartum depression be integrated into well-child visits.

USPSTF has noted that identifying women with increased risk for perinatal depression and determining ways to improve the delivery of interventions represent evidence gaps that warrant high-priority efforts. Women with postpartum depressive symptoms (PDS) are at increased risk for postpartum depression and require further evaluation to determine whether they meet the criteria for having a depressive disorder. To inform these evidence gaps, CDC used data from the Pregnancy Risk Assessment Monitoring System (PRAMS) to examine the prevalence of self-reported PDS and whether a health care provider inquired about depression during prenatal and postpartum health care visits.

Bauman BL, Ko JY, Cox S, et al. Vital Signs: Postpartum Depressive Symptoms and Provider Discussions About Perinatal Depression — United States, 2018. MMWR Morb Mortal Wkly Rep 2020;69:575–581. https://www.cdc.gov/mmwr/volumes/69/wr/mm6919a2.htm

46. Which of these is a supporting detail from the passage?
    a. Pregnant women must be screened at every visit for depression.
    b. Women who experience depression while pregnant will likely be fine postpartum.
    c. Postpartum depression impacts mother and child bonding.
    d. Depression screening can stop once the infant is six months old.

47. Which of the following is a consequence infants experience due to postpartum depression?
    a. Learning disabilities
    b. Poor motor skills
    c. Delayed language skills
    d. Behavioral problems

48. What is the main idea of the passage?
    a. Intervention is necessary for depression and anxiety in pregnant and postpartum women.
    b. Screening for depression and anxiety in pregnant and postpartum women should be prioritized.
    c. Postpartum depression is more serious than depression that occurs during the pregnancy itself.
    d. Mental health concerns contribute to deaths in pregnant women.

49. In addition to pregnant women, who else should be screened for depression?
   a. Parents or parents-to-be
   b. Children
   c. Fathers
   d. All adults

50. Based on the context of the passage, what is the meaning of *intervention* (paragraphs two and three)?
   a. An agreement between the patient and the doctor
   b. An action taken to make an improvement or change
   c. An involuntary hospitalization
   d. A new medical device used to treat a condition

Questions 51–55 are based on the following passage:

Agriculture workers had a higher prevalence than construction workers of almost all sun-protection behaviors by both industry and occupation. Prevalence of regularly seeking shade was similar across all groups (about 25%), which was lower than the national estimate of regular shade use of 37%. Although regular sunscreen use did not differ among groups by industry or occupation, all groups had a lower prevalence of use compared with the national estimate of 32%. All groups reported a higher prevalence of regular use of protective clothing compared with national estimates of use of wide-brimmed hats (14%), long-sleeved shirts (12%), and long pants or other clothing to ankles (28%). The prevalence of protective clothing use among workers in agricultural occupations was more than twice as high for use of wide-brimmed hats (29%) and long clothing (65%) and three times as high for use of long-sleeved shirts (43%) compared with national estimates.

Higher prevalence of protective clothing use may be due to injury prevention employer policies (e.g., reducing chemical exposures). However, some policies, such as requirements for construction workers to wear hard hats, could be contributing to construction workers' lower prevalence of wide-brimmed hat use compared with agricultural workers. Although wide-brim attachments for hard hats are commercially available, they are not widely used because they tend to reduce the worker's vision of overhead hazards. Neck shades that can be worn or attached to the back of hard hats, caps, or visors may be a better alternative. Among all groups, Agriculture Workers (ACWs) were more likely to use caps or visors than wide-brimmed hats, and more than half reported using them. Sunburn was common and reported by about a third of workers studied, a prevalence similar to national estimates. Sunburn during adulthood significantly increases a person's chances of developing melanoma. Although data on the anatomic sites (e.g., neck, ears) of sunburn were not available for our study, melanomas can occur on parts of the body that are not protected by caps. A combined behavioral approach (e.g., sunscreen, headwear) is important for adequate skin cancer prevention at these anatomic sites.

Results of our study indicate a need for sun-safety and skin cancer prevention efforts that target ACWs and their employers. Interventions that are highly effective at increasing sun-protection behaviors and decreasing sunburns among outdoor workers include educational, behavioral, and environmental approaches in addition to workplace policies that support sun-protection practices. For example, one study found that although exposure to an educational intervention did not increase construction workers' sun-safety knowledge, it did significantly increase sun-safety behavior, such as increasing shade use when working outdoors. Although companies may include use of personal sun-protection practices in their institutional policies, few supply sun-protection equipment, and most existing policies do not explicitly state an intent to protect employees from excessive sun exposure. However, additional studies of local government organizations found that interventions that include personal contacts and theory-based training increased the likelihood of adoption of formal sun-protection policies and that adoption of sun-safety practices is not constrained by government budget or size. More research analyzing local, state, and national sun-safety policies is needed to understand their effects in both government and nongovernment organizations.

Ragan KR, Buchanan Lunsford N, Thomas CC, Tai EW, Sussell A, Holman DM. Skin Cancer Prevention Behaviors Among Agricultural and Construction Workers in the United States, 2015. Prev Chronic Dis 2019;16:180446. https://www.ncbi.nlm.nih.gov/pmc/articles/PMC6395080/

51. Why aren't wide brimmed attachments for hard hats widely used?
    a. They are not widely available.
    b. They are cost prohibitive.
    c. They decrease visibility.
    d. They aren't as sturdy as the hard hat itself.

52. What is the subject of this passage?
    a. Protective clothing in farm workers
    b. Sun protection in agricultural and construction workers
    c. Safety for workers on construction sites
    d. The availability of protective clothing in the workplace

53. Based on the passage, educational intervention was successful in what way?
    a. It increased sun-safety behavior.
    b. It increased sun-safety knowledge.
    c. It increased the availability of protective clothing.
    d. It increased the use of sunscreen.

54. All groups reported a higher usage of which type of sun protection?
    a. Sunscreen
    b. Long-sleeve shirts
    c. Neck shades
    d. Sunglasses

55. What increased the chances of a business including sun-protection policies in the workplace?
    a. An instance of melanoma in one of the workers
    b. The presence of literature regarding sun protection and skin cancer
    c. Government regulation
    d. Personal contacts and theory-based training

Vocabulary

1. Select the meaning of the underlined word in the following sentence:

    The medication required that John abstain from alcohol.

    a. reduce
    b. stay away from
    c. limit
    d. indulge

2. What is the best synonym for the word fatigue?
    a. corpulent
    b. energized
    c. exhausted
    d. confused

3. Select the meaning of the underlined word in the following sentence:

    To allow the injury to heal, it was recommended that Roger cease high impact exercise.

    a. complete
    b. reconsider
    c. limit
    d. end

4. Bright lights may _____ migraine headaches.
    a. alleviate
    b. dilute
    c. exacerbate
    d. suppress

5. What is the best definition for the word pathogenic?
    a. disease-causing microorganism
    b. branch of medicine that studies diseases
    c. study of mental health
    d. reproduction without fertilization

6. Select the meaning of the underlined word in the following sentence:

    The doctor recommended a medication with a sublingual route of administration.

    a. inside the cheek
    b. via the rectum
    c. below the skin
    d. below the tongue

7. Despite the patient suffering strep throat more than once a year for several years, the doctors opted to leave her tonsils _____.
    a. internal
    b. intact
    c. expelled
    d. external

8. What is the best definition of the word etiology?
    a. the root of a medical condition
    b. the basis for a diagnosis
    c. the justification for a prescription
    d. a collection of symptoms

9. When the patient received the wrong medication, everyone knew who would be held _____.
    a. cursory
    b. reliable
    c. accountable
    d. labile

10. The patient didn't get out of bed today and reported feeling quite _____.
    a. convulsive
    b. insidious
    c. therapeutic
    d. lethargic

11. What is the best definition for the word hematologic?
    a. causing bruising
    b. related to blood
    c. swelling in the brain
    d. related to the skin

12. What is the best definition for otic?
    a. related to the eye
    b. over-the-counter drug
    c. related to the ear
    d. elevated risk

13. The cyclist believed his helmet meant he would be impervious to a head injury.
    a. unaffected
    b. vulnerable
    c. susceptible
    d. predisposed

14. What is the best definition for triage?
    a. nursing specialty
    b. patient prioritization
    c. patient adversity
    d. doctor training

15. Joseph was told to report any _____ effects from his medication.
   a. ambivalent
   b. contingent
   c. latent
   d. adverse

16. What is the best definition for <u>kinetic</u>?
   a. with feeling
   b. in motion
   c. potentially
   d. related to

17. The area around the incision was red and _____.
   a. insidious
   b. occluded
   c. inflamed
   d. precipitous

18. What is the best definition of <u>ubiquitous</u>?
   a. everywhere
   b. permanent
   c. translucent
   d. forgotten

19. Select the meaning of the underlined word in the following sentence:

   The doctor warned that certain foods would likely <u>exacerbate</u> the patient's stomach issues.

   a. alleviate
   b. not impact
   c. cure
   d. worsen

20. What is the best definition for <u>aegis</u>?
   a. unsupported
   b. unsupervised
   c. under protection
   d. oversimplified

21. The doctors ran multiple tests, and, after a brief conference, they were able to offer the patient a complete _____.
   a. transmission
   b. diagnosis
   c. syndrome
   d. chronology

22. What is the best definition for <u>virulent</u>?
    a. powerful
    b. manly
    c. toxic
    d. violent

23. What is the best definition for <u>manifestation</u>?
    a. indication of an illness
    b. disappearance of illness
    c. worsening of symptoms
    d. overwhelming symptoms

24. Select the meaning of the underlined word in the following sentence:

    Despite greater public awareness, genetic <u>syndromes</u> are actually quite rare.

    a. marked by defect
    b. health characteristics
    c. suppression of symptoms
    d. collection of symptoms

25. Which of the listed words is most appropriate in the following sentence?

    Even non-athletes need to be concerned with _____ levels, especially in the heat.

    a. hydration
    b. transdermal
    c. supplement
    d. therapeutic

26. What is the best definition for <u>latent</u>?
    a. lazy
    b. dormant
    c. sleepy
    d. relaxed

27. Which of the listed words is most appropriate in the following sentence?

    After striking the windshield, Michael was treated for a _____ that stretched from his chin to his scalp.

    a. trauma
    b. labile
    c. laceration
    d. mastication

28. What is the best definition for <u>flexion</u>?
    a. need for flexibility
    b. the action of bending
    c. adaptability
    d. the action of straightening

29. Select the meaning of the underlined word in the following sentence:

In addition to the prescriptions provided, the doctor recommended she take additional <u>supplements</u> to help iron absorption.

a. extra doses of given medication
b. primary medication
c. vitamin or mineral that limits efficacy
d. substance to complement or strengthen

30. Which of the listed words is most appropriate in the following sentence?

In order to evaluate the success of the surgery, the physical therapist focused on _____ movements.

a. internal
b. transdermal
c. cardiac
d. lateral

31. What is the best definition for <u>renal</u>?
a. kidney-related
b. heart-related
c. eye-related
d. vein-related

32. In order to complete the eye exam, the doctor needed to _____ her pupils.
a. distal
b. dilute
c. dilate
d. constrict

33. Select the meaning of the underlined word in the following sentence:

His discharge from the hospital was <u>contingent</u> upon his ability to walk on his own.

a. not reliant
b. dependent
c. limited by
d. scheduled

34. What is the best definition for <u>predispose</u>?
a. unwilling
b. abrupt
c. thrown away
d. lean towards

35. What is the best definition for <u>vascular</u>?
    a. airways and lungs
    b. system that carries blood
    c. related to central nervous system
    d. related to the brain

36. Which of the listed words is most appropriate in the following sentence?

Due to an inner ear infection, Raymond could not maintain _____.

    a. empathy
    b. status
    c. equilibrium
    d. depth

37. Select the meaning of the underlined word in the following sentence:

Prior to further treatment, it was necessary to <u>depress</u> the fever.

    a. reduce
    b. cure
    c. treat
    d. ignore

38. What is the best definition for <u>transdermal</u>?
    a. removal of skin
    b. below the skin
    c. over the scalp
    d. through the skin

39. What is the best definition for <u>cursory</u>?
    a. leading to seizures
    b. worsening condition
    c. hastily and poorly completed
    d. required action

40. Select the meaning of the underlined word in the following sentence:

Despite the complicated and serious diagnosis, the doctor kept his explanation <u>concise</u>.

    a. serious
    b. brief
    c. detailed
    d. superficial

41. Delivering bad news to patients and their families requires _____.
    a. empathy
    b. rationale
    c. exposure
    d. trauma

42. What is the best definition for <u>contraindication</u>?
    a. to do with concern
    b. clear course of action
    c. consistent and preferred
    d. action to avoid

43. What is the best definition for <u>audible</u>?
    a. able to be heard
    b. indiscernible
    c. unrecognizable
    d. intolerable volume

44. Select the meaning of the underlined word in the following sentence.

    One of the most important instructions for this prescription is ensuring the <u>consistency</u> of administration.

    a. durability
    b. timeliness
    c. uniformity
    d. erraticism

45. Though this medication is effective at low dosages, higher dosages may be _____.
    a. flushed
    b. toxic
    c. discrete
    d. compensatory

46. What is the best definition for <u>concave</u>?
    a. completed in secrecy
    b. hollow or depressed appearance
    c. with caution
    d. working conjointly

47. Select the meaning of the underlined word in the following sentence.

    "Any decision to discharge this patient is <u>precipitous</u>," argued the doctor.

    a. dangerous
    b. ambitious
    c. circumspect
    d. rushed

48. In triage, they decide which patients should be made a <u>priority</u>.
    a. most important
    b. concern
    c. more comfortable
    d. least important

49. Though several doctors initially disagreed, once he explained his _____, the treatment plan was approved.
    a. pathology
    b. incidence
    c. rationale
    d. exposure

50. What is the best definition for <u>chronology</u>?
    a. timeline of events
    b. study of time
    c. related to digestion
    d. a measured boundary

51. What is the best definition for <u>symmetrical</u>?
    a. having two sides
    b. uniform across an axis
    c. uneven sides
    d. disproportionate

52. What is the best definition for <u>labile</u>?
    a. inflexible
    b. reliable
    c. concerned
    d. subject to change

53. Select the meaning of the underlined word in the following sentence.

    The warning label clearly stated "do not <u>ingest</u>" because it could be toxic.

    a. touch
    b. consume
    c. inhale
    d. spill

54. The doctor's _____ concern was the patient's lack of appetite.
    a. compensatory
    b. bilateral
    c. primary
    d. impending

55. What is the best definition for <u>assent</u>?
    a. agreement
    b. rising
    c. denial
    d. possession

Grammar

1. Which of the words in the following sentence is the verb?

   We heard a lot of gossip about the new hospital wing.

   a. heard
   b. new
   c. gossip
   d. wing

2. Which of the words in the following sentence is/are the verb/s?

   The staff complained about the poorly written shift notes.

   a. shift
   b. complained, written
   c. about, poorly
   d. staff, notes

3. Identify the antecedent and pronoun in the following sentence:

   Brandy woke up early in the morning to call her friend about the test that day.

   a. Brandy, her
   b. Brandy, friend
   c. woke, day
   d. early, morning

4. Identify the missing word to complete the following sentence:

   I always _____ track of time.

   a. loose
   b. lost
   c. lose
   d. losing

5. Identify the dependent clause in the following sentence:

   If not for scheduling, Nancy would struggle to complete all her duties throughout the day.

   a. throughout the day
   b. if not for scheduling
   c. all her duties
   d. Nancy would struggle to complete

6. What conjunction works best for the sentence that follows?

The nurse does not have much time _____ he always makes time to check vitals.

a. for
b. nor
c. and
d. but

7. Which of the following is considered an independent clause?
   a. because we had Monday off
   b. which was opened in 1965
   c. sufficient medicine for the day
   d. we could not clear the floor

8. Identify the preposition in the following sentence:

The extra blankets are stored under the bed.

a. extra
b. under
c. stored
d. the

9. Which sentence uses correct capitalization?
   a. The Robert Wood Johnson Hospital ER entrance is found off Easton Avenue.
   b. The Robert Wood Johnson hospital ER entrance is found off Easton avenue.
   c. The Robert Wood Johnson Hospital ER entrance is found off Easton avenue.
   d. The Robert Wood Johnson hospital ER entrance is found off easton avenue.

10. Which one of the following sentences is grammatically correct?
    a. To many patients ignore post-care instructions, witch means we will see them again.
    b. To many patience ignore post-care instructions, which means we will see them again.
    c. Too many patients ignore post-care instructions, which means we will see them again.
    d. Too many patience ignore post-care instructions, which means we will see them again.

11. Choose the correct pronoun combination that completes the sentence that follows:

_____ and _____ carpool to work together.

a. Her, me
b. She, me
c. She, I
d. Her, I

12. Choose the best conjunction that completes the following sentence:

Please come to the staff meeting _____ you can hear all the updates.

a. so
b. because
c. while
d. until

13. Identify the adverb in the following sentence:

The new lobby has been decorated beautifully.

a. new
b. beautifully
c. decorated
d. has

14. Select the best phrase to complete the sentence that follows:

Last week, I _____ my pediatrics rotation.

a. will have completed
b. had completed
c. completed
d. have completed

15. Which word from the following sentence is considered the antecedent?

Dr. Smith shifted all her appointments until next week, so she could handle emergencies.

a. her
b. she
c. until
d. Dr. Smith

16. Fill in the sentence with missing words that best complete the idea.

I don't know _____ charts these are, but _____ not in the correct spot.

a. whose, their
b. who's, there
c. who's, they're
d. whose, they're

17. Which one of the following sentences uses the correct punctuation?
a. "Have you seen the patient in 121 yet"? the nurse asked.
b. "Have you seen the patient in 121 yet" the nurse asked?
c. "Have you seen the patient in 121 yet?" the nurse asked.
d. "Have you seen the patient in 121 yet," the nurse asked.

18. Select the best word to complete the sentence:

Bellevue Hospital is the _____ hospital in NYC.

a. biggest
b. bigger
c. most big
d. most biggest

19. Identify the indirect object in the following sentence:

In the operating room, the nurse handed the scalpel to the doctor.

a. the nurse
b. the scalpel
c. the doctor
d. operating room

20. Which of the following sentences is grammatically correct?
a. The paramedics rushed from the ambulance and right by past the triage area.
b. The paramedics had rushed from the ambulance and right by passed the triage area.
c. The paramedics have rushed from the ambulance and write past by the triage area.
d. The paramedics rushed from the ambulance and passed right by the triage area.

21. Which pronoun best replaces the word in bold?

After all, it was **Norman's** PCP who did all the complaining.

a. them
b. his
c. our
d. him

22. Identify the dependent clause in the following sentence:

Because of some bad winter storms, car accidents were on the rise and the emergency room was busy.

a. on the rise
b. the emergency room was busy
c. car accidents were
d. Because of some bad winter storms

23. Identify the verb and the verb phrase in the following sentence:

Though they were new employees, the nurses were expected to complete patient charts by the end of their shift.

a. were expected
b. were, were expected
c. were, were expected, by the end
d. were

24. Which of the listed words in the following sentence is a noun?

Nutrition is an important part of healthcare.

a. healthcare
b. important
c. an
d. of

25. Identify the adjective in the following sentence:

Despite the importance of nutrition, many patients reported the hospital food was awful.

a. despite
b. importance
c. awful
d. patients

26. Which word best completes the sentence?

Either one of the nurses _____ asked to communicate with the family.

a. was
b. were
c. is
d. had

27. Identify the subject of the following sentence:

Mary's sister sat in the waiting room while she got her x-rays.

a. x-rays
b. waiting room
c. she
d. Mary's sister

28. Which of the following sentences is correct?
a. All the nurses were expected to except the new floor rules.
b. All the nurses were expected to accept the new floor rules.
c. All the nurses were excepted to accept the new floor rules.
d. All the nurses were accepted to except the new floor rules.

29. Fill in the blank with the best word:

The patient reported that the new medication had no adverse_____.

a. affect
b. effect
c. affection
d. affliction

30. Identify the articles used in the sentence that follows:

Neither the nurse nor the doctor had an answer for the patient.

a. the, the, an, the
b. the, an
c. an
d. the, the, an

31. Which word best completes the following sentence?

If I were _____, I would avoid surgery.

a. me
b. she
c. her
d. their

32. Select the word that best completes the following sentence:

The stitches are healing _____.

a. good
b. beautiful
c. bad
d. beautifully

33. Which word in the following sentence is used INCORRECTLY?

Despite the earlier concerns, there are more operating rooms available then we expected.

a. concerns
b. despite
c. there
d. then

34. Identify the independent clause in the following sentence:

Though the call button was fine, the patient reported it was broken.

a. the call button was fine
b. Though the call button was fine
c. the patient reported it was broken.
d. it was broken.

35. Which of the listed words in the following sentence is a noun?

The new hospital wing was dedicated at a beautiful ceremony with many community leaders in attendance.

a. ceremony
b. beautiful
c. dedicated
d. many

36. Which word in the following sentence is a conjunction?

Though the storm had passed, accident victims continued to stream in, and the ER was soon overwhelmed.

a. and
b. though
c. to
d. soon

37. Select the best combination of pronouns to complete the sentence:

The nurse knows _____ time to administer the medications, but first _____ visits the supply closet to lock _____ door.

a. its, he, it's
b. it's, he, its
c. it's, his, it's
d. it's, it, it's

38. Select the best punctuation:

Veteran nurses suggest bringing the following items on your first day ____ stethoscope (if needed) and holster, scrubs, lunch, and at least 4 pens.

a. ,
b. .
c. ;
d. :

39. Which word in the following sentence is the complete verb (past tense)?

Despite the staff expanding, nurses were still expected to work extra hours.

a. expanding
b. were
c. were expected
d. work

40. Select the phrase that best completes the following sentence:

By next year, I _____ completed my nursing school entrance exams.

a. will
b. have
c. will have
d. had

41. Identify the preposition in the following sentence:

When the patients get cold, extra blankets are stored in the closet.

a. in
b. the closet
c. when
d. extra

42. Select the best word to complete the sentence:

Patients' families often feel a level of _____ when their family member is in surgery.

a. uncertainity
b. uncertainty
c. uncertainness
d. uncertain

43. Which of the following sentences has the correct subject-verb agreement?
a. The doctors were conducting a pre-surgery discussion.
b. No one in the ER were being admitted.
c. One of the nurses talk to the family.
d. Several of the patients experience problems post-surgery.

44. Which sentence is punctuated correctly?
a. Despite the fact that we were short-staffed we managed to cover all shifts.
b. Despite the fact that we were short-staffed; we managed to cover all shifts.
c. Despite the fact that we were short-staffed: we managed to cover all shifts.
d. Despite the fact that we were short-staffed, we managed to cover all shifts.

45. Which of the following sentences is grammatically correct?
a. The doctor's decision did not effect any of the patients.
b. The nurses' station was not affected by the power outage.
c. Administration didn't understand how their decision would effect the staff.
d. The researchers did not yet understand the affect of the drug.

46. Select the best word to complete the following sentence:

    There were _____ patients in the waiting room than I expected.

    a. few
    b. fewer
    c. less
    d. least

47. Which of the following sentences is grammatically correct?
    a. The patient complained that her blood was drawn too rough.
    b. The patient complained that her blood was drawn rougher.
    c. The patient complained that her blood was drawn too roughly.
    d. The patient complained that her blood draw was too roughly.

48. Find the dependent clause in the sentence that follows:

    The nurse was recognized for her quick thinking and skilled work, especially when she was assisting on surgeries.

    a. The nurse was recognized for her quick thinking
    b. when she was assisting on surgeries
    c. quick thinking and skilled work
    d. especially when she was assisting on surgeries.

49. In the following sentence, which words should be capitalized?

    st. andrew's hospital is located at 2516 e. lansing road in bellingham, washington.

    a. St. Andrew's Hospital, E. Lansing Road, Bellingham, Washington
    b. St. Andrew's, E. Lansing, Bellingham, Washington
    c. St. Andrew's Hospital, Lansing Road, Washington
    d. St. Andrew's Hospital, E. Lansing, Bellingham

50. Which word in the following sentence is an adjective?

    The hospital required that all nurses in pediatrics wear green scrubs.

    a. all
    b. green
    c. pediatrics
    d. scrubs

51. Which one of the following sentences is clearest?
    a. The nurse gave the medication to the patient that was the wrong dose.
    b. The medication that was the wrong dose was given to the patient by the nurse.
    c. The patient was given medication by the nurse that was the wrong dose.
    d. The nurse gave the wrong dose of medication to the patient.

52. Fill in the blanks with the correct words.

The nurse's review stated that she performed _____. Her handling of patient care was _____.

   a. magnificent, magnificent
   b. magnificent, magnificently
   c. magnificently, magnificent
   d. magnificently, magnificently

53. Identify the adjective in the following sentence:

While the training session seemed to last forever, and time moved slowly, it was actually pretty short.

   a. slowly
   b. short
   c. pretty
   d. forever

54. Identify the dependent clause in the following sentence:

The student, who was studying for the HESI exam, set aside 2 hours daily to practice.

   a. who was studying for the HESI exam
   b. Set aside 2 hours daily
   c. The student
   d. who was studying

55. Select the best words to fill in the blanks:

Pharmaceutical representatives _____ often _____ at the hospital.

   a. be, seen
   b. are, saw
   c. can, be seen
   d. can, be saw

Biology

1. Which of the following choices does NOT represent a primary property of life in biology?
   a. Energy processing
   b. Homeostasis
   c. Adaptation
   d. Photosynthesis

2. Based on the properties of life in biology, which of the following choices regarding a virus is correct?
   a. A virus is a living organism because it can reproduce independently and pass traits onto its offspring.
   b. A virus is a nonliving organism because it can't reproduce, adapt, and metabolize.
   c. A virus is neither a living nor a nonliving organism because it doesn't fulfill all characteristics of life.
   d. A virus is neither a living nor a nonliving organism because it can reproduce and adapt, but not metabolize.

3. Which of the given choices describes the correct biology theme discussed in the following passage?

   In a process called photosynthesis, plants acquire light energy from the sun to produce their food. In an ecosystem, plants are a source of energy or food for organisms. When an animal consumes plants and dies, decomposers such as fungi and insects break down the animals' organic matter.

   a. Stability and homeostasis of organisms
   b. Reproduction and inheritance of organisms
   c. Matter, energy, and organization of organisms
   d. Interactions with and between organisms

4. Which of the following statements regarding natural selection is INCORRECT?
   a. Increased competition will occur between populations since they produce more offspring than needed.
   b. Individuals that acquire traits that are less suited to an environment are more likely to survive.
   c. Mutations result in increased diversity and allow for natural selection to occur.
   d. Natural selection is common descent with modification.

5. Which of the following lists the correct order of some of the taxonomic categories from most to least inclusive regarding the number of organisms?
   a. Species, genus, family, order
   b. Kingdom, phylum, class, order
   c. Genus, domain, family, order
   d. Kingdom, phylum, domain, order

6. The ears of a jackrabbit help maintain constant body temperature by allowing blood to flow through the blood vessels within the rabbit's ear. Heat exchange occurs between the ear and the surrounding air. What is this type of property and the processes associated with the rabbit called?
   a. Regulation
   b. Response
   c. Evolutionary adaptation
   d. Energy processing

7. What is the primary difference between the three main kingdoms of domain Eukarya?
   a. All of the kingdoms are not multicellular.
   b. Two of the kingdoms are photosynthetic, and one kingdom ingests food.
   c. Two of the kingdoms do not contain specialized tissues, and one photosynthesizes food.
   d. One of the kingdoms consumes food by absorption, photosynthesis, and ingestion.

8. A scientific model is best described as which of the following?
   a. An informed statement that can be tested.

b. A system that allows one to control specific variables and environmental conditions.

c. A speculative idea that is made up of many concepts that join a well-supported hypothesis.

d. A model statement that describes or predicts phenomena based on repeated observations.

9. In one experiment, scientists hypothesized that the coat coloration of a mouse, within a specific environment, protected them from predation. To test the hypothesis, scientists placed white and brown mice in both a beach and inland habitat. The results are summarized in the graph and figures below.

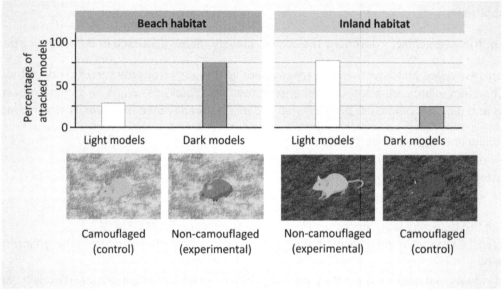

Based on the provided graphs, the hypothesis is:

a. True since the dark models were attacked more in the beach habitat and the light models were attacked more in the inland habitat.

b. False since the light models were attacked less in the beach habitat and the dark models were attacked less in the inland habitat.

c. True since the light models were attacked less in the inland habitat and the dark models were attacked less in the beach habitat.

d. False since the dark models were attacked more in the beach habitat and the light models were attacked more in the inland habitat.

10. Which of the following polar covalent bonds, indicated by a dash, will NOT form a hydrogen bond?

a. $H - F$

b. $H - Cl$

c. $H - NH_2$

d. $H - OCH_2CH_3$

11. Which of the following molecules is nonpolar?

a. NH_4^+

b. CO

c. NH_3

d. He

12. Hydrogen bonding is responsible for all EXCEPT which of the following?
    a. Providing structure and support to cellular molecules
    b. Keeping two strands of DNA connected
    c. Preserving the shape of proteins
    d. Absorbing heat by incurring a large temperature change

13. Which choice below reflects a valid property of water that is due to hydrogen bonding?
    a. Water is primarily a solute.
    b. Water has a low heat capacity.
    c. Water has a high heat of fusion.
    d. Water is an insulator.

14. As water evaporates from the leaves in plants, water obtained from the soil can move upward from the roots to leaves of the plants. This process is due to which of the following?
    a. Capillary action
    b. Cohesion
    c. Adhesion
    d. Surface tension

15. The figure below shows several possible solvation structures of water and ammonia. Which structure below represents the proper orientation of water towards ammonia?

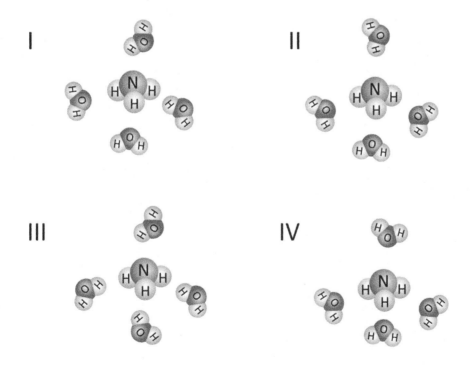

a. I
b. II
c. III
d. IV

16. Which of the following biostructures corresponds to a component of a nucleic acid?

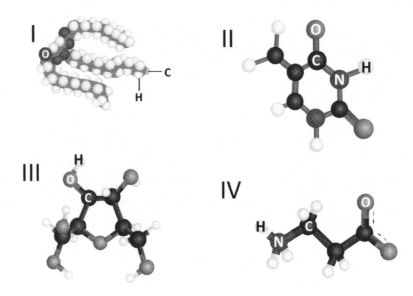

a. I
b. II
c. III
d. IV

17. Which of the following functional groups is NOT typically found in carbohydrates?
a. $R - OH$
b. $R - (CO) - O^-$
c. $R - (CO) - R$
d. $R - (CO) - H$

18. Which of the following molecular structures represent a pair of isomers?

I.

II.

III.

IV.

a. I
b. II
c. III
d. IV

19. What will be produced when a fat molecule undergoes a hydrolysis reaction?
   a. Glycerol and three fatty acids
   b. Glycerol and three molecules of unsaturated fat
   c. One molecule of saturated fat
   d. Fat molecules do not undergo hydrolysis reactions since they are not polymers.

20. If six monosaccharides undergo a condensation reaction, how many molecules of water and the disaccharide are each produced?
   a. 12
   b. 9
   c. 6
   d. 3

21. Which of the following biomolecules is an example of a pentose?

I.

$^{6'}CH_2OH$

II.

CH_2OH

III.

CH_2OH CH_2OH

IV.

$HOCH_2$ OH

a. I
b. II
c. III
d. IV

22. Which answer choice is the best reason why polysaccharides cannot pass through a cell membrane?
a. Polysaccharides are long chains that can entangle since they contain many monosaccharide subunits.
b. Polysaccharides are water-soluble and contain polar hydroxyl groups.
c. Polysaccharides are partially water-soluble and contain nonpolar hydroxyl groups.
d. Polysaccharides contain many kinked hydrocarbon chains, making it difficult to pass through.

23. Which level of protein structure is associated with the formation of an alpha and beta-sheet within a polypeptide?
a. Quaternary
b. Primary
c. Tertiary
d. Secondary

24. The figure below represents the backbone structure of one strand of DNA. The two strands within DNA are held together by hydrogen bonds. How many hydrogen bonds form between the nucleoside guanine and cytosine?

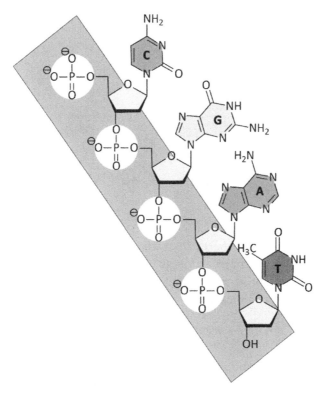

a. Three
b. Two
c. One
d. Four

25. Which of the following organelles within a cell has a catabolic function?
    a. Cytoskeleton
    b. Microbodies
    c. Ribosomes
    d. Centrioles

26. Consider the two structures below of stearic acid and glucose. Which of the following statements about the two structures shown is correct?

Stearic acid $C_{18}H_{36}O_2$

Glucose $C_6H_{12}O_6$

a. Glucose contains more chemical energy than stearic acid.
b. Stearic acid contains more mechanical energy than glucose.
c. Glucose contains more potential energy than stearic acid.
d. Stearic acid contains more chemical energy than glucose.

27. Which of the following statements is accurate regarding the role of enzymes in a metabolic pathway?
   a. The product-to-reactant activation barrier is lowered, allowing the reaction to proceed.
   b. The reactant-to-product activation barrier is lowered, which speeds up the chemical reaction.
   c. Enzymes decrease the Gibbs free energy of the products.
   d. The entropy of the reaction increases.

28. Choose the pair of terms below that correctly completes the following sentence:

   For a _____ reaction to occur, the Gibbs free energy of the system must be _____.

   a. spontaneous; negative
   b. nonspontaneous; positive
   c. spontaneous; positive
   d. nonspontaneous; negative

29. Which of the following statements correctly describes a metabolic pathway in terms of free energy?
   a. Anabolic pathways are exergonic since they require energy to build larger molecules.
   b. Catabolic pathways are exergonic since they release energy as they break down larger molecules.
   c. Anabolic pathways are endergonic since they release energy as they break down larger molecules.
   d. Catabolic pathways are endergonic since they require energy to break down larger molecules.

30. Which of the following statements best explains how ATP, through energy coupling, is used to perform work within the cell?

a. ATP condensation undergoes an exergonic reaction ($\Delta G_{ATP} = -7.3\ kcal/mol$) to drive an endergonic reaction, $\Delta G_{endergonic} = +3.4\ kcal/mol$.

b. ATP condensation undergoes an endergonic reaction ($\Delta G_{ATP} = 7.3\ kcal/mol$) to drive an exergonic reaction, $\Delta G_{exergonic} = +3.4\ kcal/mol$.

c. ATP hydrolysis undergoes an endergonic reaction ($\Delta G_{ATP} = 7.3\ kcal/mol$) to drive an exergonic reaction, $\Delta G_{exergonic} = +3.4\ kcal/mol$.

d. ATP hydrolysis undergoes an exergonic reaction ($\Delta G_{ATP} = -7.3\ kcal/mol$) to drive an endergonic reaction, $\Delta G_{endergonic} = +3.4\ kcal/mol$.

Chemistry

1. The reaction of sodium hydroxide (NaOH) and sulfuric acid (H_2SO_4) in an aqueous solution is considered what type of reaction?

$$2NaOH\ (aq) + H_2SO_4(aq) \rightarrow Na_2SO_4(aq) + 2H_2O(l)$$

a. Single displacement
b. Double displacement
c. Decomposition
d. Synthesis

2. Copper-based pigments such as copper (II) hydroxide were frequently used in ancient art. However, over time, some of the copper-based pigment that was added onto a canvas formed black spots due to the formation of copper oxide. What type of reaction is shown below?

$$Cu(OH)_2(s) \rightarrow CuO\ (s) + H_2O(g)$$

a. Single displacement
b. Double displacement
c. Decomposition
d. Synthesis

3. For the following reaction, what are the correct coefficients that give a balanced chemical equation?

$$\_\ NaI + \_Pb(C_2H_3O_2)_2 \rightarrow \_NaC_2H_3O_2 + \_PbI_2$$

a. 1, 2, 1, 2
b. 2, 1, 2, 1
c. 2, 2, 2, 1
d. 2, 1, 2, 2

4. Which of the following mixtures is not homogenous?
a. Unsweetened coffee
b. Lemonade with pulp
c. Filtered apple juice
d. Purified water

5. Which of the following mixtures is not heterogeneous?
    a. Coffee and sucrose
    b. A soup containing potatoes, carrots, and green beans
    c. Buttermilk
    d. Tomato juice

6. Suppose a solution is made by mixing 2 tablespoons of sugar and 1 cup of coffee. Table sugar is best described as what type of substance?
    a. The solute
    b. The solvent
    c. A heterogeneous mixture
    d. A homogenous mixture

7. Which of the following species represents the precipitate in the unbalanced reaction equation below?

$$\_\,NaI + \_Pb(C_2H_3O_2)_2 \rightarrow \_\,NaC_2H_3O_2 + \_PbI_2$$

    a. Sodium iodide, NaI
    b. Lead (II) acetate, $Pb(C_2H_3O_2)_2$
    c. Sodium acetate, $NaC_2H_3O_2$
    d. Lead (II) iodide, PbI_2

8. For the acid-base reaction below, which of the following species acts as a Brønsted-Lowry base?

$$HNO_3(aq) + H_2O\ (l)\ \rightarrow NO_3^-(aq) + H_3O^+(aq)$$

    a. HNO_3
    b. H_2O
    c. NO_3^-
    d. H_3O^+

9. In the phase diagram below, what phase change is indicated by the arrow?

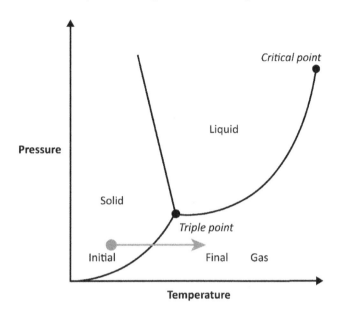

a. Sublimation
b. Freezing
c. Condensation
d. Deposition

10. Which of the following processes is an example of a chemical change?
   a. Adding liquid sugar to 1 cup of coffee
   b. Condensation of water vapor onto a cold-water bottle
   c. Heating a marshmallow until it browns
   d. The evaporation of isopropyl alcohol from someone's fingernail

11. Which of the following substances is a molecular compound?
   a. CO
   b. Cl_2
   c. Ar
   d. S_7

12. Which of the following equations does not follow the law of conservation of mass?
   a. $2C_6H_6 + 15O_2 \rightarrow 12CO_2 + 6H_2O$

   b. $2C_2H_6 + 7O_2 \rightarrow 4CO_2 + 4H_2O$

   c. $CH_4 + 2O_2 \rightarrow CO_2 + 2H_2O$

   d. $2C_8H_{18} + 25O_2 \rightarrow 16CO_2 + 18H_2O$

13. In one experiment, a balloon is filled with 300 mL of air at room temperature. The balloon is then placed over an ice bath. The volume of the balloon decreases to 50 mL. According to kinetic molecular theory, which of the following reasons explains the decrease in volume?

    a. At higher temperatures, the gas molecules inside the balloon move slower and collide with the surface with a smaller force.

    b. At lower temperatures, the gas molecules inside the balloon move faster and collide with the surface with a smaller force.

    c. At lower temperatures, the gas molecules inside the balloon move slower and collide with the surface with a greater force.

    d. At lower temperatures, the gas molecules inside the balloon move slower and collide with the surface with a smaller force.

14. In one experiment, a balloon at room temperature with a volume of 300 mL is placed in a hot-water bath at 373°K and the volume of the balloon expands. Which of the following gas laws can be used to describe the observed change?

    a. Boyle's law

    b. Charles's law

    c. Avogadro's law

    d. Gay-Lussac's law

15. Consider the redox reaction below.

$$Cu(NO_3)_2(aq) + Zn(s) \rightarrow Cu(s) + Zn(NO_3)_2(aq)$$

Which of the following half-reactions is correct?

    a. $Cu^{2+} \rightarrow Cu(s) + 2e^-$; oxidation half

    b. $Zn\ (s)\ +\ 2e^- \rightarrow Zn^{2+}$; oxidation half

    c. $Cu^{2+} +\ 2e^- \rightarrow Cu(s)$; reduction half

    d. $Zn\ (s) \rightarrow Zn^{2+} +\ 2e^-$; reduction half

16. What is the oxidization number of oxygen in lithium oxide (Li_2O)?

    a. −2

    b. −1

    c. 0

    d. +1

17. Which of the following reactants is oxidized in the reaction below?

$$Zn\ (s) + 2AgC_3H_3O_2(aq) \rightarrow 2Ag(s) + Zn(C_3H_3O_2)_2(aq)$$

    a. Silver acetate, $AgC_3H_3O_2$

    b. Zinc acetate, $Zn(C_3H_3O_2)_2$

    c. Zinc, Zn

    d. Silver, Ag

18. Which of the following reactants is the reducing agent in the reaction below?

$$Zn(s) + 2AgC_3H_3O_2(aq) \rightarrow 2Ag(s) + Zn(C_3H_3O_2)_2(aq)$$

a. Silver nitrate, $AgC_3H_3O_2$ (aq)
b. Zinc nitrate, $Zn(C_3H_3O_2)_2$ (aq)
c. Zinc, Zn (s)
d. Silver, Ag (s)

19. Which of the following species acts as an Arrhenius acid in the acid-base reaction below?

$$HClO_4 \ (aq) + KOH \ (aq) \ \rightarrow KClO_4 \ (aq) + H_2O \ (l)$$

a. $HClO_4$
b. KOH
c. $KClO_4$
d. H_2O

20. Which of the following pair of species acts as a Lewis acid for the acid-base reaction below?

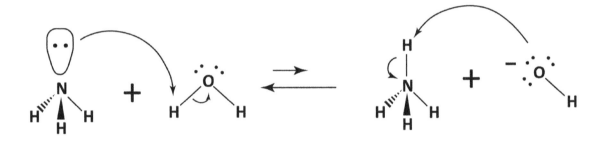

a. NH_3 and OH^-
b. H_2O and NH_4^+
c. NH_3 and H_2O
d. NH_3 and NH_4^+

21. Which of the following is considered the weakest base?
a. Barium hydroxide, $Ba(OH)_2$
b. Ammonia, $NH3$
c. Water, H_2O
d. Sodium hydroxide, $NaOH$

22. Which of the following covalent bonds is the least polar?
a. C-Br
b. C-Cl
c. C-F
d. C-I

23. A bond dipole is often drawn around a molecule to show the direction or distribution of charge. The arrow tip corresponds to the side of a molecule that is partially negative or an area that has greater electron density. The cross end (+) is the partially positive region or the area that has less electron density. In the diagram below, which of the following covalent bonds indicates the correct direction of the dipole?

a. H-O
b. C-N
c. F-C
d. H-Cl

24. Which of the following lists the elements cesium (Cs), potassium (K), gallium (Ga), and carbon (C) in order of increasing electronegativity?
    a. C < K < Ga < Cs
    b. C < Ga < K < Cs
    c. Cs < K < Ga < C
    d. Cs < Ga < K < C

25. Which of the following lists the elements neon (Ne), arsenic (As), chlorine (Cl), and tin (Sn) in order of decreasing atomic radius?
    a. Ne > Cl > As > Sn
    b. As > Sn > Cl > Ne
    c. Sn > As > Cl > Ne
    d. Ne > Sn > As > Cl

26. Which of the following lists the elements carbon (C), calcium (Ca), and germanium (Ge) in order of decreasing ionization energy?
    a. Ge > Ca > C
    b. Ca > Ge > C
    c. C > Ge > Ca
    d. C > Ca > Ge

27. Which of the following elements is associated with the most negative electron affinity?
    a. Al
    b. Tl
    c. Po
    d. S

28. Which of the following anions has a total number of 18 electrons?
   a. Mg^{2+}
   b. Br^-
   c. P^{3-}
   d. I^-

29. Which of the following elements is likely to form an anion with a 2– charge?
   a. I, iodine
   b. Mg, magnesium
   c. F, fluorine
   d. O, oxygen

30. How many protons does silver, Ag, have?
   a. 79
   b. 107
   c. 47
   d. 197

Anatomy and Physiology

1. Which kind of anatomy is devoted to the study of body structures that are visible to the naked eye, such as the liver?
   a. Systemic
   b. Microscopic
   c. Gross
   d. Developmental

2. Which structure contains two or more types of tissues that work together to carry out a specific body function?
   a. Complex cell
   b. Organ complex
   c. Tissue complex
   d. Organ

3. Which organ system responds to external stimuli, for example, pressure, in the fastest manner?
   a. Lymphatic system
   b. Circulatory system
   c. Nervous system
   d. Endocrine system

4. Which sequence is arranged from the most complex level of organization to the simplest?

   1. Cells 2. Tissues 3. Atoms 4. Organs 5. Molecules 6. Endocrine system

   a. 6-4-2-1-5-3
   b. 4-6-2-5-1-3
   c. 3-5-1-2-4-6
   d. 3-1-5-2-6-4

5. Which statement correctly explains why the anatomical position is beneficial?
   a. The anatomical position provides a common point of reference for the position of a body and helps convey anatomical relationships.
   b. The anatomical position is the most comfortable position for hospital patients, according to studies carried out at Johns Hopkins University.
   c. The anatomical position allows people to have greater blood circulation.
   d. The anatomical position is a simple diagram and is convenient for displaying on a textbook since more of the body is visible; for example, there is a greater surface area.

6. Suppose you are asked to check a person's heart rate at the carpal pulse point. Which part of the body would be the least challenging or most convenient place to check a pulse without an instrument?
   a. The posterior side of the knee
   b. The dorsal side of the wrist
   c. At the distal end of the arm
   d. At the ventral side of the wrist

7. The abdominal cavity houses the _____ and is found _____ to the vertebral cavity.
   a. kidneys and spleen, superficial
   b. Intestines and liver, posterior
   c. Liver and stomach, anterior
   d. Stomach and intestines, posterior

8. From an anatomist's viewpoint, the urinary bladder belongs to which of the following quadrants?
   a. The hypogastric region
   b. The right upper quadrant
   c. The umbilical region
   d. The left lower quadrant

9. Consider the following micrograph of epithelial kidney tubules. Which label does NOT correspond to an epithelial cell?

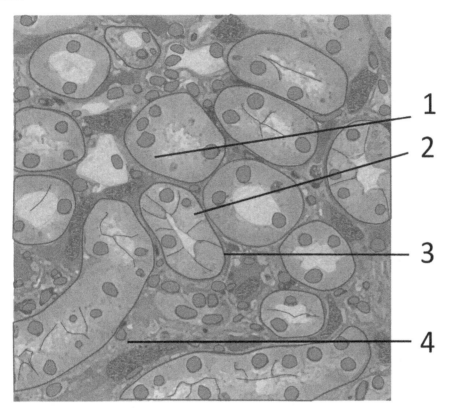

a. 3
b. 4
c. 1
d. 2

10. Which class of epithelial cells produces a lubricating mucus in the digestive tract of the stomach?
    a. Simple cuboidal epithelium
    b. Simple ciliated columnar epithelium
    c. Pseudostratified ciliated columnar (with goblet cells)
    d. Simple columnar epithelium

11. Which statement about the physical characteristics of muscle tissues is NOT true?
    a. Smooth and cardiac muscle are both involuntary and have fibers with a single nucleus.
    b. Cardiac and skeletal muscle can involuntarily undergo rapid contractions.
    c. Smooth and skeletal muscle is made up of fibers that contain a single nucleus and can undergo involuntary contractions.
    d. Cardiac muscle is different from smooth muscle in that cardiac muscle contains striations, while smooth muscle has no striations.

12. Which type of connective tissue acts as a sponge and soaks up fluid?
    a. Osseous connective tissue
    b. Dense fibrous tissue
    c. Hyaline cartilage
    d. Lamina propria

13. Which statement about the nervous system is NOT true?
    a. Neurons and nerves are found throughout the body, not just in the spinal cord and brain.
    b. Neurons protect the supporting cells in the structures of the nervous system.
    c. Cells from the nervous tissue than respond to stimuli are called neurons.
    d. Neurons cannot undergo mitosis and are formed prenatally.

14. Which type of tissue keeps the muscle tissue from separating from the bone during muscle contraction?
    a. Hyaline cartilage
    b. Osteocyte
    c. Adipose tissue
    d. Tendons

15. Which function is NOT a function of the integumentary system?
    a. Temperature regulation
    b. Synthesis of vitamins D and C
    c. Inhibition of bacteria
    d. Prevention of body dehydration

16. Dust mites feed off a layer of skin called the _____, which rubs or flakes off slowly over time.
    a. Stratum basale
    b. Epidermis
    c. Stratum spinosum
    d. Stratum corneum

17. Which statement about the structural layers of the epidermis is true?
    a. Blood vessels are located in the stratum lucidum.
    b. Cornified cells are found in the stratum spinosum.
    c. Keratin is found in the stratum granulosum.
    d. Keratin is found in the stratum basale.

18. Consider the following photomicrograph of the dermis and epidermis. In which region of the epidermis does mitosis occur continuously?

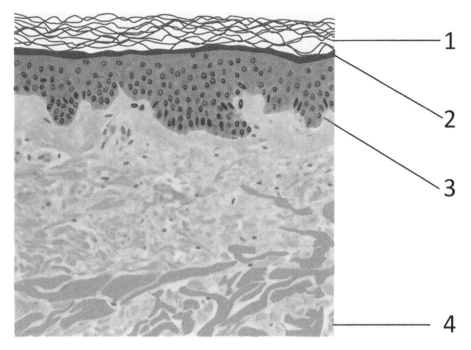

a. 2
b. 4
c. 1
d. 3

19. Suppose that the dermal papillae of the foot were "even" and lacked peg-like projections. Which statement represents a likely outcome?
   a. The epidermis will have less blood circulation, resulting in reduced friction between the flow.
   b. The epidermis of the foot will be smoother, thereby decreasing the friction between the feet and the floor.
   c. The dermis will have more capillary loops, causing the epidermis to have more ridges, thereby decreasing the friction between the feet and the floor.
   d. The dermis will have more capillary loops, causing the epidermis to have fewer ridges, thereby increasing the friction between feet and the floor.

20. As a person ages, the number of collagen and elastic fibers decreases in what specific region of the integumentary system?
   a. Reticular layer
   b. Stratum granulosum
   c. Hypodermis
   d. Stratum spinosum

21. Which of the following bone indentations would be classified as a smooth projection?
    a. The facet
    b. The groove
    c. The notch
    d. The condyle

22. Consider the following photomicrograph of an osteon. Where is a passageway that connects neighboring osteocytes?

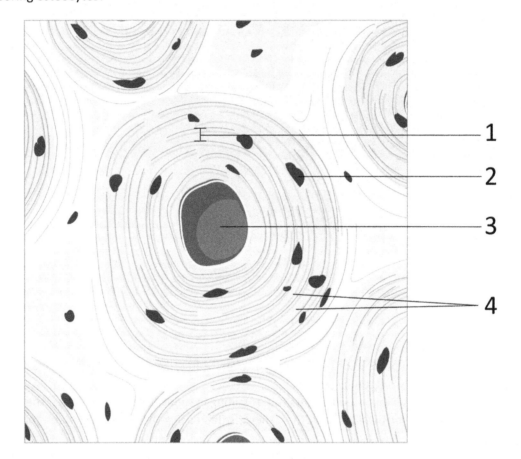

    a. 3
    b. 4
    c. 2
    d. 1

23. Which muscle type has the most elaborate connective tissue wrappings?
    a. Smooth muscle
    b. Cardiac muscle
    c. Skeletal muscle
    d. Non-striated muscle

24. Listed in order from outer to inner, the layers of connective tissue in the skeletal muscle are:
    a. Endomysium, perimysium, and epimysium
    b. Epimysium, perimysium, and endomysium
    c. Perimysium, endomysium, and epimysium
    d. Endomysium, epimysium, and perimysium

25. Which structure is not visible during muscle contraction?
    a. I band
    b. H zone
    c. Z disc
    d. A band

26. Which type of contractile protein is located in the Z disc?
    a. Actin
    b. Myosin
    c. Sarcomere
    d. Titin

27. Which statement is an example of integration in the nervous system?
    a. You see a red light.
    b. You interpret a red light to mean "stop."
    c. You feel cold.
    d. You press on the brake pedal.

28. Which effector organ is part of the somatic nervous system?
    a. A blood vessel
    b. A gland
    c. The cardiac muscle
    d. The skeletal muscle

29. Which figure best represents a microglial cell?

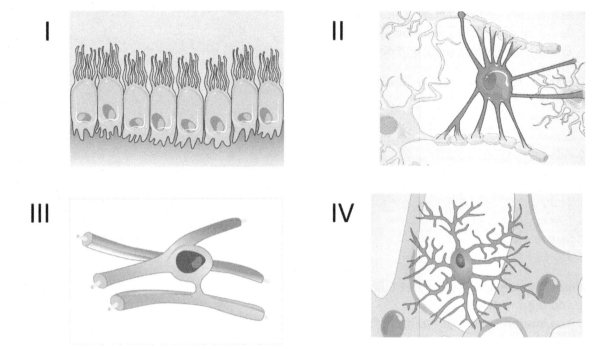

I

II

III

IV

a. 2
b. 1
c. 4
d. 3

30. Alzheimer's disease (AD) is a type of dementia that has no known treatment to slow the progression of the disease. Drug therapy has been directed toward restoring the normal function of the neurons and microglia or the cells that mediate inflammation. A recent study has shown that specific housekeeping cells of the brain have promoted the decline of neuron function in AD. Researchers discovered that these cells produced a specific toxic protein called Beta-amyloid, which was observed to accumulate in the brain of Alzheimer patients. Because the chemical environment of the brain was unregulated, the accumulation of the toxic protein led to chronic inflammation responses in the brain, thereby exacerbating AD. Which type of supporting cell does the passage likely describe?
    a. Glial cell
    b. Astrocyte
    c. Schwann cell
    d. Neuron

Answer Explanations #1

Mathematics

1. A: When adding a positive integer to a negative integer, subtract the smaller absolute value from the larger absolute value. The sign of the answer is the sign of the number with the larger absolute value. The answer is:

$$1000 - |-55| = 1000 - 55 = 945$$

2. C: When adding two negative integers, add the absolute value of both integers. The sign of the answer is always negative. The result is:

$$-(|-675| + |-246|) = -(675 + 246) = -921$$

3. B: When adding a positive integer to a negative integer, subtract the smaller absolute value from the larger absolute value. The sign of the answer is the sign of the number with the larger absolute value. The answer is:

$$-(|-431| - 99) = -(431 - 99) = -332$$

4. A: The decimals can be added vertically, after aligning the decimals and adding a 0 to 0.555 to make it 0.5550. The sum is 0.5785.

5. A: The decimals can be added vertically, after aligning the decimals and adding a 0 to 11.9 to make it 11.91. The sum is 17.31.

6. B: The decimals can be added vertically, after aligning the decimals. The whole number 18 can be rewritten as 18.000. Therefore, the sum is 18.567.

7. C: In order to add two whole numbers, add the numbers vertically, aligning the place values. First add the ones column, then the tens column, etc. The sum is 53,641.

8. D: Both addends rounded to the nearest ten-thousand place become 90,000. The estimated sum is:
$$90,000 + 90,000 = 180,000$$

9. B: 2.567 rounded to the nearest ones place becomes 3, and 4.109 rounded to the nearest ones place becomes 4. The estimated sum is $3 + 4 = 7$.

10. D: A square has four equal sides. Therefore, each side has a length of 16 meters. The perimeter of the square is the sum of the four side lengths. Therefore, the perimeter is $16 + 16 + 16 + 16 = 64$ meters.

11. B: A rectangle has two sets of equal sides. Therefore, there are two sides of length 12.6 cm and two sides of length 6.4 cm. The perimeter of the rectangle is the sum of the four side lengths. Therefore, the perimeter is:

$$12.6 + 6.4 + 12.6 + 6.4 = 38 \text{ cm}$$

12. C: Because the perimeter of a square is equal to the sum of four of its side lengths, four times the length of a side is equal to 48. It is true that $4 \times 12 = 48$. Therefore, the square has a side of length 12 cm.

13. B: In order to subtract whole numbers, align them vertically by place values. First subtract the ones column, then the tens column, etc. If the number on top is smaller, borrow from the next place value to the left. The difference is 43,881.

14. C: When subtracting integers, add the opposite. Therefore, the problem becomes:

$$-65 + (-4) = -(|-65| + |-4|) = -(65 + 4) = -69$$

15. A: When subtracting integers, add the opposite. Therefore, the problem becomes:

$$98 + 45 = 143$$

16. A: When subtracting integers, add the opposite. Therefore, the problem becomes:

$$-45 + 17 = -(|-45| - 17) = -(45 - 17) = -28$$

17. D: When subtracting decimals, align the decimals vertically. Add a 0 to the end of 14.87 to make it 14.870. Then, subtract each place value, starting with the thousandths place. The difference is 50.944.

18. B: When subtracting decimals, align the decimals vertically. Add two zeros to 4.2 to make it 4.200. Then, subtract each place value, starting with the thousandths place, borrowing if necessary. The difference is 4.146.

19. C: When subtracting decimals, align the decimals vertically. Add four zeros to 65 to make it 65.0000. Then, subtract each place value, starting with the ten-thousandths place, borrowing if necessary. The difference is 64.0001.

20. B: 95,198 rounded to the nearest ten-thousand place is 100,000. 54,987 rounded to the nearest ten-thousand place is 50,000. The estimated difference is $100,000 - 50,000 = 50,000$.

21. A: 56,999 rounded to the nearest thousand place is 57,000. 45,298 rounded to the nearest thousand place is 45,000. The estimated difference is:

$$57,000 - 45,000 = 22,000$$

22. B: 43.892 rounded to the nearest ones place is 44. 35.789 rounded to the nearest ones place is 36. The estimated difference is $44 - 36 = 8$.

23. D: In order to find how much taller the tower is, find the difference:

$$1,543 - 1,345 = 198 \text{ feet}$$

24. C: The building in New York City is $456 + 876 = 1,332$ feet tall.

25. B: Multiplication can be computed vertically. First, multiply $413 \times 4 = 1,652$. Then, multiply $413 \times 30 = 12,390$. Their sum is:

$$1,652 + 12,390 = 14,042$$

26. C: Because there are so many zeros, multiply $9 \times 7 = 63$, and then add 6 zeros. The result is 63,000,000.

27. C: A square has four equal sides. Therefore, its length and width are the same. The area of a rectangle is length times width, so the area of this square is $17 \times 17 = 289$ square feet.

28. B: The area of a rectangle is length times width. Therefore, the area of this rectangle is $8 \times 3 = 24$ square yards.

29. C: The product of two negative integers is positive: $34 \times 4 = 136$.

30. B: The product of a negative and a positive integer is negative. $45 \times 2 = 90$, and therefore, the product is -90.

31. C: The product of an even number of negative numbers is positive. Therefore, the product is:

$$3 \times 5 \times 6 \times 2 = 15 \times 6 \times 2 = 90 \times 2 = 180$$

32. A: Zero multiplied by any number is always 0.

33. B: When two decimals are multiplied, the decimal points can be ignored at first. Multiply as if there were no decimals. Then, a decimal point is placed in the result. The number of decimal places in the final answer is equal to the sum of the number of decimal points in both original factors. The number of decimal places is counted by starting at the digit in the far right and then moving to the left. $75 \times 7 = 525$. The original problem had 2 decimals. Therefore, move the decimals two places to the left, resulting in 5.25.

34. C: When multiplying decimals, ignore the decimal points, and multiply as if there were no decimals. Then, a decimal point is placed in the result. The number of decimal places in the final answer is equal to the sum of the number of decimal points in both original factors. The number of decimal places is counted by starting at the digit in the far right and moving to the left.

$$7,567 \times 241 = 1,823,647$$

The original problem had 5 decimals. Therefore, move the decimals five places to the left, resulting in 18.23647.

35. B: 5.879 rounded to the nearest ones place is 6. 19.203 rounded to the nearest ones place is 19. The estimated product is $6 \times 19 = 114$.

36. A: Both factors rounded to the nearest ten-thousands place are 20,000. The estimated product is:
$$20,000 \times 20,000 = 400,000,000$$

37. C: To find the area of a rectangle, multiply its length times its width. $8.75 \times 12 = 105$. The units are square feet.

38. C: $\frac{n}{n} = 1$ for any nonzero value n.

39. A: $\frac{0}{n} = 0$ for any nonzero value n.

40. D: In order to multiply and simplify fractions, multiply the numerators together and then multiply the denominators together. Finally, write the result in lowest terms.

$$\frac{25}{2} \times \frac{7}{6} = \frac{25 \times 7}{2 \times 6} = \frac{175}{12}$$

The answer is in lowest terms because the numerator and denominator do not share a common factor.

41. B: The numerator and denominator share a common factor of 2. Dividing this value out from each results in:

$$\frac{16}{10} = \frac{16 \div 2}{10 \div 2} = \frac{8}{5}$$

42. A: In order to multiply and simplify fractions, multiply the numerators together, multiply the denominators together, and then write the result in lowest terms

$$\frac{18}{5} \times \frac{10}{2} = \frac{180}{10}$$

The numerator and denominator share a common factor of 10. Dividing this value out from each results in:

$$\frac{180}{10} = \frac{180 \div 10}{10 \div 10} = \frac{18}{1} = 18$$

43. C: In order to multiply and simplify fractions, multiply the numerators together, multiply the denominators together, and then write the resulting fraction in lowest terms. 65 can be written as $\frac{65}{1}$.

$$65 \times \frac{2}{5} = \frac{65}{1} \times \frac{2}{5} = \frac{130}{5} = 130 \div 5 = 26$$

44. B: The area of a triangle is equal to

$$\frac{1}{2} \times b \times h,$$

where b is the base and h is the height. For this triangle, the base is 14m and the height is 10m. Therefore, the area is:

$$\frac{1}{2} \times 14 \times 10 = 70 \text{ square meters}$$

45. D: The reciprocal of a fraction is found by interchanging the numerator and the denominator. Therefore, flip the fraction to obtain $\frac{5}{14}$.

46. B: To divide by a fraction, multiply times that fraction's reciprocal.

$$\frac{15}{4} \div 5 = \frac{15}{4} \times \frac{1}{5} = \frac{15}{20} = \frac{3}{4}.$$

47. A: To divide by a fraction, multiply times its reciprocal.

$$\frac{5}{8} \div \frac{15}{4} = \frac{5}{8} \times \frac{4}{15} = \frac{20}{120} = \frac{1}{6}$$

48. C: The LCD is the LCM of the two denominators 6 and 15. The LCM is the smallest number that is a multiple of both numbers, which is 30.

49. B: Because the denominators are the same, add the numerators and keep the denominator as 17.

$$\frac{15}{17} + \frac{2}{17} = \frac{17}{17} = 1$$

50. D: To add fractions with different denominators, the fractions must be expressed as equivalent fractions with the LCD as their denominators. The LCD is 24, which is the LCM of 8 and 6. Therefore,

$$\frac{1}{8} + \frac{1}{6} = \frac{1}{8} \times \frac{3}{3} + \frac{1}{6} \times \frac{4}{4} = \frac{3}{24} + \frac{4}{24} = \frac{7}{24}$$

51. A: To subtract fractions with different denominators, the fractions must be expressed as equivalent fractions with the LCD as their denominators. The LCD is 75, which is the LCM of 25 and 15.

$$\frac{18}{25} - \frac{14}{15} = \frac{18}{25} \times \frac{3}{3} - \frac{14}{15} \times \frac{5}{5} = \frac{54}{75} - \frac{70}{75} = -\frac{16}{75}$$

52. C: To convert to an improper fraction, multiply the whole number times the denominator and add the numerator to that product. Then, write that result over the original denominator.

$$6\frac{1}{7} = \frac{6 \times 7 + 1}{7} = \frac{43}{7}$$

53. D: To convert to a mixed number, divide. The quotient is the whole number, and the remainder is the numerator. Therefore,

$$\frac{76}{9} = 76 \div 9 = 8R4 = 8\frac{4}{9}$$

54. B: To multiply a mixed number, convert it to an improper fraction first.

$$4\frac{1}{3} \times \frac{3}{8} = \frac{13}{3} \times \frac{3}{8} = \frac{39}{24}$$

55. C: To add mixed numbers, convert them to improper fractions first.

$$4\frac{1}{2} + 1\frac{1}{12} = \frac{9}{2} + \frac{13}{12}$$

Because these fractions have different denominators, they must be expressed as equivalent fractions with the LCD, 12, as their denominators.

$$\frac{9}{2} + \frac{13}{12} = \frac{9}{2} \times \frac{6}{6} + \frac{13}{12} = \frac{54}{12} + \frac{13}{12} = \frac{67}{12}$$

Reading Comprehension

1. B: The very first sentence of the text reads *"Fluoride use is one of the main factors responsible for the decline in prevalence and severity of dental caries and cavities (tooth decay) in the United States."* While Choice *A* and Choice *C* are discussed, there is no noted correlation in the passage.

2. D: The text notes, *"However, ingestion of too much fluoride while teeth are developing can result in visibly detectable changes in enamel structure such as discoloration and pitting (dental fluorosis)."* There is no mention in the passage or evidence to suggest that Choice *A* or Choice *B* is correct. While the passage notes that children under the age of two do not need fluoride, there is more to toothpaste than just fluoride. Therefore, Choice *C* is not the best option.

3. A: The researchers analyzed answers from caregivers regarding toothbrushing in the children the caregivers supervise. While the data was gathered regarding both children and adolescents, neither was consulted, nor was anyone observed first-hand, so Choices *B*, *C,* and *D* are incorrect.

4. B: Contextual clues, such as the contrasting information regarding a developed swallowing reflex, informs the reader that a child over a certain age can control whether to swallow or not, thereby avoiding unintentional ingestion. Choices *A*, *C*, and *D* do not correctly define *inadvertent*.

5. C: The passage notes that brushing should begin at the appearance of a child's first tooth, usually around six months of age, not eight to ten months as Choice *C* suggests. Choices *A*, *B*, and *D* were details included in the passage.

6. C: According to the text, "If nothing else is done in the United States beyond what is being done now, simulated growth trajectories that model today's children show that over half (59% of today's toddlers and 57% of children aged two to nineteen) will have obesity at age thirty-five." Choices *A*, *B*, and *D* are not true.

7. B: There are three primary challenges identified. The first challenge is genetic and biological components. While Choice *A*, fast food, might contribute, it is not one of the factors mentioned in this study. Though they might be part of a larger discussion on the issue, neither Choice *C* nor Choice *D* are discussed in this specific article either.

8. D: Increasing walkability in a neighborhood might have a positive impact on a child's nutrition and physical activity habits. In fact, the passage notes that traffic, Choice *B*, is a problem. Choice *A* and Choice *C* are not mentioned.

9. D: According to the passage, "Obesity is defined as a body mass index (a person's weight in kilograms divided by the square of height in meters) of 30.0 or higher." Choices *A*, *B*, and *C* do not correctly define obesity.

10. A: The first half of the sentence suggests a reason why we might see different obesity rates in specific children. The second half of the sentence, by way of comparison, suggests that racial and ethnic demographics have an impact as well. Therefore, *disparities* mean differences, and they allow researchers to account for why some children have a greater chance of becoming obese (parental, racial, ethnic differences). Choices *B*, *C*, and *D* are not appropriate substitutions for the word *disparities*.

11. B: According to the text, "The approximate two-thirds decline in adult cigarette smoking prevalence that has occurred since 1965 represents a major public health success." This indicates that Choice *B*, decreased, is correct and Choices *A*, *C*, and *D* are incorrect.

12. A: According to the text, "The prevalence of adult e-cigarette use increased from 2.8% in 2017 to 3.2% in 2018" and "the prevalence of e-cigarette usage among persons aged eighteen to twenty-four years is higher than that among other adult age groups, and e-cigarette use in this age group increased from 5.2% in 2017 to 7.6% in 2018." This quote confirms that Choice *A* is correct, and Choices *B*, *C*, and *D* are incorrect.

13. B: As the focus of the text (it's overall message) is reducing smoking among both adults and adolescents, one can infer from the references to smoking cessation programs that *cessation* means to end or quit. *Cessation* does not mean beginning, continuing, or assisting, rendering Choices *A*, *C*, and *D* inaccurate.

14. C: When considering the limitations, the report does not comment on the age group of the individuals reporting their smoking status. It lists the following as limitations: "responses were self-reported and were not validated by biochemical testing [...] NHIS is limited to the noninstitutionalized U.S. civilian population [...] the NHIS Sample Adult response rate of 53.1% might have resulted in nonresponse bias." Therefore, Choices *A*, *B*, and *D* are all included in the study limitations.

15. D: The article notes that proven measures include implementation of tobacco price increases, comprehensive smoke-free policies, high-impact antitobacco media campaigns, barrier-free cessation coverage, and comprehensive state tobacco control programs, combined with regulation of the manufacturing, marketing, and distribution of all tobacco products. The list does not include raising the smoking age (Choice *A*), banning e-cigarettes (Choice *B*), or punitive fines (Choice *C*), though all have been part of the larger discussion.

16. A: According to the text, skipping meals is a great way to reduce calories, but there is an impact on the quality of one's diet when doing so. While Choice *B* is true, it doesn't reflect the full idea and misses part of the conclusion. Choice *C* is brought up as a potential impact of skipping meals but is not the focus of the text. Choice *D* doesn't reflect the research nor is that advice mentioned in the text.

17. D: Researchers did gather "detailed information about the types (Choice *A*) and amounts (Choice *B*) of food consumed in two non-consecutive days, as well as when each food was eaten (Choice *C*) and if it was part of a meal or a snack," but no information was gathered on where meals or snacks were eaten.

18. B: The article establishes early on that skipping meals may be a beneficial strategy to losing weight and/or preventing weight gain and "influencing dietary quality," so the initial premise is that it is okay to skip a meal. Therefore, Choice *D* is not correct. Then, the final conclusion in the article is that skipping *dinner* reduces caloric intake the most with the least impact on diet quality. Therefore, Choice *B* is the correct answer, and skipping lunch, Choice *A*, or breakfast, Choice *C*, is not correct.

19. C: There is not any discussion of the weight loss impact of skipping a meal. All of the other data is presented in the text selection, making Choices *A*, *B*, and *D* incorrect.

20. C: Dietary elements such as refined grains, sodium, and empty calories are part of the HEI along with food groups. Choice *A* and Choice *B* are both food groups and already covered. Choice *D* is not mentioned as part of the HEI.

21. A: According to the text, "In general, these studies have found that greater availability of fast-food restaurants and lower prices of fast-food restaurant items are related to poorer diet." Choices *B*, *C*, and *D* have nothing to do with access to fast food and cheap fast-food prices.

22. D: According to the text, "Access to full-service restaurants shows either no relationship or a positive relationship with healthy dietary intake." Full-service restaurants do not show a significant decrease in healthy diets, greater likelihood of fast-food restaurants in the area, or poor store access in the vicinity, making Choices *A*, *B*, and *C* incorrect.

23. B: According to the text, "The Glasgow study used a pre/post study design to assess change in shopping and food intake behaviors surrounding a new store opening." Choices *A*, *C*, and *D* were not measured in the Glasgow study.

24. C: The Glasgow study "shows that some of the increase in fruit and vegetable intake among sampled individuals could be due to overall increased consumption of these foods in both the control and study area—not due to the better accessibility to the store in the study area." Choices *A*, *B*, and *D* do not account for the increase in fruit and vegetable consumption.

25. D: While one study showed the increase in fruit and vegetable consumption was significant, the other did not. Therefore, Choice *A* is incorrect. Neither Choice *B* or Choice *C* is discussed in relation to the new store opening. However, "Results of both studies showed that shopping behavior was affected by the openings of new stores—that is, a significant number of sampled individuals from the neighborhood switched their shopping to the new store."

26. A: According to the text, "This trend provides a stark reminder that sepsis is likely to arise as a secondary confounder of any health security threat." Choice *B* includes the qualifier *every*, which is inaccurate and, therefore, incorrect. There is no evidence, in this article, to support Choice *D*. Choice *C* is incorrect based on the information presented in the first few sentences of the selection.

27. B: BARDA, which develops countermeasures, focuses on health security threats including "chemical, biological, radiological, nuclear, pandemic, and emerging infectious diseases." While natural disasters, Choice *A*, might be impacted by health issues, it's not included in that list. Similarly, while important, Choices *C* and *D* are not included in the scope of their work.

28. A: According to the text, diagnostic capabilities exist (Choice *B*), but are not enough. Instead, what would help is our ability to "identify COVID-19 patients who are on the path to sepsis." Thus, Choice *A* is the best option. The focus of the passage does not include information about treatment (Choice *C*), but instead focuses on diagnostic and preventative measures. Though the passage notes that many Americans are unaware of sepsis, it doesn't not discuss a public education program as part of the improvements needed. Thus, Choice *D* is incorrect.

29. C: The sentence suggests a range of ages where the spectrum spans a lifetime, starting with newborns to the elderly. The suggestion of the range is the first clue to the meaning. Further, if one analyzes the word itself, it includes the prefix *neo-*, which means new, and *nates* (as in natal), which means born, making newborns the correct answer choice. Choices *A*, *B*, and *D* all inaccurately define *neonates*.

30. B: According to the text, "sepsis technologies are agnostic to the source of infection, validating their use builds real solutions to any emerging infectious disease outbreak." Unfortunately, COVID-19 patients are unlikely to see immediate relief due to the time needed for research (Choice *A*). There is no mention of government funding (Choice *C*). Finally, while decreased hospitalizations may be an outcome, we do not yet have that evidence (Choice *D*).

31. C: According to the text, "that number is expected to increase to nearly twenty million by 2026 because nearly half of cancer survivors live longer than ten years." While Choice *A*, there are more cancer diagnoses; Choice *B*, we have identified new cancers; and Choice *D*, treatments have gotten better, may all be true, there is no specific data or detail in this text to support these claims.

32. D: According to the text, pain "can be caused by cancer itself (e.g., tumor pressing on nerves, bones, or organs), surgery, treatment and treatment side effects (e.g., peripheral neuropathy, mouth sores, radiation mucositis), or other procedures and tests." While metastasis (the spreading of cancer), Choice *A*, may cause the same complications, it's not referred to here. Similarly, Choices *B* and *C* are not mentioned in this text.

33. C: The primary focus of this paragraph is multiple aspects of pain as it relates to cancer survivors. Choice *A*, cancer, is too broad. Choice *B* is also too broad, and not the focus of the paragraph (though it does come up in supporting details). Choice *D* is related but is not the focus of the passage.

34. B: In the final paragraph of the text, the writers note that one of the primary obstacles to addressing this issue is that patients are often unaware and, therefore, do not report concerns about physical pain. Choice *A* is not discussed, though provider participation in educational needs and the need for provider training in how pain manifests in patients are noted. Choice *C* is incorrect because the first paragraph details, fairly specifically, all of the potential causes for physical pain post-cancer. Similarly, Choice *D* is incorrect because the final paragraph focuses on the need for education.

35. C: In the third paragraph, the text suggests that co-existing conditions may make the pain worse and harder to treat. Additionally, with analysis of the word itself, *co-* means with (as in cooperate), so two conditions exist with one another. Choice *A* is incorrect as cancer is the original diagnosis/condition. Choice *B* may be true but is not correct. Choice *D* is also not correct as the meaning is conditions that exist simultaneously rather than one preceding another.

36. A: The main idea is that more services need to be provided for mental health care for adults with arthritis. While Choice *B* is true, it is not the primary focus of this passage. The focus is on patients with arthritis. This is too broad, though other conditions are mentioned. Choice *C* is incorrect, though tele-medicine is discussed, it is not the main idea. Finally, Choice *D* is a supporting detail for the main idea, but not the main idea itself.

37. B: Shortages in mental health care providers means we need to include community and clinical approaches. While Choices *C* and *D* may be part of the solution, they fall under the umbrella of the recommendation to include both community and clinical approaches. Choice *A* is not mentioned in this text and is, therefore, incorrect.

38. B: According to the research presented, "persons with chronic conditions who reported current depression were three times more likely to have a reduced adherence to medical treatment recommendations." There is no evidence in this passage to suggest that they were more (Choice *D*) or less (Choice *A*) likely to seek initial care. Choice *C* is the opposite of what is reflected in the research and is, therefore, incorrect.

39. C: According to the passage, "Home-based supports, such as the use of community health workers, can support culturally appropriate care and further patient engagement in treatment goal-setting and self-management. Using community health workers can result in greater improvements in participant behavior and health outcomes." There is no mention of Choice *A* or Choice *B* in the text. While Choice *D* might be an outcome based on the other factors, it is not mentioned in this text.

40. A: According to the research, "states with high prevalence of frequent mental distress were geographically clustered, with eight of the ten states in the highest quintile in the Appalachian and southern states." Neither Choice B nor Choice C is mentioned in terms of demographic information regarding the states (population or population density). Finally, the research notes that the states were "geographically clustered" and, therefore, close together, which means Choice D is incorrect.

41. D: According to the text, "binge drinking contributes a substantial proportion of all alcohol consumption in the United States." Choice A is incorrect because the passage notes, "binge drinking increased significantly by 12% from 2011 to 2017." Further, it has increased significantly among non-Hispanic whites, but we have no data about whether the prevalence of it is lowest among this group, so Choice B is incorrect. The final paragraph of the passage reports, "persons living in states with more restrictive alcohol policies are also less likely to binge drink," so Choice C is also incorrect.

42. C: Factors identified in the article include "lower education and income levels" and "the majority of persons reporting prescription opioid misuse are also adults who reported binge drinking." While Choices A, B, and D might all be factors, none of them are discussed in this particular research.

43. D: According to the text, "examining the total number of binge drinks consumed by adults who reported binge drinking is a relatively new way to assess binge drinking." While the other methods mentioned in Choices A, B, and C might be valuable, they are not mentioned in this passage.

44. A: According to the research, "persons living in states with more restrictive alcohol policies are also less likely to binge drink and experience alcohol-attributable harms, including motor vehicle crash deaths, alcoholic liver cirrhosis, and alcohol-involved homicides and suicides than are persons living in states with less restrictive alcohol policies." While Choices B, C, and D may be true, there is no evidence in the passage to support those claims.

45. B: The fourth paragraph highlights the fact that the reduction of binge drinking is vital to the decrease of excessive drinking in general. Additionally, as the study in general establishes the need to reduce frequency, prevalence, and intensity of binge drinking. While Choice A is correct, it is a supporting detail in the passage, and not the main idea. Choice C is incorrect because the passage only establishes that binge drinking contributes significantly to overall alcohol consumption in the U.S. but does not say that binge drinking is a majority of alcohol consumption. Choice D is also incorrect because it is a contributing factor and a supporting detail.

46. C: Research reports, "Postpartum depression is associated with lower rates of breastfeeding initiation, poorer maternal and infant bonding, and increased likelihood of infants showing developmental delays." Further, according to the text, pregnant women *should* be screened at least once during the perinatal visits and during postpartum visit. It doesn't say that they *must* be screened at every visit. Therefore, Choice A is incorrect. Based on the information provided in the passage, women are at risk for depression both during pregnancy and after birth and there is no indication that depression ends once a woman gives birth. This makes Choice B incorrect. Choice D is incorrect as the passage suggests screening should continue through well-child visits with no age cutoff indicated.

47. D: Choice D is correct. According to the text, "Left untreated, postpartum depression can adversely affect the mother's health and might cause sleeping, eating, and behavioral problems for the infant." While the passage mentions potential developmental delays, none of the other choices are mentioned specifically in the passage as possible consequences for the infant and cannot, therefore, be claimed.

48. A: The main idea of the passage is to address the severity of postpartum depression and need for intervention. Choice *B* and Choice *D* are supporting details and contribute to the main idea, but they are not the main idea itself. Choice *C* is incorrect as it is not stated in the passage at all.

49. D: "The United States Preventive Services Task Force (USPSTF) recommends that all adults be screened for depression, including pregnant and postpartum women." While Choice *A* and Choice *C* are included in adults, they are too narrow a response based on the recommendation. Further, while children should be screened as well, that is not discussed; therefore, Choice *B* is also incorrect.

50. B: The definition of the word *intervention* refers to a medical program or action made in effort to improve an outcome or patient's treatment/life. The text recommends interventions as a course of treatment or as part of the treatment of depression. While a conversation between a doctor and patient (Choice *A*) might be part of an intervention, an intervention is not the agreement itself. Further, while interventions might include a hospitalization, that's not the meaning of the term (Choice *C*). And finally, while an intervention might include the use of a new device, not all do, so Choice *D* is also incorrect. An intervention is the act of coming between two things (the depression and the patient, as *inter* means "between").

51. C: According to the passage, wide-brimmed attachments for hard hats "are not widely used because they tend to reduce the worker's vision of overhead hazards." There is no mention of their availability (Choice *A*), their cost (Choice *B*), or their sturdiness (Choice *D*).

52. B: Sun protection in agricultural and construction workers is the subject of the passage. While the passage discusses protective clothing (Choice *A*), safety for construction workers (Choice *C*), and the availability of protective clothing (Choice *D*), they are all noted in the context of the overall subject of the passage which is, specifically, sun protection in agricultural and construction workers.

53. A: According to the text, "although exposure to an educational intervention did not increase construction workers' sun-safety knowledge, it did significantly increase sun-safety behavior, such as increasing shade use when working outdoors." As noted, Choice *B* is incorrect. Choice *C* is also incorrect as the research found that despite policies, "few supply sun-protection equipment." Choice *D* is incorrect as noted in the first paragraph: both groups of workers showed less use of sunscreen than the national average.

54. B: The research reports, "All groups reported a higher prevalence of regular use of protective clothing compared with national estimates of use of wide-brimmed hats (14%), long-sleeved shirts (12%), and long pants or other clothing to ankles (28%)." While sunscreen is discussed, it's lack of usage is noted in the passage, so Choice *A* is incorrect. Similarly, neck shades are mentioned as an option, but not one currently in popular use. Therefore, Choice *C* is incorrect. Finally, sunglasses are not mentioned at all, so Choice *D* is incorrect.

55. D: According to the studies, "interventions that include personal contacts and theory-based training increased the likelihood of adoption of formal sun-protection policies." There is no mention of Choice *A* or Choice *B* in the passage. Finally, while the passage mentions education, there is no mention of literature availability or evidence that literature successfully motivates employers or workers to include sun-protection gear and policies, so Choice *C* is also incorrect.

Vocabulary

1. B

2. C

3. D

4. C

5. A

6. D

7. B

8. A

9. C

10. D

11. B

12. C

13. A

14. B

15. D

16. B

17. C

18. A

19. D

20. C

21. B

22. C

23. A

24. D

25. A

26. B

27. C

28. B

29. D

30. D

31. A

32. C

33. B

34. D

35. B

36. C

37. A

38. D

39. C

40. B

41. A

42. D

43. A

44. C

45. B

46. B

47. D

48. A

49. C

50. A

51. B

52. D

53. B

54. C

Grammar

1. A: *Heard* is the only verb, or word denoting an action; therefore, Choice *A* is the correct answer. Choice *B, new,* is an adjective, Choice *C, gossip,* is a noun, and Choice *D, wing,* is a noun.

2. B: *Complained* and *written* are both verbs; therefore, Choice *B* is correct. *Shift,* choice *A,* is an adjective that modifies *notes; about* and *poorly,* choice *C,* are adverbs; finally, *staff and notes,* choice *D,* are nouns.

3. A: Choice *A* includes a pronoun (*her*) and an antecedent (*Brandy*). Therefore, Choice *A* is the correct answer.

4. C: Choice *C, lose,* is in the present tense; therefore, it is the correct answer. *Loose* means baggy or not tight, so Choice *A* is not correct. Choice *B, lost,* is the past tense of the verb *lose*, and since the word *always* is an indication that the speaker's losing track of time is an ongoing issue, past tense is not the correct tense. Choice *D, losing,* is also incorrect. To be correct, *losing* would need a helping verb; hence, the sentence should read, *I am always losing track of time.*

5. B: Only Choice *B* is a dependent clause that also functions as an introductory element. It would need the rest of the sentence to make sense. Choices *A*, *C*, and *D* are all types of phrases (prepositional, adverb, subject + verb phrases, respectively), but are not full clauses.

6. D: Choice *D* is the coordinating conjunction that sets up the correct relationship between the two parts of the sentence. The sentence structure sets up a contradiction (*not enough time, but time for...*). Choice *A, For,* implies causal relationship, Choice *B, nor,* implies that something negative will follow, and Choice *C, and,* implies connection.

7. D: Choice *D* is correct as it is the only clause/phrase that can stand on its own as a complete sentence. Choice *A* starts with *because,* which suggests a cause-and-effect relationship; we have the *cause* (*Monday off*), but we do not have the *effect*. Choice *B* leaves us wondering what was opened; hence, the information is incomplete. Choice *C* also does not include all the information. The sentence is missing its subject; it does not specify what pertained to the *sufficient medicine for the day*; therefore, this choice is also incomplete.

8. B: Only Choice *B*, which tells us location, is a preposition. *Extra* (Choice *A*) is an adjective that modifies *blankets*. *Stored* (Choice *C*) is a verb. *The* (Choice *D*) is an article.

9. A: *Robert Wood Johnson Hospital* is a proper noun as it is the name of a hospital. *ER,* is an abbreviation. The name of a street (*Easton Avenue*) is a proper noun too; therefore, only Choice *A* includes all the correct capitalized words.

10. C: *Too* in this sentence is an adverb meaning a large quantity; therefore, Choice *C* shows the correct usage of the word. Choices *B* and *D* are incorrect because the word *patients* pertains to people in a hospital; therefore, the word *patience* (one's ability to wait) does not belong in the sentence. Choice *A* uses the word *witch* (which pertains to a person performing sorcery) in place for the correct word *which*.

11. C: The sentence states who carpools to work together. This means that the subjects in the sentence must be subject pronouns and must answer the question *who/what.* Choice *C* offers the subject pronouns *She* and *I,* and is, therefore, the correct answer.

12. A: The relationship between the two sentence parts is cause and effect, like in *come to the meeting so this can happen...*; therefore *Choice A* is the best option.

13. B: Adverbs modify or describe verbs. Choice B *beautifully* describes how the lobby was decorated; therefore, it is the adverb in the sentence.

14. C: The phrase *last week* states that the event happened in the past. This means the verb that the sentence requires must be in the simple past tense as in Choice *C, completed.*

15. D: The pronoun in this sentence is *she*, which refers to *Dr. Smith*, the subject of the sentence. The word *her* takes the place of the antecedent, Dr. Smith (*Choice D*).

16. D: The word *who's* is a contraction of the words *who* and *is*, which do not fit correctly in the sentence. The word *their* denotes possession, and *there* pertains to a place. *They're* is a contraction of the words *they* and *are.* So, the correct sentence is *I don't know whose charts these are, but they are not in the correct spot* (Choice *D*).

17. C: Choice *C* is correct because it uses the required quotation marks for a direct quote, and the appropriate end sentence punctuation. Choice *A* misplaces the end punctuation by putting it outside the quotes. Choice *B* does not have any punctuation to end the question directly quoted. Choice *D* incorrectly puts a comma where a question mark is necessary.

18: A: Choice *A* is correct as the word *biggest* is the superlative adjective describing the highest degree. Choices *C* and *D* are both incorrect because of the inclusion of the word *most*, which is not required for this superlative. Choice *B* creates an incomplete idea, and is therefore, incorrect.

19: C: An indirect object is whomever or whatever is affected by the subject's action. In this sentence, the nurse is the subject. She hands *the scalpel **to** the doctor.* Therefore, the doctor is the indirect object, so Choice *C* is correct.

20. D: Choice *D* is correct as it uses the correct verb tense (simple past) as well as the correct spelling of the word *passed.* In Choice A, *past* is incorrect. In Choice B, *had rushed* suggests something else happens because of the verb tense. While the verb in Choice C is correct, the word *write* is not.

21. B: *Norman* is a singular name that acts as part of the subject. Therefore, the best pronoun to replace *Norman* would be *his* as it is the singular subject pronoun.

22. D: Choice *D* is correct as it is an incomplete thought. What happened *because of bad winter storms*? The clause requires the rest of the sentence and the phrases that make it up (Choices *A, B, C*), to complete the idea.

23. B: Choice *B* is the only choice that includes the linking verb *were* and the verb phrase *were expected.* While Choice *C* includes those, it also includes an extra phrase, which includes words that are NOT verbs.

24. A: Choice *A* is the only noun in the list. Choice *B* is an adjective. Choice *C* is an article. Choice *D* is a preposition.

25. C: Choice C is correct as the word *awful* describes the *food*. Choice A, *despite,* is a preposition. Choice B is a noun (and part of the prepositional phrase). Choice D is a noun.

26. A: *Either* is a singular indefinite pronoun; therefore, the verb must be singular. The word *asked* is in past tense, which tells us the helping verb should also be in past tense. Therefore, Choice A is correct.

27. D: The subject states who or what is performing the action in the sentence. The phrase *Mary's sister sat* states both who and what was done; therefore, Choice D is the correct answer.

28. B: The word *accept* means to take or receive something offered. *Expect* means likelihood that something will happen, and *except* means to leave out. Therefore, *the nurses were expected to accept the new rules*. Thus, Choice B is correct.

29. B: *Affect* is a verb that means to impact feelings or emotions, or to have an impact. *Effect* is a noun that means a change or consequence. *Affection* is also a noun that describes what we feel when we like someone. Finally, *affliction* is something that affects us badly. So, Choice B is the correct choice.

30. A: The three articles in the English language are *the, a,* and *an*. Choice A includes all the articles found in the sentence, so it is correct.

31. C: The subject of the sentence is the speaker, *I*. The sentence requires a singular object pronoun, *her*, so Choice C is correct.

32. D: Because the word *healing* is a verb, the correct answer must be an adverb. Choice D is the only adverb among all the options.

33. D: The word *then* is an indicator of time. The sentence offers a comparison between what was expected and what is reality; thus, it requires the word *than* instead of *then*.

34. C: Choice C is correct because it is the only part of the sentence that can stand on its own. It contains a subject, a verb, and a complete idea. While Choice A is an independent clause, it is a part of a dependent clause in the sentence.

35. A: Choice A is the only noun in the list; therefore, it is the correct choice. Choice B is an adjective. Choice C is a verb. Choice D is an adverb.

36. A: Conjunctions are words that connect phrases and clauses within a sentence; therefore, Choice A, *and*, is correct.

37. B: Choice B is correct as the sentence should read: *The nurse knows it's (it is) time to administer medications, but first he visits the supply closet to lock its (possessive) door.*

38. D: A colon sets a list apart from the rest of the sentence without interrupting the main clause, so a colon is the appropriate punctuation.

39. C: A complete verb includes the helping verb and the main/action verb. Therefore, *were* (helping verb) and *expected* (main verb) complete the verb phrase, so Choice C is correct.

40. C: The phrase *next year* states that the action will happen in the future. This means that the sentence requires helping verbs (*will have*) that indicate future tense with the main verb *completed*. Therefore, Choice C is correct.

41. A: Prepositional phrases can provide more information about location in regard to the subject, *extra blankets.* Choice *A*, which reveals that *the blankets are stored **in** (the closet),* is the preposition in the sentence.

42. B: Choice *B* is the correct answer as it is spelled correctly, and it is in the correct form (as a noun).

43. A: Choice *A* includes a plural subject and a plural verb, whereas Choices *B* and *C* use singular subjects with plural verbs, and Choice *D* uses a plural subject and singular verb.

44. D: *Despite the fact that we were short-staffed* is an introductory clause that is dependent on the rest of the sentence. Dependent clauses are off-set by a comma, so Choice *D* is correct.

45. B: Choice *B* includes the correct possessive form of *nurses'* and the correct use of *affected* as a verb. In Choice *A*, *effect* is used incorrectly; it should be the verb *affect.* In Choice *C*, it should be *affect* as a verb not *effect.* Finally, in Choice *D*, *affect* should be the noun *effect.*

46. B: The word *than* in the sentence shows that there is a comparison happening, which means it requires a superlative form. Of all the choices, only Choice *B* is a superlative that indicates *not as many* in comparison.

47. C: This sentence looks to answer how the blood was drawn, which means it needs an adverb. Only Choice *C* includes the appropriate adverb, *roughly,* so it is the correct answer.

48. D: Choice *D* is correct—*the nurse was recognized for her quick thinking and skilled work* is an independent clause. The dependent clause (*especially when she was assisting on surgeries*) gives more information on her *quick thin*king and *skilled work*—part of the independent clause—but cannot stand on its own as a complete idea.

49. A: Choice *A* is correct as *St. Andrew's Hospital, E Lansing Road*, and *Bellingham, Washington* are all proper nouns.

50. B: Adjectives are words that describe or modify nouns. Therefore, the only adjective in this sentence is *green.* The correct answer is Choice *B*.

51. D: Choice *D* is correct as it is the easiest to follow given the information included. Choices *A*, *B*, and *C* all have misplaced modifiers.

52. C: The first blank must be a word that modifies the verb *performed*, so the correct choice would be an adverb. However, the second blank is for a word that modifies *care*, a noun, so it should be an adjective. Choice *C* offers *magnificently* as an adverb and then *magnificent* as an adjective. Thus, it is the correct choice.

53. B: Only Choice *B* is an adjective. Choice *A* is an adverb that describes how time moved. Choice *C* is an adverb because the word *pretty* modifies the adjective *short*. Choice *D* is also an adverb as it modifies how the session lasted.

54. A: *Also,* in this case, is called a non-essential element since it can be removed from the sentence without changing the meaning. The phrase *who was studying for the HESI exam* is an incomplete thought that is dependent on information from the main clause, so it is a dependent clause. Therefore, Choice *A* is correct.

55. C: Choice *C* offers the correct verb conjugation for this sentence. Choice *A*, Choice *B*, and Choice *D* do not include correct subject-verb agreement.

Biology

1. D: Photosynthesis is not necessarily a characteristic that defines a living organism. For example, mammals within the Kingdom Animalia ingest food from plants/animals and don't photosynthesize their food. Choices *A, B,* and *C* are all characteristics of life.

2. C: It is generally accepted that viruses are not quite living or dead. Viruses have free forms of RNA/DNA that they can't reproduce or replicate by themselves. Instead, viruses invade living organisms to replicate. By hijacking the host cell's machinery, viruses will replicate themselves. Living organisms tend to take actions that reflect the characteristics of life. For instance, an animal will look for food, or a plant will sprout its roots to look for water. A virus doesn't have self-sustaining actions and is inert unless it comes in contact with a cell. Choice *A* is incorrect since viruses can make copies of themselves, but not independently. Choice *B* is incorrect because viruses can only reproduce if they are given a host cell. In addition, a virus doesn't have a metabolism; they steal energy from their host. Viruses can adapt to antibiotics. Choice *D* is incorrect because a virus cannot fulfill all characteristics of life, such as self-replication. A virus does not grow in size and doesn't have an energy-producing system.

3. D: The passage describes how plants, animals, and fungi interact with one another. Plants need sunlight to produce carbohydrates such as sugars. Animals such as cows must consume plants to survive. Humans consume animals and plants to acquire energy and perform work. Fungi will decompose dead organisms and return nutrients to the soil.

4. B: To increase the likelihood of survival, individuals must acquire traits that are well suited to their environment. Choices *A* and *D* are incorrect because they accurately reflect Darwin's observations. Choice *C* is incorrect because mutations can be described as traits or changes in the genetic code. These changes may occur to ensure the survival of organisms within a specific environment.

5. B: A useful mnemonic to remember the correct order of taxa, from most to least inclusive (domain, kingdom, phylum, class, order, family, genus, species) is: **D**ear **K**ing **P**hilip **C**ame **O**ver **F**or **G**rape **S**oda." The most general category is the domain, while the least inclusive is species. Choice *A* is incorrect since it lists the taxa from least to most inclusive. Choices *C* and *D* are incorrect since the domain is the most inclusive.

6. A: Blood flow throughout the blood vessels of the jackrabbit's ears can be controlled or regulated to maintain body temperature. At a temperature of around 30°C (86 °F), the jackrabbit cools down by releasing heat from its ears. Blood carrying heat will flow from the body to the ears. Heat is dissipated around the blood vessels of the jackrabbit's ears. Its ears act as radiators, much like a radiator that is found in a car. Water is also retained and is not lost as sweat or panting. Choice *B* is incorrect; it is a property that describes the response to an environmental stimulus. For example, a Venus flytrap closes when an insect lands on it. Choice *C* is incorrect since evolutionary adaptation describes a trait that is suited to a certain environment. For example, penguins developed large flat wings to swim in the water better. Choice *D* is incorrect and involves the consumption of a food source to perform work.

7. D: Protists are unique in that they absorb, photosynthesize, or ingest food. Fungi absorb food, and plantae photosynthesize food. Kingdom Animalia are heterotrophs that ingest food and rely on other organisms for nourishment. Choice *A* is incorrect because all multicellular organisms are eukaryotes.

Choice *B* is incorrect because there are two kingdoms (animalia and protists) that can ingest food. Choice *C* is incorrect since there are two kingdoms (plantae and protists) that can photosynthesize food.

8. B: Scientific models allow scientists to control certain conditions not possible in a natural environment. Choice *A* is incorrect because it is the definition of a hypothesis. Choice *C* is incorrect because it describes a theory. Choice *D* is incorrect because it is the definition of a scientific law.

9. A: The hypothesis is true since the dark model mice were attacked in the beach habitat more because they cannot camouflage well against a white, sandy background. Additionally, the light model mice in the inland habitat are attacked more often since they cannot camouflage well against a brown background. Choice *B* is incorrect because the hypothesis should be labeled as 'true' for the provided statement. Choice *C* is incorrect because light model mice were attacked more in the inland habitat. Choice *D* is incorrect because the hypothesis should be 'true.'

10. B: Hydrogen chloride will not form a hydrogen bond; rather, it will form a weaker bond type called a dipole-dipole bond. Hydrogen bonds form with hydrogen and a slightly negative atom, such as oxygen, nitrogen, and fluorine. The difference in electronegativity between hydrogen and chlorine is $\Delta EN = |2.1 - 3.0| = 0.9$ making it a relatively weaker type of polar covalent bond than other choices. For example, HF has an $\Delta EN = |2.1 - 4.0| = 1.9$, H-NH$_2$ has an $\Delta EN = |2.1 - 3.0| = 0.9$, and H-OCH2CH3 has an $\Delta EN = |2.1 - 3.5| = 1.4$. NH$_3$ and HCl have the same value, but ammonia can hydrogen bond because the nitrogen atom is smaller than the chlorine atom. Because nitrogen is relatively smaller, it can form a stronger dipole-dipole called a hydrogen bond. The slightly negative chlorine atom of one HCl molecule will be attracted to the slightly positive hydrogen of another HCl molecule. A weaker dipole-dipole bond will form.

11. A: Ammonium contains four polar N-H bonds that are arranged tetrahedrally. The nitrogen atom in ammonium is relatively more electron-deficient, as indicated by the positive charge around the molecule. Even though nitrogen is electron-deficient due to its electron sharing with another hydrogen atom, nitrogen is still more electronegative than hydrogen. The direction of the dipole is directed from the slightly positive hydrogen to the slightly negative nitrogen. All dipoles are directed from the corners of a tetrahedron to the nitrogen. Consequently, all the individual dipoles cancel out, thereby making the overall molecule nonpolar. Choice *B*, carbon monoxide, is incorrect and polar since there is one dipole directed from the slightly positive carbon towards the more electronegative oxygen. Choice *C*, ammonia, is incorrect and is nonpolar. The electron geometry is tetrahedral with three N-H dipoles. The electron distribution is uneven because there are now three dipoles that point towards the nitrogen atom, thereby making the molecule polar. Choice *D* is incorrect because helium is not a molecule but an atom.

12. D: The hydrogen bonds that connect water molecules allow water to absorb heat without incurring a large temperature change. Coastal cities are typically cooler than inland cities because water can take in large amounts of heat. The high heat capacity of water allows organisms to maintain internal changes and prevent large temperature increases. Choices *A* and *B* are similar and true, and therefore incorrect. DNA is a type of biological or cellular molecule that is held together by hydrogen bonds. For example, guanine in one strand of DNA will hydrogen bond to the cytosine nucleotide base found on the second strand. Choice *C* is incorrect because hydrogen bonds allow proteins to stay folded. Hydrogen bonding is responsible for maintaining the secondary protein structure.

13. D: Water acts as an insulator because ice water found on ponds or lakes keeps liquid water below from freezing. As a result, aquatic organisms can survive. Choice *A* is incorrect since water acts mostly as a solvent. Choice *B* is incorrect since water has a high heat capacity. Choice *C* is incorrect since water has a high heat of vaporization (not fusion/melting).

14. A: Capillary action is attributed to the intermolecular forces between liquid water and the surrounding polar-solid surfaces. As water evaporates from a leaf, the water column moves upward as a result of cohesive and adhesive forces. Surface tension, which is due to the cohesion within water, and adhesive forces between water molecules and transport vessels, will cause water to move upward. Without cohesive and adhesive forces, the plant would dry up and die.

15. B: Figure II correctly indicates three hydrogen bonds that form between the slightly negative oxygen atom of water and the slightly positive hydrogen atom of ammonia. These hydrogen bonds (O-H) bonds are located at the base of the solvation structure. At the top, there is one hydrogen bond between the slightly positive hydrogen and the slightly negative nitrogen atom.

16. B: Structure II represents thymine, a type of base found in DNA. Choice *A* is incorrect and represents a fatty acid (triglyceride) since it contains a long hydrocarbon chain bonded to an ester group (C-(C=O)-O-C-). Choice *C* is a carbohydrate called fructose, a naturally-occurring sugar found in fruit. Carbohydrates tend to contain hydroxyl (-OH) groups). Choice *D* is an amino acid found in proteins. The amino acid contains an amine (NH_2 or NH_{23}) and a carboxyl (-COOH or -COO-) group.

17. B: R–(CO)–O⁻ represents a carboxylic acid group typically found in amino acids and proteins. Carbohydrates tend to have hydroxyl, ketone, and aldehyde groups. Choice *A* represents an alcohol group, choice *C* is a ketone group, and choice *D* is an aldehyde group.

18. C: Structure III represents a pair of isomers. Both molecules contain the same number of atoms but with a different bonding arrangement. The structure on the left inset is a ketone, and the structure on the right is an aldehyde. Choice *A* and Choice *B* are both incorrect. Both are similar structures since the left inset structures contain eight hydrogen atoms, and the right inset structures contain six hydrogen atoms. Choice *D* is incorrect since the left inset structure contains three oxygen atoms and the right structure four oxygen atoms.

19. A: Triglycerides are examples of fat molecules that can undergo hydrolysis reactions to produce glycerol and three fatty acids. Three molecules of water are required to break down the fat molecule. Choice *B* is incorrect because the hydrolysis of a fat molecule produces three fatty acids. Fat molecules may be unsaturated or saturated. Choice *C* is incorrect since glycerol is produced in a hydrolysis reaction. Choice *D* is incorrect because fat molecules can undergo hydrolysis reactions. However, lipids, such as fat molecules, are not technically polymers.

20. D: Consider the following reaction below for the production of a disaccharide from two monosaccharide (monomer) subunits.

$$2\ monosaccharide \overset{condensation}{\rightleftharpoons} 1\ disaccharide + 1\ water$$

The general stoichiometric equation indicates that for every two molecules of monomer subunits, one disaccharide and one molecule of water are produced. Because the problem indicates that six monosaccharide units are present, the reactants must be multiplied by a factor of three to have six monosaccharide subunits.

$$3 \times \left[2\ monosaccharide \overset{condensation}{\rightrightarrows} 1\ disaccharide + 1\ water \right]$$

Consequently, by the conservation of mass, the product side must be multiplied by three to give three molecules of a disaccharide and three molecules of water. Therefore, the balanced chemical reaction is:

$$6\ monosaccharide \overset{condensation}{\rightrightarrows} 3\ disaccharide + 3\ water$$

Three disaccharides and three molecules of water are created during a condensation reaction.

21. D: A pentose is a monosaccharide that contains five carbon atoms. Selection IV, represents deoxyribose, a molecule with five carbon atoms. Choice *A* represents a sugar molecule (glucose) that contains six carbon atoms. Choice *B* represents a sugar molecule (galactose) that contains six carbon atoms. Choice *C* represents a sugar molecule (fructose) containing six carbon atoms. Choices *A, B,* and *C* are all incorrect because they are hexoses, which are sugar molecules that contain six carbon atoms.

22. B: Polysaccharides contain many polar hydroxyl groups that can undergo hydrogen bonding, thereby making them water-soluble. Choice *A* is a true statement but does not explain why the polysaccharide will not pass through the lipid membrane. Choice *C* is incorrect because, as stated before, polysaccharides are water-soluble and contain polar hydroxyl groups. In general, the membrane of a cell is semi-permeable and is composed of a phospholipid bilayer. Because the polysaccharide is hydrophilic, it will not pass through a lipid because the lipid is mostly hydrophobic. Choice *D* is incorrect because the hydrocarbon chains are not kinked. The outer layer of the membrane is hydrophilic, but the inner layer is hydrophobic. The head of the phospholipid is polar and points towards the inner cell or outer cell. The tail ends of the phospholipid are nonpolar since they are composed of two unkinked hydrocarbon chains. These chains are tucked away from the aqueous environment inside and outside the cell.

23. D: Hydrogen bonding between amino acids occurs at the secondary level and causes the polypeptide to form an alpha helix or a beta-pleated sheet. Choice *A* is incorrect because the quaternary structure is the level where two or more polypeptides interact to carry out a specific function. Choice *B* is incorrect because the primary level is associated with linear sequencing of amino acids (determined by genes within DNA). Choice *C* is incorrect because the tertiary structure is level where amino acids within a side chain interact (covalent bonding such as disulfide linkages), fold, and conform to the 3-D shape of a protein.

24. A: When two strands of DNA come together, three hydrogen bonds are created between the complementary bases of guanine and cytosine. Within the guanine, the oxygen atom on the carbonyl (C=O) bond will form a hydrogen bond to a specific hydrogen atom on cytosine. The hydrogen atom, on the N-H bond of guanine, will form a hydrogen bond to the nitrogen atom on cytosine. A second hydrogen atom, on the N-H bond of guanine, will form a hydrogen bond to the oxygen atom located on the carbonyl group (C=O) of cytosine.

25. B: Microbodies are organelles within the cell's cytoplasm that facilitate the breakdown of fats, alcohols, and amino acids (catabolic). Choice *A* is not the best answer since the cytoskeleton, made from protein filaments/tubules, provides mechanical support to the cell during cell division and maintains the shape and internal organization of the cell. Choice *C* is incorrect because ribosomes are responsible for the assembly of polypeptides from amino acids. Choice D is incorrect since centrioles are cylindrical organelles that help with cell division by forming spindle fibers to separate the chromosomes.

26. D: Stearic acid is a fatty acid that contains a saturated hydrocarbon chain. The number of chemical bonds (e.g., C-H bonds) is greater than glucose; therefore, stearic acid will have more potential or chemical energy. Choice A is incorrect because glucose is a type of sugar/monosaccharide that contains fewer chemical bonds compared to stearic acid. Choice B is incorrect because mechanical energy is a type of kinetic energy. Choice C, like Choice A, is incorrect because stearic acid has more potential energy. Lipids generally have more stored chemical energy than carbohydrates since they contain more reduced hydrogens or hydrogens bonded to a less electronegative atom such as carbon. For example, when the body metabolizes a lipid or carbohydrate during cellular respiration, the general reaction is:

$$C_xH_yO_z + nO_2 \rightarrow mCO_2 + H_2O$$

Because lipids provide more hydrogen atoms per carbon, they will have more chemical energy.

27. A: An enzyme will speed up a chemical reaction by lowering the reactant to product activation barrier. Choice B is incorrect because the product to reactant activation barrier (reverse reaction) should be greater than the forward reaction. Enzymes act as catalysts since they increase the reaction rate by lowering the reactant to product barrier allowing the reaction to move forward. Choice C is incorrect because the Gibbs Free energy (ΔG) remains unchanged and is not altered by an enzyme, only the activation barrier. Choice D is not necessarily true and depends on the reactants and products. For example, if the two molecules are combined to form one molecule, then the disorder (entropy) decreases.

28. A: The correct statement is, "For a <u>spontaneous</u> reaction to occur, the Gibbs free energy of the system must be <u>negative</u>." In the study of metabolism, energetically favorable (spontaneous) processes occur when the Gibbs free energy is negative ($-\Delta G$). The energy that is released from a chemical reaction can be used to perform work within the cell. For example, the overall reaction of cellular respiration is spontaneous and will have negative free energy.

$$C_6H_{12}O_6 + 6O_2 \rightarrow 6CO_2 + 6H_2O \ \Delta G = -686 \ kcal/mol$$

A spontaneous process is one where the entropy of the system is increasing. There are seven molecules on the left-hand side and twelve molecules on the equation's right-hand side.

29. B: Catabolic pathways such as those involved in cellular respiration are exergonic processes since they release free energy as complex molecules (glucose) and are broken down into simple ones (carbon dioxide and water). Choice A is incorrect because anabolic processes are endergonic and require energy to build larger molecules. Photosynthesis is an example of an anabolic pathway. Choice C is incorrect because anabolic pathways are endergonic since they require energy to build larger molecules. Choice D is incorrect because catabolic pathways are exergonic and release energy as larger molecules are broken down.

30. D: ATP combines with a water molecule (hydrolysis) to form adenine diphosphate (ADP) and an inorganic phosphate group. The spontaneous reaction releases free energy and is therefore exergonic. To drive an endergonic reaction, the net free energy of the coupled system must be negative.

$$\Delta G_{net} = \Delta G_{ATP} + \Delta G_{exergonic} = -7.3\frac{kcal}{mol} + 3.4\frac{kcal}{mol} = -3.9 \ kcal/mol$$

Since the overall net free energy is negative, the reaction is spontaneous. In the cellular synthesis of glutamine, an amino acid, the reaction is coupled with ATP hydrolysis. Choices A and B are incorrect since ATP combines with water (hydrolysis). Choice C is incorrect since ATP hydrolysis is exergonic.

Chemistry

1. B: The reaction is an acid-base or neutralization reaction that involves the exchange of cations and anions. Because there are two cations and anions involved in the exchange, the reaction a is a double displacement: $AB + CD \rightarrow AD + CB$ whereby sodium ($Na^+ = A$) combines with sulfate ($SO_4^{2-} = D$), and a proton ($H^+ = C$) combines with hydroxide ($OH^- = B$) to form a sodium sulfate salt ($Na_2SO_4 = AD$) and water ($2H_2O = CB$).

2. C: The blue pigment used in old Renaissance paintings, called copper (II) hydroxide ($Cu(OH)_2$), decomposes to copper (II) oxide (black product) and water (H_2O). Because the reactant breaks down into two products, it is a decomposition reaction: $A \rightarrow B + C$ where $A = Cu(OH)_2$, $B = CuO$, and $C = H_2O$.

3. B: The acetate ion ($C_2H_3O_2^-$) is a molecular compound that is kept together when balancing equations. Because there are two moles of acetate in lead (II) acetate ($Pb(C_2H_3O_2)_2$), start by placing a coefficient of 2 in front of sodium acetate ($NaC_2H_3O_2$). There are now two moles of sodium in $NaC_2H_3O_2$, so place a coefficient of 2 in the front of sodium iodide (KI) on the reactant side to balance sodium (Na) in $NaC_2H_3O_2$. Two moles of iodide (I^-) are present in NaI and lead (II) iodide (PbI_2), so a coefficient of 1 is placed before PbI_2. One mole of lead (Pb) is present in $Pb(NO_3)_2$, like PbI_2, so a coefficient of 1 is placed in front of $Pb(C_2H_3O_2)_2$. The correct order of coefficients must be 2, 1, 2, 1. Note that coefficients of 1 are not typically written.

$$2\,NaI\ (aq) + Pb(C_2H_3O_2)_2\ (aq) \rightarrow 2NaC_2H_3O_2(aq) + PbI_2\ (s)$$

4. B: Freshly squeezed lemonade contains small bits of pulp that will not uniformly spread out. The composition of unsweetened or black coffee (caffeine), filtered apple juice (sugar and tartaric acid), and purified water (minerals) are uniform and not pure solutions.

5. A: Coffee with sugar (sucrose), when mixed uniformly in small amounts, is primarily homogenous. The soup is a heterogeneous mixture because some vegetables are denser and will collect at the bottom, with some less dense vegetables on top. If the number and type of vegetables in each spoonful were counted, the tallies would vary. Tomato juice is heterogeneous because it contains visible suspended particles. Buttermilk has particles of butterfat and is, therefore, heterogeneous.

6. A: A solution is a type of homogeneous mixture that has two or more components. The solute is sugar because it is the substance with less mass. The solvent is the substance with the larger mass (water or coffee). Therefore, addition of sugar to black coffee forms a homogenous mixture because sugar is evenly distributed within the mixture. The sugar-coffee mixture is considered an unsaturated solution because the solubility of sugar in water at room temperature is approximately 2 g/mL (200 g per 100 mL of water). Two tablespoons of sugar have roughly 25 g, and 1 cup of water is approximately 237 g or 237 mL (25 g/237 mL = 0.105 g/mL, which is < 2 g/mL).

7. D: The aqueous reaction of NaI and $Pb(C_2H_3O_2)_2$ forms a precipitate or solid substance, $PbI_2\ (s)$. The solution is initially colorless and clear, but when the two aqueous reactants are mixed, a yellowish cloudy precipitate, PbI_2 (s), will form immediately. Lead (II) iodide is insoluble, but sodium acetate is a soluble ionic compound.

8. B: A Brønsted-Lowry base is a species that will accept a hydrogen proton, H^+. For the reaction that is shown, water (H_2O) acts as a base by accepting H^+ from nitric acid, HNO_3, and produces the hydronium ion (H_3O^+). Nitric acid is the Brønsted-Lowry acid.

9. A: The arrow points from a solid (initial state) to a gas (final state). This phase change or transition is called *sublimation* and is a physical process in which the solid or fixed molecules transition to a gas phase. In a sublimation process, the liquid phase is bypassed. When a piece of dry ice (solid carbon dioxide) is brought to room temperature (1 atm), it will sublime and convert to gaseous carbon dioxide. Therefore, the meaning behind "dry ice" comes from the fact that a liquid state is not observed.

10. C: The addition of liquid sugar cane to coffee will not change the chemical structure of sugar. However, if the sugar were caramelized or brown, done by cooking, the chemical structure of sugar would change. Water condensing on a cold-water bottle is a process in which water vapor from the air undergoes a gas to liquid phase change as it touches the cold surface. The phase transition is physical, and the structure of water remains unchanged. Marshmallows are made up of sugar, and when roasted or browned, the marshmallow changes from white to brown or black. Therefore, the color change means that the sugar molecules undergo a chemical reaction with heat and a structural change in chemical composition. The evaporation of rubbing alcohol (isopropyl alcohol) from someone's fingernail is a liquid to gas phase change.

11. A: Carbon monoxide is a molecular compound because it contains at least two different elements: C and O. Chlorine gas is a molecular element and has two atoms that are of the same element. Argon, Ar, is neither a molecular element or a compound and is a monatomic gas (particles consisting of single atoms). Cyclo-heptasulfur, S_7, is an allotrope of sulfur and can be described as a molecular element.

12. B: The correct balanced equation for the combustion of ethane, C_2H_6, is:

$$2C_2H_6 + 7O_2 \rightarrow 4CO_2 + 6H_2O$$

Six moles of water (coefficient of 6) should be produced instead of four moles (coefficient of 4). The law of conservation of mass means that both sides of the equation should have equal masses. For example, there are 4 carbon atoms, 12 hydrogen atoms, and 14 oxygen atoms on the reactant side. If a coefficient of 4 was used, there would be 4 carbon atoms, 8 hydrogen atoms, and 12 oxygen atoms on the product side. If the correct coefficient of 6 was used ($6H_2O$), there would be 12 hydrogen atoms and 14 oxygen atoms, and the law of conservation would be followed.

13. D: Based on kinetic molecular theory, the average kinetic energy of a gaseous particle is dependent on its absolute temperature. As the temperature increases, the gas particles will move faster (greater average velocity) and collide with a greater force within the balloon (F = mass × acceleration). Consequently, because more force is exerted (pressure = force/area), the pressure inside the balloon increases and causes the volume to increase. If the temperature is decreased, the kinetic energy of the gas decreases, and so does its average velocity. As a result, the gas particles will collide within the balloon with a smaller force or pressure. The volume of the balloon decreases.

14. B: Charles's law describes the relationship between volume and absolute temperature at a constant external pressure and a fixed number of moles.

$$\frac{V_1}{T_1} = \frac{V_2}{T_2}$$

Suppose the initial temperature (room temperature) is approximately 298°K ($T_1 = 298\ K$). The initial volume was given as $V_1 = 300\ mL$ and the final temperature as $T_2 = 373\ K$. The estimated volume of the balloon can be determined by rearranging the equation from above. However, it's expected that the calculated volume will be greater because Charles's law says that as the temperature increases, so does the volume of the gas. Therefore, the value of V_2 should be greater than V_1.

$$V_2 = T_2 \times \frac{V_1}{T_1} = (373\ K) \times \frac{300\ mL}{298\ K} = 376\ mL$$

15. C: The reaction equation in Choice A is not correct because $Cu^{2+} \rightarrow Cu(s)$ corresponds to a reduction half. Although Zn undergoes oxidation, the reaction equation shown for Choice B is not written correctly and should have the electrons placed on the product side. Choice C is written correctly and corresponds to a reduction half-reaction. The reaction equation for Choice D is written correctly but corresponds to an oxidation half-reaction.

$$Cu^{2+} + 2e^- \rightarrow Cu\ (s); \text{reduction half}$$

$$Zn\ (s) \rightarrow Zn^{2+} + 2e^-; \text{oxidation half}$$

$$\text{Net reaction: } Cu^{2+} + Zn\ (s) \rightarrow Cu\ (s) + Zn^{2+}$$

16. A: Group IA metals have an oxidation number that's equal to their group number. For example, the oxidation number for lithium (Li) is equal to +1. Lithium oxide is a neutral compound, so the total oxidation number is $2(+1) = 1(x_0) = 0$, where x_0 is equal to the oxidation number of oxygen. Solving the equation would give a value of $x_0 = -2$.

17. C: Zinc has an oxidation number equal to 0 because the reactant is solid. There are two acetate ions that each have a charge of 1−, so the oxidation number of solid zinc in ($Zn(C_3H_3O_2)_2\ (aq)$) is +2. Zinc is oxidized because its oxidation number changes from 0 to +2 ($Zn\ (s) \rightarrow Zn^{2+}(aq)$) and loses electrons in the process. The silver ion initially has a charge of +2 and undergoes a reduction to form solid silver:

$$Ag^+\ (aq) \rightarrow Ag\ (s)$$

18. C: A reducing agent reduces another reactant by providing electrons but causes that agent to be oxidized. In contrast, an oxidizing agent oxidizes the other reactant by removing its electrons, causing that "agent" to become reduced in the redox process. Silver nitrate ($AgC_3H_3O_2\ (aq)$) acts as the oxidizing agent because it oxidizes zinc. The oxidation number of zinc changes from 0 to +2:

$$Zn\ (s) \rightarrow Zn^{2+}\ (aq) + 2e^-$$

Silver acetate dissociates into the silver ion and acetate ion. The oxidation number of the silver ion $Ag^+\ (aq)$ will change from +1 to 0, thereby becoming reduced in the process:

$$Ag^+\ (aq) + e^- \rightarrow Ag\ (s)$$

Solid zinc, Zn (s), is oxidized and acts as the reducing agent because it provides electrons to the silver ion.

19. A: A substance that produces H^+ ions is called an Arrhenius acid. Perchloric acid initially dissociates to form a proton or a hydronium ion.

$$HClO_4 \ (aq) \rightarrow H^+ \ (aq) + ClO_4^- \ (aq)$$

or

$$HClO_4 \ (aq) + \ H_2O \ (l) \rightarrow H_3O^+ \ (aq) + ClO_4^- \ (aq)$$

Potassium hydroxide then reacts with the proton or hydronium ion to produce potassium perchlorate and water. Strong acids, such as perchloric acid, are strong electrolytes that dissociate to the right to produce hydrogen ions (H^+).

20. B: A Lewis acid is a species that accepts an electron pair, whereas a Lewis base is the species that donates a pair of electrons. When the reaction proceeds to the right, ammonia (NH_3) donates an electron pair (two electrons) from one orbital and shares them (one curved arrow) with one proton from water, H_2O. During the reaction, the electrons that were once shared between H and O travel to an oxygen atom to produce the hydroxide ion, OH^-. The reaction is reversible and can proceed in the reverse direction whereby the hydroxide ion (OH^-) acts as a Lewis base by donating its electron pair to ammonium (NH_4^+). Water and the ammonium ion both act as Lewis acids, whereas the ammonia and hydroxide ions act as Lewis bases.

21. C: Group IA and IIA metals that are bonded to hydroxide ion, OH^-, are considered strong bases. Based on the table that lists strong acids and bases, water and ammonia must be the possible answer choices. Which base is weaker? Ammonia or water? Consider the reaction of ammonia and water shown below.

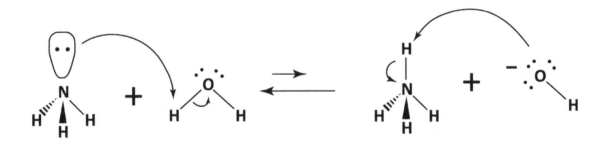

The reaction proceeds slightly to the right but more toward the reactant side. Ammonia and hydroxide ions both act as bases. However, the hydroxide ion is a stronger base because the reaction proceeds toward the reactant side. On the reactant side, the water molecule is amphoteric, meaning it can act as an acid or base, depending on the reaction equation (e.g., perchloric acid reacts with water). In the reaction above, water acts as a Lewis acid instead because the oxygen atom is more electronegative than nitrogen and is less likely to share its electrons. Because water is more likely to release a proton to ammonia, it will preferably act as a Lewis acid and less like a Lewis base. The nitrogen in ammonia contains a lone pair and is a stronger base because it's more likely to share its electrons than the oxygen atom in water. Therefore, the weakest base is water.

22. D: Bond polarity results when electrons are not shared equally between a chemical bond containing two different atoms. The greater the differences in the electronegativity value between each atom, the greater the bond polarity. The electronegativity value of an element will increase from left to right along a row on the periodic table but decrease top to bottom within a column. Each answer choice contains a halogen that is bonded to a carbon atom. Therefore, we can make a qualitative conclusion as to which bond is the least polar. Fluorine is the most electronegative element, and the electronegativity values decrease going down group VIIA:

$$F > Cl > Br > I$$

Iodine is the least electronegative. A carbon-iodine bond is expected to be the least polar. For a quantitative answer, it's best to calculate the difference in electronegativity (ΔEN), given an EN table, to determine the least polar bond.

$$\Delta EN(C - Br) = |2.5 - 2.0| = 0.5$$

$$\Delta EN(C - Cl) = |2.5 - 3.0| = 0.5$$

$$\Delta EN(C - F) = |2.5 - 4.0| = 1.5$$

$$\Delta EN(C - I) = |2.5 - 2.5| = 0.0$$

The C-I has a difference of 0, thereby making it nonpolar or the least polar bond.

23. D: Chlorine is more electronegative than hydrogen, so the electron cloud will lean more toward the chlorine atom. The electron cloud or density around the hydrogen atom will be less compared to chlorine. Chlorine will be polarized negative, and hydrogen will be polarized positive. The bond dipole underneath H-Cl shows the correct direction with the cross end on the side of the hydrogen atom and the arrow tip on the side of the chlorine atom.

24. C: Recall that the electronegativity value for an element increases from left to right along a row and bottom to top within a group. Cesium, Cs, is less electronegative than potassium, K, because it is farther down the group (IA). Potassium, K, is less electronegative than gallium, Ga, because it's to the left of gallium. Carbon, C, is more electronegative than gallium, Ga, because it is located one column to the right of Ga and two rows up.

25. C: The atomic radius of Sn > Ge and Ge > As. Therefore, Sn > As. The atomic radius of As > P and P > Cl. Therefore, As > Cl. The atomic radius of Cl > F and F > Ne, making Cl > Ne. Consequently, the order of decreasing atomic radius is Sn > As > Cl > Ne.

26. C: When moving from the lower left to the upper right along the periodic table, the ionization energy increases. Along a row, as the atomic number (Z) increases, so does the ionization energy. Down a column, the ionization energy tends to decrease because the effective nuclear charge decreases. The carbon atom has greater ionization energy than germanium because it is two rows above. Germanium will have a larger first ionization energy than calcium because it is located to the right of calcium. There is an exception in ionization energy when moving across a row from group IIA to IIIA. Gallium, Ga (group IIIA, ns^2np^1), has a smaller ionization energy than calcium (group IIA, ns^2np^0). The smaller ionization energy in group IIIA elements is due to the ease of electron removal from the np^1 orbital.

27. D: Sulfur has the most negative value. Electron affinities (EAs) become more negative when moving left to right along a row on the periodic table. EAs will become more positive when moving down a column for a given group. Therefore, the EA value for aluminum (Al) is more negative than thallium (Tl). Sulfur (S) has an EA value that is more negative than polonium (Po). Because sulfur is located to the right of aluminum, the EA value will be more negative.

28. C: Bromine, phosphorous, and iodine are nonmetals that will gain electrons to form an anion. First, look at each neutral element and find the number of electrons by using the atomic number. For example, magnesium is a metal that has 12 protons and must have 12 electrons to be neutral. However, the answer choice indicates that magnesium exists as a cation with a 2+ charge. The magnesium cation has two fewer electrons, so the total number of electrons is $16 - 2 = 14$. Each nonmetal anion should have additional electrons that are equal to its charge. For example, neutral P has 15 electrons and P^{3-} has 3 additional electrons. The total number of electrons is determined by combining the number of electrons from a neutral atom and the extra electrons from the anion: $15 + 3 = 18$ electrons. Neutral bromine, Br, has 35 electrons, and the bromide anion, Br^- (one extra electron), has 36 electrons ($35 + 1 = 36$). Lastly, neutral iodine has 53 electrons, and I^- has 54 electrons ($53 + 1 = 54$).

29. D: An anion is a negatively-charged element that forms when the neutral element undergoes reduction (electron gain). Metals such as magnesium are more likely to undergo oxidation to obtain a noble gas configuration. Magnesium will form a 2+ charge. Halogens such as iodine and fluorine are nonmetals that will tend to gain one electron to form the respective anions. The charges for fluoride and iodide anions are both 1–, and the reduction of both halogens gives a stable noble gas electron configuration. Oxygen will tend to lose two electrons (reduction) to form an anion with a 2– charge, thereby obtaining a stable neon-like electron configuration.

30. C: Silver has an atomic number (Z) equal to 47. The number located at the top within each element block corresponds to the atomic number and is equal to the number of protons.

Anatomy and Physiology

1. C: Choice *C* is the correct answer since gross anatomy is the study of large structures that can be observed with the human eye. The liver is an example of a large body structure that is visible to the naked eye. Other examples of large body structures include the heart, the lungs, and the kidneys. Choice *A* is incorrect since systemic anatomy refers to the study of structures that comprise a discrete body system. These structures work together to carry out a unique body function (for example, the skeletal muscles in the body). Choice *B* is incorrect because microscopic anatomy is the study of structures on a microscopic scale. Histology involves the study of tissues using a microscope. Choice *D* is incorrect since developmental anatomy is the study of how cells, organs, and tissues in the body undergo a change starting from a germ cell to a parent to its offspring. Developmental anatomy is a field of embryology that covers prenatal and postnatal development.

2. D: Choice *D* is the correct answer choice. An organ is made up of two or more tissues that work together to perform a certain function for the body. For example, the skin (the largest organ in the body) is made up of two layers, the epidermis and the dermis. The epidermis contains tightly packed epithelial cells (tissue), and the dermis is made up of dense, irregular connective tissues that cover the hair follicles, the blood vessels, and the sweat glands. The epidermis acts as a waterproof barrier and prevents infection. The dermis supplies the epidermis with blood. The dermis also contains phagocytes or cells that consume toxins or impurities such as bacteria. Choice *A* is incorrect since a cell is the smallest unit of a living organism, just above the chemical level of structural organization. Choice *B* is incorrect because an organ complex is a group of organs that work together. Choice *C* is incorrect since a tissue complex is a collection of tissues that are associated with each other.

3. C: Choice *C* is correct. The nervous system is a fast-acting control system that responds to external and internal changes. Examples of external changes or stimuli include temperature and pressure changes. Sensory receptors allow for the changes to be detected, and messages are sent through the central nervous system. These messages are sent by electrical signals that are known as nerve impulses. The central nervous system (CNS) consists of the brain and spinal cord. As messages are sent, the CNS assesses the information and responds by initiating body effectors such as glands or muscles. Choice *A* is incorrect since the lymphatics system acts to remove interstitial fluid by returning the fluid to the blood and functions in immunity by cleansing the blood. Choice *B*, the circulatory or cardiovascular system, is not correct since its role is to transport nutrients through the blood through pumping with the heart. Choice *D* is incorrect because the endocrine system is responsible for regulating cell growth, reproduction, and metabolism. Each process is regulated by the secretion of hormones via the glands.

4. A: Choice *A* is correct. The order from most to least complex is endocrine system, organs, tissues, cells, molecules, and atoms. The endocrine system, an organ system, is the most complex system in this list. Organs are less complex than organ systems; they are made up of different types of tissues, and tissues are made up of similar cells. Cells are composed of molecules. For example, the cell wall is composed of a phospholipid bilayer that contains a hydrophobic and hydrophilic region. These phospholipid bilayers consist of molecules that have a hydrocarbon tail and polar head group. Molecules are made up of atoms such as hydrogen, carbon, and nitrogen. Atoms are the lowest and simplest level of the structural organization chain.

5. A: Choice *A* is the correct statement since the anatomical position provides a framework for representing anatomical relationships. When describing the position or location of body parts, another body part is used as a frame of reference. Regardless of the body's position, most terminology refers to the anatomical position and is useful to avoid confusion. Choice *B* is incorrect; there are no studies that demonstrate the anatomical position is the most comfortable. In fact, most people would find that lying in the anatomical position is rather uncomfortable. (Give it a try!) Choice *C* is incorrect since there is no evidence to suggest that the anatomical position would provide a person with better circulation, and the answer choice makes no reference to how the body is positioned in space. A person can be upside down or prone on the floor and still be in the anatomical position. In each scenario, the blood circulation will vary. While Choice *D* is a reasonable answer, it is not the primary reason for using the anatomical position. Other body positions (for example, a position where the wrists are facing backward), can be shown for display, but the anatomical position's purpose is to provide a point of reference.

6. D: Choice *D* is correct since the ventral side of the arm refers to the side of where the radial artery is located. The pulse is taken by placing your index, middle, and ring finger over the radial artery. The carpal or wrist is part of the upper limbs. The posterior term refers to the backside of that body structure. For example, the posterior side of the knee refers to behind the knee. The posterior side of the wrist means behind the wrist. A pulse is typically taken on the ventral or front side of the wrist. The radial artery is found on the ventral side of the wrist. Choice *A* is incorrect since the posterior side of the knee, or the back of the knee, is the most challenging place to take a pulse. The posterior side of the knee contains the popliteal pulse, which is an important vital sign that can help determine the severity of knee or femur injury. Choice *B* is incorrect since the radial artery is not on the dorsal side of the wrist. Choice *C*, the distal end of the arm, would correspond to your fingertips. Taking the heart rate at the fingertip typically requires an instrument such as a fingertip pulse oximeter. There are advantages to taking the pulse at the fingertips. In 2013, a professor at the University of Iowa developed a technique for measuring the stiffness of an aorta. The method works by placing an instrument called a transducer on a finger that contains the brachial artery. Therefore, Choice *C* is not the best answer choice since it requires an instrument.

7. C: The abdominal cavity houses the liver, intestines, and stomach. The abdominal cavity is anterior to the spinal cavity. In other words, the abdominal cavity is toward the front of the body. For Choice *A*, the kidneys and spleen are located in the abdominal cavity, but they are not superficial to the spinal cavity. An organ that is superficial to the vertebrae would be above or more external to the vertebrae. For example, the dorsal plates on a stegosaurus are superficial to the vertebrae. Choice *B* is not correct since the abdominal cavity is not at the backside of the body (posterior); the spinal cavity is at the dorsal or backside of the abdominal cavity. Choice *D*, like Choice *B*, contains organs that are found in the abdominal cavity, but these organs are not posterior to the spinal cavity, so Choice *D* is incorrect.

8. A: Anatomists separate the abdominopelvic region into nine quadrants. The urinary bladder is located in the pubic or hypogastric region. Therefore, Choice *A* is the correct answer. Choices *B* and *D* are not the best choices since they refer to an abdominopelvic region that is divided into four quadrants. The urinary bladder is found in the right lower quadrant and lower left quadrant. Choice *C* correctly uses the nine-quadrant naming convention. However, the umbilical region refers to a region where the small intestine is located. The urinary bladder is found underneath the umbilical region.

9. B: Choice *B* is the correct answer choice (label 4) since it represents connective tissue. Connective tissue supports the epithelial tissue and is visible throughout the micrograph. Notice that the location of the connective tissue (label 4) is slightly more outside the cell compared to the basement membrane (label 3). Therefore, this area must not be part of the epithelium since it has a different shape (is not cuboidal). Choice *A*, label 3, refers to the basement membrane, a structureless material secreted by the epithelial cells. The cuboidal cells sit on the basement membrane. Choice *C*, label 1, and Choice *D*, label 2, are pointed toward the same type of epithelial cells called simple cuboidal.

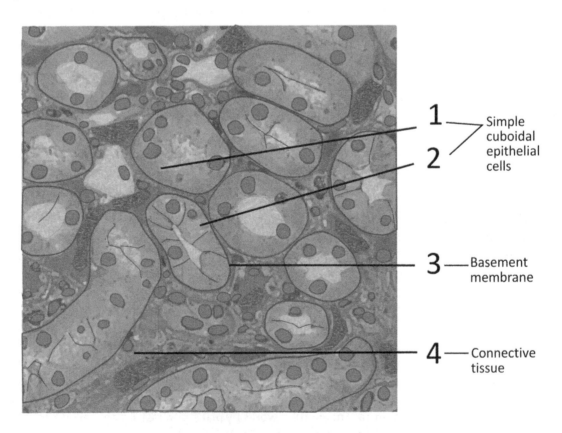

1 — Simple cuboidal epithelial cells

2 —

3 — Basement membrane

4 — Connective tissue

10. D: All the answer choices are types of simple epithelial tissue. The simple columnar epithelium (Choice *D*) is the correct answer choice since it lines the digestive tract in addition to the gallbladder and the excretory ducts of some glands. The simple cuboidal epithelium (Choice *A*) covers the surface of the ovaries and is found on the lining of kidney tubules. It is also found in the pancreatic ducts and salivary ducts. The simple ciliated columnar epithelium lines the uterine tubes and parts of the respiratory tract (Choice *B*). The passage indicates that the epithelial tissue contains goblet cells. Choices *C* and *D* both contain goblet cells. These cells create a lubricating mucus. The pseudostratified ciliated columnar type lines the auditory tubes and respiratory passages (Choice *C*). An abundant amount of mucus is typically needed in the respiratory tract.

11. C: The table below lists the three types of muscles and their corresponding traits.

Muscle Type	Structure and function	Location
Smooth	Found on the walls of hollow internal organs (e.g., the intestine).	The fibers are spindle-shaped and elongated. Each fiber has a single nucleus. Muscle contraction is slow and involuntary.
Skeletal	Found along the bones and joint of the skeleton/tendons.	The fibers are striated, cylindrically shaped, and arranged in slender bundles called fasciculi. Muscle contraction is both involuntary and voluntary (for example, joints of a skeleton).
Cardiac	Only along the wall of the heart.	Striated fiber with one nucleus. The fibers are branched and have intercalated discs. Muscle contraction is rapid/rhythmic and involuntary.

Choice *C* is the correct answer because skeletal muscles are the only type of multinucleated muscle fibers. Skeletal muscle cells are multinucleated due to the fusion of several myoblasts. Because these cells are multinucleated, large amounts of proteins and enzymes can be produced. Skeletal muscles are constantly undergoing contractions, so they require more energy. Consequently, muscle fibers (along the skeleton) generate more heat. For example, during exercise, the skeletal muscles break down more ATP and produce more heat.

12. D: The correct answer is Choice *D*. Lamina propria is a soft type of areolar connective tissue that is found underneath the mucosal epithelium. It is a fluid matrix that appears to be empty when viewed through a microscope. This tissue provides a reservoir of water and salts to nearby tissues. It's a fluid tissue and can soak up excess fluid like a sponge when inflamed. In a condition known as edema, the tissue becomes puffy or swells because it soaks up fluid. Choice *A* is incorrect since osseous tissue or bone tissue is composed of bone cells (osteocytes) inside cavities or pits (lacunae). This tissue is relatively hard since its matrix contains calcium salts and collagen fibers. Choice *B* is incorrect because dense fibrous tissue, as its name implies, is dense because it's crowded with fibroblasts between the collagen fiber matrix. Choice *C* is incorrect because hyaline cartilage contains an abundance of collagen fibers embedded in a rubbery matrix that does not uptake fluid but can solidify over time. For example, a skeleton of a fetus is made up of hyaline cartilage. After a baby is born, much of that cartilage is replaced by bone.

13. B: Choice *B* is correct because neuroglia, or glial cells, are the supporting cells that assist neurons. Neurons respond to stimuli as Choice *C* states. Neuroglia are specialized cells in the nerves, brain, and spinal cord that support and protect the nervous system. A neuron photomicrograph illustrates how the nuclei of the neuroglia are abundant and widely dispersed. These specialized cells act as an insulating medium for the delicate neurons.

14. D: Choice *D* is the correct answer choice. Tendons are a tough type of fibrous connective tissue. They connect the muscle to the bone and can withstand tension or contraction. Choice *A* is incorrect since hyaline cartilage is found throughout a few parts of the body. It makes up the trachea and connects the ribs to the breastbone. This cartilage is most abundant in the skeleton of a fetus. Choice *B* is incorrect and refers to a type of bone cell found in bone tissue. Choice *C*, adipose tissue, or fat, is a type of loose connective tissue. It is found underneath the skin and provides protection for organs like the kidneys, which are cushioned by fat capsules.

15. B: Choice *B* is correct. Our bodies cannot produce or store vitamin C. Vitamin C has many functions, which include wound healing; stimulation of the immune system; and maintenance of the teeth, cartilage, and bones. Therefore, it is important to consume vitamin C daily from food sources. The daily recommended amount of vitamin C for an adult is about 65 to 90 mg. Answer choices *A*, *C*, and *D* are all functions of the integumentary system.

16. D: Choice *D* is the correct answer choice. The stratum corneum makes up the outer coat of our body and protects deeper cells from water loss and hostile environments. These types of cells are dead and contain membranous sacs that are filled with keratin. The stratum corneum flakes off our skin and is commonly known as dandruff. Choice *A*, the stratum basale, is incorrect since it is the most underlying structure of the epidermis. Choice *B* is incorrect since the epidermis is made up of the stratum corneum, the stratum granulosum, stratum spinosum, and the stratum basale. Choice *C* is the stratum spinosum and is deep to the stratum corneum but is superficial to the stratum basale.

17. C: The correct statement is Choice *C*. Keratin is the fibrous protein that is found in the epidermis. In the keratinocytes it takes the form of bundled filaments. It is used to form specialized tissues (for example, hair and nails). Keratinocytes produce keratin; they migrate from the stratum spinosum and become the granular cells that are found in the stratum granulosum. There are typically one or more layers of these granular cells that contain shriveled nuclei.

18. D: The correct answer is Choice *D*. The stratum basale is the structural layer that contains stem cells, where mitosis occurs. The basale layer connects to the dermis along a wavy or corrugated border. It looks somewhat similar to a wavy river on a map. Choice *A* is incorrect and points to the stratum granulosum. Choice *C* is incorrect and points to the stratum corneum, the layer that contains membranous sacs containing keratin and glycolipids in an extracellular space. Choice *D* points to a region of the dermis called the reticular layer, the deepest skin layer. The reticular layer is made up of dense irregular tissue, sweat glands, oil glands, blood vessels, and pressure receptors called lamellar corpuscles.

19. B: Choice *B* is the correct answer choice. The papillary dermis is made up of loose areolar connective tissue that contains fingerlike projections called papillae. The papillae contain networks of blood capillaries. These nipple-like extensions appear as epidermal or papillary ridges (called fingerprints) at the surface of the skin. If the dermal papillae of the foot were even and lacked peg-like projections, then the papillary layer would not have any indentations. Since the dermis is connected to the epidermis, then the epidermal surface would be smoother and lack ridges. Because there is less surface area at the epidermal surface, the friction between your feet and the smooth surface would be reduced. Therefore, your ability to grip the floor with your feet would be decreased, making it easier to slip (because the surface is smoother). Choice *A* is incorrect; the epidermis is avascular because capillaries are found in the dermal layer. Choice *C* is incorrect because if your epidermis had more ridges, then the friction would increase (not decrease). Choice *D* is incorrect because if there were fewer ridges, then the friction between your feet and floor would decrease (not increase). Note that Choices *C* and *D* assume that an "even" dermal papillae would contribute to more capillary loops. However, this statement is contradictory since these "loops" contribute to whorled ridges on the epidermal surface, thereby resulting in an epidermal surface that would have more ridges.

20. A: Choice *A* is the correct answer choice. The reticular layer, in addition to the papillary layer, is part of the dermal layer and is made up of collagen and elastic fibers. Over time the number of elastic and collagen fibers decreases, resulting in less structural support in the dermal layer. Consequently, the epidermal surface becomes more ridged or wrinkled. Choices *B* and *D* are incorrect since they are part of the epidermal layer and do not contain collagen or elastic fibers. Choice *C*, the hypodermis, is found deep to the dermal layer and is composed of adipose tissue that stores fat.

21. A: The correct answer choice is Choice *A*, the facet. Indentations are a type of bone marking that can be categorized as projections or depressions. The facet is a type of projection that forms a joint. It is located at the end of a rib and has a smooth, flat surface. For example, the superior costal facet (the head of the rib) makes contact with the body of the thoracic vertebrae. Choices *B* and *C* are incorrect since they are classified as depressions. Choice *B*, the groove, is a depression found in the inner mandible that lies near the lower molars. Choice *C*, the notch, is also found on the upper border of the mandible. Choice *D*, the condyle or condylar, is a round projection that lies adjacent to the mandibular notch. Like a facet, it helps to form joints.

22. D: Choice *D*, or label 1, the lamellae, is the correct answer choice. Lamella are arranged in concentric circles and contain collagen fibers in a parallel array. Choice *A*, or label 3, corresponds to the Haversian canal. These are the tubes or canals located at the center of the osteon. Choice *B*, or label 4, refers to the Canaliculus or canaliculi. The canaliculi are small channels or ducts that connect to the osteocytes thereby allowing nutrients to be supplied to these cells. Choice *C*, or label 2, is the lacunae, which are small cavities that are situated between the lamellae. Under a microscope, the lacunae appear as oblong spaces and opaque spots.

23. C: Choice *C* is correct since skeletal muscles contain several types of connective tissue. The fascicle is a bundle of muscle fiber cells wrapped together. The perimysium wraps and contains several fascicles. The epimysium, the toughest overcoat, covers the perimysium. Choices *A* and *B* are incorrect. Both smooth muscle and cardiac muscle contain one protective covering, called the endomysium, and they are less elaborate than the skeletal muscle. Choice *D* is incorrect and equivalent to Choice *A*. Smooth muscle, Choice *A*, is a type of muscle that has no striations.

24. B: The correct answer is Choice *B*. The correct order of layers, outer to inner, is the epimysium, perimysium, and the endomysium. The figure below illustrates the three different sheaths of the skeletal muscle fibers. Note that the term "endo" means "inner" or "within." The term "peri" means around or about, and "epi" means "over." The three connective tissue layers of the skeletal muscle are essential for integrity and support, especially when these muscles are contractive or moving in a voluntary manner. The cardiac and smooth muscles don't have several layers of connective tissue; as they are involuntary, they do not undergo fast contractions and are not subjected to large forces.

25. B: The correct answer choice is Choice B, the H zone. The H zone is the light zone at the center of the sarcomere as illustrated in the microscope (muscle relaxed). During contraction, the H zone, located at the center of the A band disappears, causing the Z discs to come closer to the thick filaments. The H zone disappears since the actin and myosin filaments overlap with each other completely. Choice A, the I band, is incorrect since the I bands are still visible but have reduced in length. Choice C is incorrect because the Z disc is still visible in the microscope image. Choice D, the A band, is also incorrect since it is still visible in the microscope image and does not change in length or changes minimally.

26. A: The correct answer is Choice A. Actin is a contractile protein that makes up the thin filaments in the sarcomere. The thin filaments are attached to the Z disc or Z line. Choice B, the protein myosin, is incorrect since these are bundled molecules that make up the thick filaments. Choice C, a sarcomere, is the entire contractile structure (which is made of the contractile proteins actin and myosin) and is not the correct answer choice. Choice D is incorrect. Titin is a protein that is greater than one micrometer in length and acts as a molecular spring. Titin keeps myosin molecules in place and gives muscle its elasticity. Although titin is attached to the Z disc or line, it is considered an elastic protein.

27. B: The correct answer is Choice B. Your nervous system integrates the red light as a signal to stop. Choices A and C are incorrect since these are examples of sensory input. Sensory receptors monitor changes that include, for instance, a change in color, temperature, or pressure. Choice D is incorrect and refers to the results of the integration process that lead to motor output. The brain interprets red as "stop"; therefore, you press your foot (motor output) on the brake pedal to stop.

28. D: The skeletal muscle, Choice D, is the correct answer choice. The somatic nervous system is one subdivision of the efferent or motor division. The somatic system allows voluntary control of our skeletal muscles, except for skeletal muscle reflexes. Choice A is incorrect; a blood vessel is an example of a smooth muscle and is part of the autonomic subdivision and sympathetic nervous systems. Smooth muscles, such as blood vessels, are involuntarily controlled. Choice B is incorrect since a gland is an effector organ that belongs to the autonomic and sympathetic nervous systems. Choice C, the cardiac muscle, is part of the autonomic and parasympathetic nervous systems.

29. C: The microglia is represented by selection 4, so Choice C is the correct answer. Microglia are spiderlike phagocytes and are next to neuron cells. Choice A, selection 2, is incorrect and represents an astrocyte that contains swollen ends that cling to neurons and wrap around blood capillaries. These swollen ends are not seen in the microglia cells. Choice B, selection 1, is incorrect and represents several ependymal cells that line the brain and spinal cord. These cells contain cilia, unlike other glial cells, that face the fluid-filled cavity. Choice D, selection 3, is incorrect and represents an oligodendrocyte. These cells contain myelin sheaths that wrap around the nerve fibers.

30. B: Choice B is the correct answer choice. Astrocytes have a significant role in controlling the chemical environment in the brain, mainly since they are anchored to the blood capillaries and neurons. Therefore, astrocytes have a definite function in neuronal support and protection. Researchers have highlighted how astrocytes can play a role in the handling of excess protein. Astrocytes are involved in the transport of proteins and the removal of toxic byproducts that move across the blood-brain barrier.

A large body of evidence that indicates astrocytes play a role in the secretion of amyloid-beta or "beta-amyloid 42." Beta-amyloid can promote chronic inflammation and neuronal death in the brain. Astrocytes normally reduce the amount of toxic or excess proteins. However, these proteins can react with the astrocyte and reduce its function. For example, when a certain threshold of the toxic protein is reached, it causes the death of surrounding astrocytes and neurons, thereby resulting in the formation of plaques. Consequently, as neurons are injured or die throughout the brain, neuron networks fall apart, and brain regions shrink in size. In the final stage of Alzheimer's, called brain atrophy, there is a significant loss in brain volume. Choice *A* is incorrect because it refers to several types of glial cells such as the oligodendrocyte. Choice *C* is incorrect since the Schwann cell's major function is to protect the nerve fibers by forming a myelin sheath. Choice *D* is incorrect because the neuron is not a supporting cell.

Practice Test #2

Mathematics

1. Write 0.081 as a fraction.
   a. $\dfrac{81}{100}$
   b. $\dfrac{81}{1000}$
   c. $\dfrac{81}{10000}$
   d. $\dfrac{8.1}{100}$

2. Write 33.75 as a fraction.
   a. $\dfrac{3375}{100}$
   b. $\dfrac{135}{1000}$
   c. $\dfrac{135}{4}$
   d. $\dfrac{3375}{1000}$

3. Write $\dfrac{567}{1000}$ as a decimal.
   a. 0.567
   b. 5.67
   c. 0.0567
   d. 56.7

4. Write $\dfrac{56790}{100}$ as a decimal.
   a. 5.679
   b. 56.79
   c. 567.9
   d. 5679

5. Which number is the largest?
   a. -5.678
   b. -5.6781
   c. -5.677
   d. -5.681

6. Round 8.56789 to the nearest thousandths place.
   a. 8.567
   b. 8.568
   c. 8.5679
   d. 8.57

7. Which number is the largest?

    a. 1.219

    b. 1.2189

    c. 1.2191

    d. 1.2192

8. Round -6.899 to the nearest hundredth.

    a. -6.89

    b. -6.9

    c. -6.99

    d. -7

9. Round 15.7890 to the nearest one.

    a. 15

    b. 20

    c. 15.8

    d. 16

10. Write $\frac{17}{25}$ as a decimal.

    a. 0.17

    b. 0.68

    c. 0.25

    d. 0.1725

11. Write $\frac{2}{9}$ as a decimal.

    a. 0.2

    b. 0.22

    c. 0.222

    d. $0.\overline{2}$

12. Write $\frac{7}{24}$ as a decimal, rounding to the nearest hundredth.

    a. 0.292

    b. 0.29

    c. 0.2917

    d. 0.2916

13. Express the ratio 18 to 40 in fraction form.

    a. $\frac{18}{40}$

    b. $\frac{40}{18}$

    c. $\frac{9}{20}$

    d. $\frac{20}{9}$

14. Mike traveled 565 miles in 9.5 hours. What was his speed in miles per hour? Round to the nearest tenth.

    a. 60 mph

    b. 59.4 mph

    c. 59.5 mph

    d. 0.1 mph

15. Which is the best buy?

    a. 16 ounces of coffee for $8.99

    b. 24 ounces of coffee for $11.99

    c. 32 ounces of coffee for $16.99

    d. 40 ounces of coffee for $20.99

16. Solve the proportion $\frac{x}{7} = \frac{5}{54}$.

    a. $\frac{35}{54}$

    b. $\frac{54}{35}$

    c. 35

    d. 54

17. Solve the proportion $\frac{9.1}{y} = \frac{3}{2.1}$.

    a. 0.69

    b. 6.37

    c. 3.73

    d. 11.2

18. A 12-pound ham contains 15 servings of meat. How many pounds of ham should be purchased for a dinner party in which 60 servings are needed?

    a. 24

    b. 36

    c. 38

    d. 48

19. On a map, 0.5 in. represents 75 mi. Mike needs to drive 90 mi to pick up his grandmother. How many inches on the map would represent this distance?

    a. 0.6

    b. 0.4

    c. 0.75

    d. 2

20. A biologist wants to estimate the number of fish in a lake. On a single day, the biologist catches 214 fish, tags them, and returns them back into the lake. On another day, 92 fish are caught, and 18 of them are tagged. Using the same proportion, approximately how many fish are in the lake? Round your answer to the nearest whole number.

    a. 1,094

    b. 41

    c. 42

    d. 8

21. A building casts a shadow that is 14 ft long. At the same time of day, a tree that is 12 ft tall casts a shadow that is 4 ft long. What is the height of the building?
    a. 5 ft
    b. 36 ft
    c. 42 ft
    d. 12 ft

22. The following two triangles are similar. Find the missing side length a.

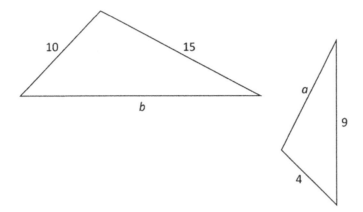

    a. 4
    b. 6
    c. 8
    d. 12

23. How many inches are in 9.5 ft?
    a. 114 in.
    b. 108 in.
    c. 120 in.
    d. 95 in.

24. How many yards are in 6 miles?
    a. 10,560 yd
    b. 31,680 yd
    c. 10,000 yd
    d. 17,520 yd

25. How many meters are in a kilometer?
    a. 100
    b. 1,000
    c. 10,000
    d. 100,000

26. Complete the following conversion: 56.78 cm = ___ mm.
    a. 0.5678
    b. 5.678
    c. 567.8
    d. 5,678

27. Complete the following conversion: 34,598 cm = ____ km.
    a. 3.4598
    b. 0.34598
    c. 0.034598
    d. 34.598

28. How many cm are there in 3 ft? Round your answer to the nearest tenth.
    a. 91
    b. 7.6
    c. 91.4
    d. 16.8

29. Complete the following conversion: 18 gal = _____ oz.
    a. 1,502
    b. 1,024
    c. 2,304
    d. 3,712

30. How many quarts are in 8,490 cups?
    a. 2,122.5
    b. 2,123
    c. 2,122
    d. 4,245

31. How many cc of an oral medicine are in 750 mL of that same medicine?
    a. 75
    b. 7.5
    c. 7,500
    d. 750

32. How many liters are in 7,500 milliliters?
    a. 7.5
    b. 75
    c. 75,000
    d. 0.75

33. How many pounds are in 4 tons?
    a. 4,000
    b. 6,000
    c. 8,000
    d. 10,000

34. How many ounces are in 8 pounds?
    a. 16 ounces
    b. 64 ounces
    c. 0.5 ounces
    d. 128 ounces

35. Complete the following conversion: 89,452 g = _____ kg.
  a. 8.9452
  b. 89.452
  c. 894.52
  d. 8,945.2

36. Complete the following conversion: 675.2 g = _____ mg.
  a. 0.6752
  b. 67.52
  c. 67,520
  d. 675,200

37. What is the freezing point of water?
  a. 0°F
  b. 0°C
  c. 32°C
  d. 100°C

38. Convert 214°F to Celsius. Round to the nearest tenth.
  a. 101°C
  b. 101.1°C
  c. 417.2°C
  d. 417°C

39. Convert 45°C to Fahrenheit.
  a. 7°F
  b. 7.2°F
  c. 114°F
  d. 113°F

40. Write the number 3,786 in Roman numerals.
  a. MMMDCCLXXXVI
  b. MMDCCLXXXVI
  c. MMMCCLXXVI
  d. MMMCCCLXXVI

41. Write the number 2,765 in Roman numerals.
  a. MMDCLXV
  b. MDCCLXV
  c. MMDCCLXV
  d. MDCCCLXV

42. What is 8:45 p.m. in military time?
  a. 0845
  b. 08:45
  c. 1245
  d. 2045

43. Convert 1530, a military time, to standard time.
    a. 3:30 a.m.
    b. 3:30 p.m.
    c. 2:30 p.m.
    d. 5:30 p.m.

44. A doctor orders a nurse to administer 375 mg of an oral medication one time a day to her patient. One tablet of this medication is equal to 150 mg. How many tablets should she give the patient each day?
    a. 2
    b. 3
    c. 2.5
    d. 4

45. A doctor's order to a patient is for her to receive 125 mg of a cough syrup p.o. once a day. The label on the medicine states that the syrup is 25 mg/ml. How many ml should the patient be receiving each day?
    a. 3
    b. 4
    c. 5
    d. 6

46. Convert 0.00005 to a percent.
    a. 0.005%
    b. 0.05%
    c. 0.5%
    d. 5%

47. Convert 0.04% to a decimal.
    a. 0.4
    b. 0.004
    c. 0.04
    d. 0.0004

48. What is 95% of 1,895?
    a. 2,229.4
    b. 1,800.25
    c. 2,000
    d. 1,795

49. 45% of what value is 38?
    a. 17.1
    b. 50
    c. 84.$\overline{4}$
    d. 92.2

50. 65 is what percent of 140? Round your answer to the nearest tenth of a percent.
    a. 4.6%
    b. 0.5%
    c. 46.4%
    d. 6.5%

51. If $x = 5$ and $y = 7$, evaluate $5x^3 - 4y^2$.
    a. 429
    b. 1,615
    c. -71
    d. 821

52. Solve the equation $8x + 5 = 69$ for x.
    a. 5
    b. 6
    c. 7
    d. 8

53. Solve the equation $12(x - 9) = 120$ for x.
    a. 10
    b. 1
    c. 11
    d. 19

54. Solve the equation $1.1y + 7.2 = 18.2$ for y.
    a. 1
    b. 10
    c. 100
    d. 5

55. If $x = 2$ and $y = 4$, evaluate $2x^2 + 8y^3$.
    a. 136
    b. 516
    c. 520
    d. 736

Reading Comprehension

Questions 1–5 are based on the following passage:

Although the number of movies with tobacco incidents remained stable during 2010–2018, the number of tobacco incidents within these movies increased, including a 120% increase in PG-13 movies. Although the number of PG-13 fictional movies with tobacco incidents declined substantially during 2010–2018, the number of PG-13 biographical dramas with tobacco incidents approximately tripled. The total number of PG-13 movies in both these genres with tobacco incidents approximately doubled since 2010; approximately 80% of all tobacco incidents in 2018 occurred in PG-13 biographical dramas. These findings suggest that the increasing number of youth-rated biographical dramas with tobacco incidents has negated previous progress made in reducing tobacco incidents in youth-rated fictional movies.

All major motion picture companies have policies to reduce tobacco depictions in youth-rated movies; however, Disney and Viacom were the only companies with no tobacco use in youth-rated movies in 2018. Paid placement of tobacco brands is prohibited in media such as movies, television, and video games by the 1998 Master Settlement Agreement between states and tobacco companies. Public health groups have suggested interventions to reduce tobacco imagery in movies, such as the Motion Picture Association of America assigning an R rating to any movie with tobacco imagery, unless it portrays an actual historical figure who used tobacco or depicts the negative effects of tobacco use. Research suggests that such an R rating, in coordination with additional interventions, could help eliminate tobacco incidents in youth-rated movies and reduce youth cigarette smoking by an estimated 18%.

Establishing the impact of youths' exposure to tobacco imagery through movies (as well as original programming on television, streaming and on-demand services, and social media) and the effects of this exposure on youths' tobacco use is important. A recent survey of streaming content popular with young persons and analysis of two full seasons of fourteen programs identified at least one tobacco incident in 86% of programs, even as tobacco incidents have begun to decline in fictional theatrical feature films. Reducing the reach of tobacco incidents in streaming and other media platforms is essential to protect youths from exposures that can normalize tobacco use. Continued research will be necessary to understand how this exposure affects youth tobacco initiation and use.

Tobacco related incidents in youth-rated movies remained common, particularly in biographical dramas. The majority of persons using tobacco in these biographical dramas were fictional figures, not historical. Studios could limit tobacco use in biographical dramas to real persons who actually used tobacco. Other evidence-based solutions could be implemented by producers and distributors of youth-rated entertainment to reduce the public health risk caused by exposure to on-screen tobacco imagery. For example, assigning all movies with tobacco incidents an R rating could eliminate tobacco product imagery from youth-rated films, which could further reduce initiation of tobacco product use among U.S. youths.

Tynan MA, Polansky JR, Driscoll D, Garcia C, Glantz SA. Tobacco Use in Top-Grossing Movies — United States, 2010–2018. MMWR Morb Mortal Wkly Rep 2019;68:974–978.DOI: http://dx.doi.org/10.15585/mmwr.mm6843a4

1. Public groups have suggested an R rating for movies that include any tobacco use unless:
   a. The tobacco user is the "bad guy"
   b. The tobacco user is unlikeable
   c. The tobacco user is a historical figure who used tobacco
   d. The tobacco user is over the age of twenty-one

2. What is the main idea of this passage?
   a. Tobacco usage in movies should be banned to decrease smoking in young Americans.
   b. Movies depicting tobacco usage should be rated R to decrease exposure to tobacco incidents.
   c. Most television programs and movies targeting youths include incidents of tobacco usage among main characters.
   d. Increases in tobacco usage in youth-rated movies has negated progress and must be addressed to decrease youth smoking.

3. Tobacco incidents from 2010-2018 tripled in what kind of films?

    a. Biography

    b. Comedy

    c. Horror

    d. Action

4. According to the passage, what is the danger of failing to limit youth exposure to tobacco incidents in film/television?

    a. It will be featured in more movies/shows.

    b. There is no specified danger to be concerned with.

    c. It normalizes tobacco usage.

    d. Movies/television will soon include vaping.

5. How many motion picture companies have formalized an effort to decrease tobacco use in films marketed towards teens and children?

    a. Two

    b. All

    c. None

    d. Only Disney

Questions 6–10 are based on the following passage:

Cancer survivors aged eighteen to sixty-four years in the United States had higher annual out-of-pocket expenditures and were more likely to report higher out-of-pocket burden than were persons without a cancer history. Further, approximately one-fourth of cancer survivors reported having material financial hardship, and one third reported having psychological financial hardship associated with cancer, its treatment, or late and lasting effects of treatment. These findings are consistent with other evidence suggesting that cancer survivors experience substantial financial difficulties coping with the costs of health care.

In 2009, the American Society of Clinical Oncology's Cost of Care Task Force identified the critical role of oncologists in addressing out-of-pocket costs of cancer care with their patients. Subsequently, in 2013, the National Academies of Science, Engineering, and Medicine (NASEM) described affordable health care as a component of high-quality cancer care. In 2014, NASEM highlighted the issue of rising cancer drug costs and patient access to affordable and effective drug therapies. The 2018 President's Cancer Panel report, Promoting Value, Affordability, and Innovation in Cancer Drug Treatment, further emphasized the importance of affordability. These reports and findings from the current study reflect the growing evidence that financial hardship might negatively affect survivors' health and well-being.

Access to health insurance coverage has been identified as essential to providing affordable cancer care by the American Society of Clinical Oncology and NASEM. Substantial evidence links health insurance coverage with positive health outcomes among cancer survivors. In this study, uninsured cancer survivors had lower out-of-pocket spending than did survivors with private insurance coverage, but that spending represented a larger proportion of family income. Lack of health insurance coverage was also strongly associated with both material and psychological financial hardship. Many cancer survivors with private insurance coverage even reported borrowing money, being unable to cover their share of medical care costs, going into debt, or filing for bankruptcy.

This report used the most recent national data available to present evidence of substantial out-of-pocket expenditure, out-of-pocket burden, and financial hardship among cancer survivors aged eighteen to sixty-four years. The number of Americans with a history of cancer is projected to increase in the next decade, and the economic burden associated with living with a cancer diagnosis will likely increase as well. The findings in this report might lead to increased awareness in all sectors of the public health and medical community that the rising cost of cancer care is a major barrier to survivors' well-being. Efforts at the provider, practice, employer, payer, state, and federal levels are needed to develop and implement evidence-based and sustainable interventions (e.g., including systematic screening for financial hardship at cancer diagnosis and throughout the cancer care trajectory, integrating discussions about the potential for adverse financial consequences of treatments in shared treatment decision-making, and linking patients and survivors to available resources) to minimize financial hardship for cancer survivors.

Ekwueme DU, Zhao J, Rim SH, et al. Annual Out-of-Pocket Expenditures and Financial Hardship Among Cancer Survivors Aged 18–64 Years — United States, 2011–2016. MMWR Morb Mortal Wkly Rep 2019;68:494–499. DOI: http://dx.doi.org/10.15585/mmwr.mm6822a2

6. Cancer patients with private insurance coverage reported which of the following?
    a. Full coverage for treatment
    b. Filing for bankruptcy
    c. Better overall standard of care
    d. Difficulty communicating with insurers

7. The findings in this report will hopefully do which of the following?
    a. Raise awareness about the lack of health care options for cancer survivors.
    b. Raise awareness about the projected increase in the number of Americans with history of cancer.
    c. Raise awareness about the economic hardships faced by cancer survivors to encourage interventions.
    d. Help cancer survivors find funding sources to cover out of pocket expenses related to treatment.

8. Approximately what percentage of cancer survivors reported material financial hardship?
    a. 50%
    b. 66%
    c. 75%
    d. 25%

9. Based on the passage, what type of screening should be completed in conjunction with cancer diagnosis?
    a. Genetic/family history
    b. Insurance eligibility
    c. Financial hardship
    d. Medical history

10. Based on context, in the final paragraph, final sentence, what does the word *adverse* mean?
    a. Harmful
    b. Minimal
    c. Measured
    d. Immense

Each year during 2012–2016, an estimated average of 34,800 human papillomavirus (HPV)-attributable cancers were diagnosed in the United States, and 92% (32,100) were attributable to the HPV types targeted by 9vHPV. Previous annual estimates of cancers attributable to the types targeted by 9vHPV were 28,500 for 2008–2012, 30,000 for 2010–2014, and 31,200 for 2011–2015. The higher estimates in more recent years are, in part, due to an aging and growing population and increases in oropharyngeal, anal, and vulvar cancers.

HPV vaccination is an important component of cancer prevention, yet only about half of adolescents are up-to-date on this vaccine. The Advisory Committee on Immunization Practices recommends routine HPV vaccination at ages eleven or twelve years and catch-up HPV vaccination for all persons through age twenty-six years. Catch-up vaccination is not recommended for all adults aged older than twenty-six years because the benefit of HPV vaccination decreases in older age groups; however, vaccination based on shared clinical decision-making can be considered for some persons aged twenty-seven to forty-five years who are not adequately vaccinated. In 2018, HPV vaccination coverage varied by state, and no state met the Healthy People 2020 objective for HPV vaccination (receipt of two or three doses of HPV vaccine by 80% of adolescents aged thirteen to fifteen years). State efforts to meet the Healthy People 2020 objective for HPV vaccination could reduce geographic disparities in HPV-associated cancer incidence in the future.

Cervical cancer is the only HPV-associated cancer for which screening is routinely recommended. Recommendations state that women aged twenty-one to sixty-five years be screened regularly for cervical precancers and cancers. Women aged twenty-one to twenty-nine years should be screened with the Papanicolaou (Pap) test every three years. Women aged thirty to sixty-five years can be screened with one of three strategies: Pap test every three years, HPV test every five years, or both a Pap and HPV test every five years. Regardless of screening strategy, all abnormal test results require follow-up of abnormal results and appropriate treatment. The Healthy People 2020 target for cervical cancer screening coverage is 93%; however, in 2015 only 81% of women aged twenty-one to sixty-five years reported receiving a Pap test within the past three years; coverage was lower among Asians, Hispanics, non–U.S. born, and uninsured women.

Progression from persistent HPV infection to precancers and eventually invasive cancer occurs over many years, so it might be too soon to see the effects of HPV vaccination on invasive cancers. However, several studies have demonstrated the population-level impact of HPV vaccination in the United States, including a reduction in the prevalence of vaccine-type HPV infection and rates of high-grade cervical precancers in women aged less than twenty-five years. Cervical cancer rates declined 1.6% per year during 1999–2015, largely because of screening, although decreases among the youngest age group of women might be due in part to HPV vaccination.

Among the 43,999 HPV-associated cancers that occur each year in the United States, an estimated 34,800 are attributable to HPV, including 32,100 attributable to HPV types targeted by 9vHPV. During 2018, only half of adolescents were up to date on HPV vaccination. Surveillance for HPV-associated cancers using population-based cancer registries with high-quality data and the assessment of HPV-attributable cancers can be used to monitor the long-term impact of HPV vaccination and current cervical cancer screening strategies in the United

States. The examination of state-level data enables states to plan for and monitor the impact of vaccination and cervical cancer screening.

Senkomago V, Henley SJ, Thomas CC, Mix JM, Markowitz LE, Saraiya M. Human Papillomavirus–Attributable Cancers — United States, 2012–2016. MMWR Morb Mortal Wkly Rep 2019;68:724–728. DOI: http://dx.doi.org/10.15585/mmwr.mm6833a3

11. What number of adolescents are up to date on HPV vaccines?
    a. Less than 10%
    b. More than 75%
    c. About half
    d. Almost none

12. How many states met the Healthy People 2020 objective for HPV vaccination?
    a. Five
    b. None
    c. Almost half
    d. All

13. Regular screening is routinely recommended for which cancer associated with HPV?
    a. Oropharyngeal
    b. Cervical
    c. Vulvar
    d. Anal

14. Why are catch-up vaccinations not recommended for adults twenty-six and older?
    a. The efficacy has not been studied completely.
    b. The chances of exposure have increased significantly.
    c. Too much time between the first and second doses renders it ineffective.
    d. The benefit decreases the older one gets.

15. What is the topic of this passage?
    a. HPV
    b. Cancer
    c. Screenings
    d. Vaccinations

Questions 16–20 are based on the following passage:

Obesity negatively affects children's health because of its associations with cardiovascular disease risk factors, type 2 diabetes, asthma, fatty liver disease, victimization stemming from social stigma and bullying, and poor mental health (e.g., anxiety and depression). Children who are overweight or obese in early childhood are approximately four times as likely to be overweight or obese in young adulthood as their normal weight peers. Obesity prevalence is especially high among children from low-income families. In 2010, the overall upward trend in obesity prevalence turned downward among children aged two to four years enrolled in the Special Supplemental Nutrition Program for Women, Infants, and Children (WIC), a program of the U.S. Department of Agriculture (USDA); prevalence decreased significantly in all racial/ethnic groups and in thirty-four of the fifty-six WIC state or territory agencies during 2010–2014. A more recent study among young children enrolled in WIC reported that the overall obesity prevalence decreased from 15.9% in 2010 to 13.9% in 2016 and statistically significant decreases were observed in all age, sex, and racial/ethnic subgroups. However, this study did not provide obesity trends at the state level. In collaboration with USDA, the Center for Disease Control (CDC) used data from the WIC Participant and Program Characteristics (WIC PC) to update state-specific trends through 2016. During 2010–2016, modest but statistically significant decreases in obesity prevalence among children aged two to four years enrolled in WIC occurred in forty-one (73%) of fifty-six WIC state or territory agencies. Comprehensive approaches that create positive changes to promote healthy eating and physical activity for young children from all income levels, strengthen nutrition education and breastfeeding support among young children enrolled in WIC, and encourage redemptions of healthy foods in WIC food packages could help maintain or accelerate these declining trends.

Adjusted obesity prevalence decreased by greater than three percentage points in seven WIC state or territory agencies (Guam, New Jersey, New Mexico, Northern Mariana Islands, Puerto Rico, Utah, and Virginia); the largest significant decrease was in Puerto Rico, where adjusted obesity prevalence among WIC beneficiaries aged two to four years decreased by 8.2 percentage points from 2010 to 2016. Only three WIC state agencies reported significant increases in obesity prevalence across all years; adjusted obesity prevalence increased by 0.5 percentage points in Alabama, 0.6 percentage points in North Carolina, and 2.2 percentage points in West Virginia.

Pan L, Blanck HM, Park S, et al. State-Specific Prevalence of Obesity Among Children Aged 2–4 Years Enrolled in the Special Supplemental Nutrition Program for Women, Infants, and Children — United States, 2010–2016. MMWR Morb Mortal Wkly Rep 2019;68:1057–1061. DOI: http://dx.doi.org/10.15585/mmwr.mm6846a3external icon

16. What impact did WIC have on obesity?
    a. Obesity prevalence in children decreased.
    b. Obesity prevalence in children increased.
    c. Obesity prevalence in children decreased then increased.
    d. There was no way to track this data.

17. Which of these is a change recommended to accelerate the obesity trend seen with WIC thus far?
    a. Increase the number of children eligible
    b. Strengthen nutrition education
    c. Expand the program to include older children as well
    d. Provide nutrition coaches to regions to work with WIC families

18. What is the main idea of this passage?
    a. Obesity is an issue in American children.
    b. WIC is a program that provides healthy food for women and children.
    c. Young children benefit most from the WIC program.
    d. WIC has successfully decreased obesity levels in children and could do more.

19. WIC is a program sponsored by whom?
    a. USDA (United States Department of Agriculture)
    b. CDC (Center for Disease Control)
    c. It is its own entity (WIC is WIC)
    d. HHS (Health and Human Services)

20. Obesity is associated with which health issue?
    a. Increased cancer risk
    b. Type 1 Diabetes
    c. Fatty liver disease
    d. Osgood-Schlatter disease

Questions 21–25 are based on the following passage:

To reach the Million Hearts 2022 goal of preventing one million acute cardiovascular events over five years, substantial progress is needed in reducing Cardiovascular Disease-related (CVD) risk factors. To achieve needed progress, Million Hearts 2022 has set clinical targets of 80% performance on the ABCS of CVD prevention: **a**spirin when appropriate, **b**lood pressure control, **c**holesterol management, and **s**moking cessation. At the community level, a 20% reduction in the prevalence of combustible tobacco product use and of physical inactivity and a 20% reduction in mean daily sodium intake are targeted. These indicators, along with cardiac rehabilitation participation, are the focus of Million Hearts 2022; progress in reaching indicator targets has been shown to have a substantial effect on preventing acute cardiovascular events.

The data in this report serve as a baseline for Million Hearts 2022. These findings suggest that in addition to universal strategies aimed at the entire population with and at risk for CVD, there is a need to focus action on high-burden, high-risk subsets of the population. For example, opportunities for risk factor prevention and management among younger adults are of particular importance given the increase in heart disease mortality observed from 2010 to 2015 among adults aged thirty-five to sixty-four years in approximately half of U.S. counties. Compared with adults aged greater than sixty-five years, younger adults were less likely to be using aspirin or taking a statin when indicated and were more likely to use combustible tobacco and have an elevated daily sodium intake. Furthermore, only approximately half of adults aged thirty-five to sixty-four years with hypertension have their blood pressure (BP) under control. If the population deficits for each risk factor in this analysis (e.g., 9.0 million persons who are not taking aspirin as recommend) are summed, they represent approximately 213 million opportunities for better risk factor prevention and management, many of which might be present in the same person. More than half of these opportunities are among adults aged thirty-five to sixty-four years.

Additional demographic disparities in risk factor prevalence present opportunities to develop and implement culturally and linguistically tailored and effective interventions. For example, compared with whites, Hispanics were less likely to use aspirin for secondary prevention or take a statin when indicated, Blacks were less likely to have their blood pressure under control, and persons of other racial/ethnic groups, including American Indians and Alaska Natives, were more likely to use combustible tobacco products. Other studies confirm the existence of these disparities.

Included in the Million Hearts 2022-recommended clinical strategies are self-measured blood pressure monitoring with clinical support, standardized treatment protocols, reduced out-of-pocket costs and adherence approaches for medications, clinician-driven tobacco assessment and treatment, increasing awareness of the effect of particle pollution (including tobacco smoke, automobile or diesel exhaust, and wood smoke) on persons with known heart disease, and using clinical data to identify persons with undiagnosed conditions. Community-based strategies include comprehensive smoke-free policies, evidence-based tobacco cessation campaigns, sodium reduction strategies, built environment approaches to increase physical activity, increased access to places for physical activity, and peer support programs. Public and private partners, such as the Agency for Healthcare Research and Quality's EvidenceNOW initiative, state and local departments of health, the National Association of Community Health Centers, and Target: BP from the American Heart Association and the American Medical Association, are actively implementing these strategies.

Heart disease and stroke are leading causes of death in the United States; their risk factors are prevalent in the general population and are particularly high among certain subgroups. Evidence-based strategies for preventing acute cardiovascular events exist, with 213 million opportunities for better risk factor prevention and management. It will require a concerted national implementation effort to prevent one million acute cardiovascular events by 2022.

Wall HK, Ritchey MD, Gillespie C, Omura JD, Jamal A, George MG. Vital Signs: Prevalence of Key Cardiovascular Disease Risk Factors for Million Hearts 2022 — United States, 2011–2016. MMWR Morb Mortal Wkly Rep 2018;67:983–991. DOI: http://dx.doi.org/10.15585/mmwr.mm6735a4external icon

21. The data in this study suggests that we need to focus CVD reduction strategies on high-risk high-burden subsets like which of the following?
    a. Seniors over sixty-five
    b. Sedentary adults of all ages
    c. Young adults aged twenty-one to thirty-three
    d. Middle-aged adults aged thirty-five to sixty-four

22. Million Hearts 2022 has identified two primary community level targets. Which of the following is one of these target?
    a. 50% reduction in combustible tobacco products
    b. 20% reduction in sodium
    c. 80% increase in physical activity
    d. 50% increase in health monitoring

23. Risk factors are noted across multiple demographics and include groups which are:
    a. Less likely to exercise
    b. Less likely to monitor sodium intake
    c. Less likely to take aspirin as a preventative
    d. Less likely to know family history of heart disease

24. The Million Hearts 2022 campaign has identified both community and clinical strategies. Which of the following is among the clinical strategies?
    a. Supervised exercise programs
    b. Reduced out-of-pocket costs
    c. Sodium-free nutrition support
    d. Cholesterol reduction programs

25. What is the main idea of this passage?
   a. Cardiovascular disease is one of the leading killers in the U.S. and many opportunities exist for prevention and management.
   b. The Million Hearts 2022 Campaign is an important initiative and one that deserves support from the medical community.
   c. Younger Americans need to be far more aware of the risks associated with cardiovascular disease.
   d. The best approach to manage cardiovascular issues is both clinical and community based.

Questions 26–30 are based on the following passage:

E-cigarettes were introduced to the U.S. market in 2007. In 2018, 20.8% of high school students reported current e-cigarette use. E-cigarette use is markedly lower among U.S. adults than among youths; in 2018, only 3.2% of adults currently used e-cigarettes, with higher prevalence among persons aged eighteen to twenty-four years (7.6%) and twenty-five to thirty-four years (5.4%) than among older age groups. Approximately three-fourths of patients in this investigation were aged less than thirty-five years. In the general U.S. adult population, current e-cigarette use is slightly higher among males than females for both adults and youths; in the present investigation, approximately seven in ten cases occurred in males. In this investigation, 62% of patients were aged eighteen to thirty-four years; this is consistent with the age group with highest reported prevalence of marijuana use in the preceding thirty days in the United States.

Tetrahydrocannabinol (THC)-containing and nicotine-containing products were the most commonly reported substances used in e-cigarettes, or vaping products, by patients. Specific data on use of THC in e-cigarettes, or vaping products, in the general population is limited; among U.S. middle and high school students in 2016 who had ever used an e-cigarette, 30.6% reported using THC in an e-cigarette (33.3% among males and 27.2% among females). Among adults who reported using marijuana in 2014, 9.9% reported consuming it via a vaporizer or other electronic device (11.5% among men and 7.8% among women). In a recent study of college students, approximately 75% of those who had used substances other than nicotine in e-cigarettes reported using marijuana or THC-containing products in an e-cigarette. Because information about substance use in this investigation was self-reported, the information is not available for some cases because of the time required for completing and reporting patient interviews, inability to conduct interviews (e.g., patient refusal, loss to follow-up, persons who were too ill or died before they could be interviewed), and missing data for certain variables (e.g., patient refusal to answer certain questions). In addition, patients might not always know what substances they use or might be hesitant to reveal use of substances that are not legal in their state.

Continued monitoring of patient case counts and characteristics, as well as substances used with e-cigarette, or vaping, products, is critical to informing the ongoing investigation and helping to identify the cause. CDC and state health departments continue to collect and analyze epidemiologic data to better understand what types of devices and products patients are using (e.g., cartridges and e-liquids), the source of products or location where they were obtained, and the patterns (e.g., duration and frequency) of specific product use. Given the vast number of chemicals used in e-cigarette or vaping products, it is important to link epidemiologic data with findings from laboratory analyses of products and clinical specimens from patients. Federal, state, and private laboratories are working to collect and analyze products obtained from patients with lung injury associated with e-cigarette or vaping use. In addition,

CDC, clinical, and public health laboratories are collecting clinical specimens for future targeted analyses of substances identified in product samples.

Perrine CG, Pickens CM, Boehmer TK, et al. Characteristics of a Multistate Outbreak of Lung Injury Associated with E-cigarette Use, or Vaping — United States, 2019. MMWR Morb Mortal Wkly Rep 2019;68:860–864. DOI: http://dx.doi.org/10.15585/mmwr.mm6839e1

26. From the time e-cigarettes were introduced, approximately how long did it take before 20% of high school students reported use?
    a. Five years
    b. Eight years
    c. Two years
    d. Eleven years

27. Based on the passage, why are laboratory analyses of products important to research?
    a. In order to connect products to distribution companies
    b. In order to begin to identify product chemicals
    c. In order to match product chemicals to epidemiologic data
    d. In order to identify THC content in marijuana vaping devices

28. Research studies often have limitations. One here is the inability to conduct interviews. Which of the following is one reason given for that limitation?
    a. Patient age of consent
    b. Patient incarceration
    c. Patient ineligibility
    d. Patient refusal

29. Based on this passage, e-cigarette use is highest among which group?
    a. Young men
    b. Older men
    c. Young women
    d. Older women

30. What is the primary concern with e-cigarettes according to this passage?
    a. Marijuana usage
    b. Lung injury
    c. Growth in e-cigarette usage
    d. Nicotine dependence

Questions 31–35 are based on the following passage:

The 2017 age-standardized prevalence of arthritis was highest in Appalachia and the Lower Mississippi Valley; prevalence of severe joint pain and physical inactivity among adults with arthritis were highest in southeastern states. Estimates for all three outcomes in 2017 were similar to those in 2015. Except for age, urban-rural status, and sexual orientation, sociodemographic patterns for prevalence of severe joint pain and physical inactivity were similar and offer potential targets for interventions designed to reduce arthritis pain.

Joint pain is often managed with medications, which are associated with various adverse effects. The 2016 National Pain Strategy advises that pain-management strategies be multifaceted and individualized and include nonpharmacologic strategies, and the American College of Rheumatology recommends regular physical activity as a nonpharmacologic pain reliever for arthritis. Although persons with arthritis report that pain, or fear of causing or worsening it, is a substantial barrier to exercising, physical activity is an inexpensive intervention that can reduce pain, prevent or delay disability and limitations, and improve mental health, physical functioning, and quality of life with few adverse effects. Physical Activity Guidelines for Americans recommends that adults, including those with arthritis, engage in the equivalent of at least 150 minutes of moderate-intensity aerobic physical activity per week for substantial health benefits. Adults who are unable to meet the aerobic guideline because of their condition (e.g., those with severe joint pain) should engage in regular physical activity according to their abilities and avoid physical inactivity. Even small amounts of physical activity can improve physical functioning in adults with joint conditions. Most adults with arthritis pain can safely begin walking, swimming, or cycling to increase physical activity.

Arthritis-appropriate, evidence-based, self-management programs and low-impact, group aerobic, or multicomponent physical activity programs are designed to safely increase physical activity in persons with arthritis. These programs are available nationwide and are especially important for those populations that might have limited access to health care, medications, and surgical interventions (e.g., those in rural areas, those with lower income, and racial/ethnic minorities). Physical activity programs including low-impact aquatic exercises (e.g., Arthritis Foundation Aquatic Program) and strength training (e.g., Fit and Strong!) can help increase strength and endurance. Participating in self-management education programs, such as the Chronic Disease Self-Management Program, although not physical activity–focused, is also beneficial for arthritis management and results in increased physical activity. Benefits of the Chronic Disease Self-Management Program include increased frequency of aerobic and stretching/strengthening exercise, improved self-efficacy for arthritis pain management, and improved mood. Adults with arthritis can also engage in routine physical activity through group aerobic exercise classes (e.g., Walk with Ease, EnhanceFitness, Arthritis Foundation Exercise Program, and Active Living Every Day).

Effective, inexpensive physical activity and self-management education programs are available nationwide and can help adults with arthritis be safely and confidently physically active. This report provides the most current state-specific and demographic data for arthritis, severe joint pain, and physical inactivity. These data can extend collaborations among CDC, state health departments, and community organizations to increase access to and use of arthritis-appropriate, evidence-based interventions to help participants reduce joint pain and improve physical function and quality of life.

Guglielmo D, Murphy LB, Boring MA, et al. State-Specific Severe Joint Pain and Physical Inactivity Among Adults with Arthritis — United States, 2017. MMWR Morb Mortal Wkly Rep 2019;68:381–387. DOI: http://dx.doi.org/10.15585/mmwr.mm6817a2

31. Which of the following is an issue with medications for joint pain?
    a. They are addictive.
    b. They have bad side effects.
    c. They are expensive.
    d. They are minimally effective.

32. Adults who, due to pain, cannot meet exercise guidelines should do which of the following?
    a. Not exercise and avoid strenuous activity
    b. Exercise through the pain
    c. Avoid physical inactivity
    d. Medicate prior to exercise

33. What is the main idea of this passage?
    a. Physical exercise is a good nonpharmacologic strategy for managing arthritis pain.
    b. Arthritis is a crippling condition that impedes one's ability to exercise.
    c. Regionally, arthritis is a bigger issue in the southeast.
    d. Many programs exist to help get patients with arthritis moving.

34. Exercise programs for patients with joint pain/arthritis should be:
    a. Low-impact
    b. Solitary to avoid overdoing it
    c. High-intensity
    d. Strength-based

35. What population is identified as those most in need of exercise programs?
    a. Former athletes
    b. Those with no exercise background
    c. Those who report the highest level of pain
    d. Those in rural areas

Questions 36–40 are based on the following passage:

An estimated 24% of U.S adults with chronic obstructive pulmonary disease (COPD) have never smoked. Among persons who never smoked, an estimated 26%–53% of COPD can be attributed to occupational exposures. Previous studies have shown that occupational exposures to dust and toxins, as well as biologic and social differences, and genetic factors were associated with increased risk for COPD among persons who never smoked. Therefore, identifying occupational risk factors is needed for preventing and reducing COPD among workers. This study, which provides industry- and occupation-specific COPD prevalence estimates among 106 million persons who never smoked and were employed any time in the past twelve months, found that two-thirds of those with COPD were women. Women who had never smoked had higher COPD prevalence than did men regardless of their sociodemographic characteristics. Within-group variations were observed among sex, race, and ethnicity, with the highest prevalence among non-Hispanic black women and non-Hispanic white men.

National surveys have shown that exposure to vapors, gas, dust, fumes, grain dust, organic dust, inorganic dust, ammonia, hydrogen sulfide, diesel exhaust, environmental tobacco smoke, and chemicals increases the risk for COPD morbidity and mortality among persons who have never smoked. For example, exposure to coal mine dust or respirable crystalline silica among workers in the mining industry has been associated with COPD and other pulmonary diseases. In this study, office and administrative support workers (including secretaries, administrative and dental assistants, and clerks), protective service workers, and information industry workers (including publishing, telecommunications, broadcasting, and data processing workers) had the highest COPD prevalence. Workers in these industries can be exposed to organic and inorganic dusts, isocyanates, irritant gases, paper dust and fumes from photocopiers, chemicals, oil-based ink, paints, glues, isocyanates, toxic metals, and solvents, all of which are known respiratory irritants and have been associated with bronchitis, emphysema, and COPD. In addition, workplace exposures to environmental tobacco smoke can be associated with COPD.

In this report, although the pattern of responses to all three COPD-related questions among those who ever smoked and those who never smoked was similar (e.g., highest proportions with COPD were among those who were diagnosed with chronic bronchitis), chronic bronchitis was nineteen times more frequently reported than emphysema among those who never smoked, compared with 3.5 times among those who ever smoked. These results are similar to those previously reported that a substantial proportion of COPD among the nonsmoker population might be explained by chronic bronchitis.

The findings of high COPD prevalence among workers who never smoked corroborates findings that occupational exposures, in addition to smoking, might be associated with development of COPD. Higher COPD prevalence in certain industries and occupations underscore the importance of continued surveillance, identification of potential workplace exposures, collection of detailed occupational history, performance of pulmonary function testing, and assessment of environmental tobacco smoke exposure for early diagnosis and treatment of COPD among workers. Efforts to reduce adverse workplace exposures (including exposure to dust, vapors, fumes, chemicals, and indoor and outdoor air pollutants) and promote research to characterize the many contributing risk factors in COPD are needed to reduce the prevalence of COPD.

Syamlal G, Doney B, Mazurek JM. Chronic Obstructive Pulmonary Disease Prevalence Among Adults Who Have Never Smoked, by Industry and Occupation — United States, 2013–2017. MMWR Morb Mortal Wkly Rep 2019;68:303–307. DOI: http://dx.doi.org/10.15585/mmwr.mm6813a2external icon

36. What is the main idea of this passage?
    a. Some occupations have more medical hazards than others and should be avoided.
    b. Smokers are more likely to get COPD than nonsmokers.
    c. There is a need to identify occupational risk factors to prevent and reduce COPD.
    d. People with COPD are more likely to have bronchitis and emphysema.

37. COPD is often associated with coal mining, but what other occupations are at high risk according to this research?
    a. Hospital workers
    b. Information industry workers
    c. Professional athletes
    d. Construction workers

38. What significant commonality did the research find among both smokers and nonsmokers who had COPD?
    a. Emphysema
    b. Exposure to dust
    c. Chronic bronchitis
    d. Children of smokers

39. Respiratory irritants in the workplace have been associated with COPD and what else?
    a. Lung cancer
    b. Asthma
    c. Sinus infections
    d. Emphysema

40. Based on context, in the first sentence of the final paragraph, what does the word *corroborates* mean?
    a. Diminishes
    b. Confirms
    c. Contradicts
    d. Underscores

Questions 41–45 are based on the following passage:

> Delays in receipt of appropriate care lead to worse outcomes among heart attack victims. Although this nationally representative survey indicates improvement in the percentage of adults who know the signs and symptoms of a heart attack and to call 9-1-1 if they witness someone having a heart attack, in 2017, approximately half of respondents (50.2%) knew all five common heart attack signs and symptoms, and disparities in awareness and response exist among all demographic groups and by cardiovascular disease (CVD) risk status.
>
> Data from fourteen states reporting in the 2005 BRFSS found that 85.8% of respondents had the knowledge to call 9-1-1 as the first action when witnessing a heart attack and 31% were aware of all five heart attack symptoms. Although the percentage of persons with this knowledge was higher in this study than in the 2005 BRFSS, disparities by sex, race/ethnicity and level of education persisted. Both the BRFSS data and estimates from this report identify a need for increased awareness regarding the signs and symptoms of one of the most common important health events that can occur in persons in the United States. Recognizing this need, the U.S. Department of Health and Human Services *Healthy People 2020* (HP2020) program included objectives specifically calling for an increase in the awareness of heart attack signs and symptoms and the appropriate response. Using the 2008 NHIS data as the HP2020 baseline, the target for awareness of five common heart attack symptoms was set at 43.6% (10% increase from the 2008 adjusted prevalence of 39.6%), and the target for knowing to call 9-1-1 if someone is having a heart attack was set at 93.8% (2% increase from 91.8%). Although data from the current study indicate that in 2017 these goals for awareness of heart attack symptoms (50.2%) and calling 9-1-1 (94.9%) were met overall, estimates for certain subpopulations remained below the HP2020 target, including racial/ethnic minorities and adults with less than a high school education.
>
> Many educational efforts have historically been undertaken to promote increased awareness about and response to a heart attack. For example, CDC and other federal agencies, such as the National Heart, Lung and Blood Institute and principal nonfederal partners, such as the American Heart Association, have promoted awareness of and response to heart attacks through public health messaging campaigns and improved early identification of heart attack symptoms when entering the emergency response system. Despite these promotion efforts, general knowledge about the symptoms of a heart attack remain suboptimal. Consistent messaging campaigns should be complemented with regular contact with a health care provider because screening and evaluation might lead to early intervention.

Because of the high prevalence and significant health impact of heart attacks, awareness of the major signs and symptoms of a heart attack and the appropriate response to the event should be common knowledge among all adults. However, the suboptimal knowledge among U.S. adults identified in this study, especially among racial/ethnic minority groups, those with lower levels of education, and those with more CVD risk factors, highlight a need for enhanced and focused educational efforts. Clinical, community, and public health efforts are needed to continue to systematically improve the awareness of heart attack symptoms throughout the United States.

Fang J, Luncheon C, Ayala C, Odom E, Loustalot F. Awareness of Heart Attack Symptoms and Response Among Adults — United States, 2008, 2014, and 2017. MMWR Morb Mortal Wkly Rep 2019;68:101–106. DOI: http://dx.doi.org/10.15585/mmwr.mm6805a2external icon

41. What is the main idea of this passage?
    a. Awareness of the symptoms and response to a heart attack should be common knowledge, so we need to educate adults.
    b. The first action to take when one witnesses someone experiencing a heart attack is to call 9-1-1.
    c. There are five common symptoms, or signs, of a heart attack.
    d. Failure to immediately care for or help heart attack victims results in more severe outcomes.

42. According to the research, approximately what percentage of respondents knew the five common symptoms of a heart attack?
    a. 10%
    b. 25%
    c. 80%
    d. 50%

43. Messaging campaigns about the symptoms of a heart attack have failed in the past. What should they be partnered with to be more successful?
    a. Publicly available classes
    b. Regular contact with a physician
    c. A hotline number
    d. Information in school health class

44. Which of the following is a subpopulation that scored worse at remembering the symptoms of a heart attack and to call 9-1-1 first?
    a. Seniors who had not experienced a heart attack
    b. Middle-aged adults
    c. Adults with less than a high school education
    d. Adults with few risk factors

45. The article suggests the best organizations and groups to raise awareness include which of the following?
    a. Clinical
    b. Individual
    c. Institutional
    d. Educational

Nonsmoking workers residing in states with comprehensive smoke-free laws reported significantly lower prevalence of frequent exposure to workplace second-hand smoke (SHS). Moreover, SHS exposure among nonsmoking workers also significantly varied by industry. During 2013–2014, one in four U.S. nonsmokers reported exposure to SHS, and an estimated 41,000 deaths among nonsmoking adults were associated with SHS exposure. Furthermore, workplace SHS exposure has been recognized as one of the top occupational hazards that contributes substantially to the prevalence of occupational cancer among nonsmokers. During 2000–2015, the number of states with smoke-free laws that prohibited smoking in indoor areas of worksites, restaurants, and bars increased from zero to twenty-seven. In this report, workers residing in states with smoke-free laws in all three venue categories were least likely to report frequent exposure to workplace SHS. Previous studies have revealed that the absence of a policy restricting or prohibiting smoking at the worksite put workers at higher risk for workplace SHS exposure. Despite the considerable progress in implementation of smoke-free laws over the past two decades, this analysis found that even in states with smoke-free laws in three categories of venues, 8.6% of nonsmoking workers reported frequent workplace SHS exposure. This finding suggests that certain workplaces might be outside the scope of most smoke-free laws.

Based on National Health Interview Survey data for 2014–2016, 34.3% of workers in the construction, 30.4% of workers in the mining, and 30.2% of workers in the transportation industries used some form of tobacco. Higher smoking prevalence among workers employed in these industries might lead to exposure of their nonsmoking coworkers to SHS. Previous findings of higher tobacco use and SHS exposure among workers in the construction industry are consistent with current findings. The industry subcategories with the highest prevalence of reported SHS exposure in this study and the industry category with the highest number of exposed workers (construction) include outdoor workplaces and other settings that are unlikely to be protected by smoke-free laws. A recent study determined that indoor workers who reported working at a worksite having a 100% smoke-free policy had significantly lower odds of smoking combustible tobacco than did those reporting a partial or no smoke-free policy. Enhanced and sustained efforts to protect nonsmoking workers through comprehensive smoke-free laws and implementation of smoke-free workplace policies by employers can benefit public health.

Workplace SHS exposure is harmful for workers' health. In this study, nonsmoking workers residing in states without comprehensive smoke-free laws and those employed in certain industries were more likely to be frequently exposed to workplace SHS. National Institute for Occupational Safety and Health encourages employers, especially those in industries with high prevalence of SHS exposure, to implement workplace-specific smoke-free policies to complement state and local smoke-free laws to help reduce SHS exposure among workers and protect workers' health.

Su C, Syamlal G, Tamers S, Li J, Luckhaupt SE. Workplace Second-hand Tobacco Smoke Exposure Among U.S. Nonsmoking Workers, 2015. MMWR Morb Mortal Wkly Rep 2019;68:604–607. DOI: http://dx.doi.org/10.15585/mmwr.mm6827a2external icon

46. What is the subject of this passage?
    a. Smoke-free policies
    b. Second-hand smoke in the workplace
    c. Second-hand smoke deaths
    d. Nonsmoking workers

47. What has put workers at higher risk of the impact of second-hand smoke?
    a. The industry they work in
    b. Smoking areas at the workplace
    c. Absence of a smoke-free policy
    d. Working predominantly indoors

48. The research names three industries where exposure to second-hand smoke may be most prevalent based on the high number of tobacco users. Which of the following is one of those industries?
    a. Food service
    b. Healthcare
    c. Transportation
    d. Landscaping

49. What type of policy decreased the likelihood of individuals using combustible tobacco products?
    a. 100% smoke-free
    b. No policy
    c. Designated smoking areas
    d. This was not part of the scope of the research.

50. Exposure to smoke from co-workers and others in the workplace is:
    a. A top workplace complaint
    b. A top occupational hazard
    c. A top reason individuals can't quit smoking
    d. A top reason for leaving a workplace

Questions 51–55 are based on the following passage:

The American Academy of Pediatric Dentistry (AAPD) provides guidance on preventive dental services and anticipatory guidance for children. For children aged two to six, AAPD recommends that dental health care personnel provide sealants for caries-susceptible primary molars and permanent molars, premolars, and anterior teeth; children should be reassessed at recall appointments to determine the need for new sealants or maintenance of existing sealants. In addition, the American Dental Association supports the use of sealants and encourages dentists to speak to their patients or parents about them. For parents of young children, especially those who are poor or from racial/ethnic minorities, initiating these discussions as early as possible could better prepare parents for sealant placement. However, because dental care is reduced among low-income and racial/ethnic minority families and among parents with only very young children, relying on dental professionals to provide sealant information is problematic.

School nurses and pediatricians could help increase knowledge of dental sealants. School sealant programs are a successful and cost-effective strategy to increase sealant receipt among children who typically lack access to clinical dental care. A major barrier to successful implementation of these programs is low consent rates, which might be influenced by parental lack of sealant knowledge. Our finding that parents with only children younger than six have less knowledge of sealants is consistent with a recent study in Maryland that conducted a focus group of low-income parents or caregivers of children aged six and younger and pregnant women. That study found that very few of the participating parents had heard of dental sealants.

Although prevalence of dental sealants has increased, they are still underutilized among children at risk for untreated caries. There are corresponding disparities in knowledge of the preventive purpose of sealants. The dental community remains a major source of information on the preventive benefits of sealants. Further efforts by dental professional organizations and public health organizations to develop oral health promotion and education programs to reach low-income and racial/ethnic minority parents and parents with only young children could reduce disparities in sealant knowledge and untreated dental caries.

Junger ML, Griffin SO, Lesaja S, Espinoza L. Awareness Among US Adults of Dental Sealants for Caries Prevention. Prev Chronic Dis 2019;16:180398. DOI: http://dx.doi.org/10.5888/pcd16.180398external icon

51. AAPD recommends sealants for children two to six for which type of teeth?
    a. Canine
    b. Incisors
    c. None
    d. Premolars

52. What is the primary barrier to successful implementation of school sealant programs?
    a. Low consent rates
    b. Lack of access to schools
    c. Not enough dentists
    d. Too expensive

53. Why is relying on dentists to inform and educate patients regarding sealants ineffective?
    a. Many see sealants as an attempt to make a profit.
    b. Dental care is reduced among the populations that need the information.
    c. Dental professionals are already overwhelmed with patients.
    d. Sealants are underutilized, so many dentists don't even use them.

54. Based on the research, which community is least likely to have heard of dental sealants?
    a. Parents of teenagers
    b. Low-income parents
    c. Parents with a history of dental disease
    d. School nurses

55. What is the main idea of this passage?
    a. More programs to provide dental sealants are needed across the U.S.
    b. Dentists need to be more proactive in educating their patients.
    c. More education about dental sealants is needed among communities who might benefit.
    d. Sealants are a great preventative dental treatment to be used in children.

Vocabulary

1. Select the word that best fits in the following sentence:

    The doctor stressed that Richard would need to strictly _____ to his instructions for a full recovery.

    a. restrict
    b. infer
    c. retain
    d. adhere

2. Select the meaning of the underlined word in the following sentence:

    The doctor was sure to discuss <u>potential</u> side effects of the medication.

    a. possible
    b. impossible
    c. dangerous
    d. insignificant

3. What is the best definition for <u>neurovascular</u>?
    a. related to blood vessels in the brain
    b. related to the skeletal system
    c. related to the central nervous system
    d. the system of veins, capillaries, and arteries

4. The doctor explained that the splint was not just to stabilize and protect, but also to _____ movement.

    a. retain
    b. restrict
    c. constrict
    d. initiate

5. Select the meaning of the underlined word in the following sentence:

    Despite having completed rotations in each department, Rosa was <u>ambivalent</u> about where she wanted to work.

    a. certain
    b. troubled
    c. unsure
    d. angry

6. Select the meaning of the underlined word in the following sentence:

Through his tone, I was able to infer that the situation was much worse than he let on.

a. interpret body language
b. misunderstand communication
c. conclude through information or reasoning
d. explain to another

7. What is the best definition for vital?
a. unnecessary
b. lifelike
c. lethal
d. essential

8. What is the best definition for discrete?
a. disconnected
b. secretive
c. removed
d. forcible

9. Select the meaning of the underlined word in the following sentence:

Julia's skin was flushed where she had been stung.

a. puffy and bruised
b. covered in hives
c. warm and red
d. raised and hard

10. Curtis has a lot of questions and concerns about his _____ surgery.
a. deteriorating
b. preexisting
c. impending
d. therapeutic

11. What is the best definition for occluded?
a. darkened
b. blocked
c. overdeveloped
d. extended

12. After checking the CT scan results, the doctor assured the patient that the bleeding was only _____.
a. external
b. insidious
c. distal
d. posterior

13. While the doctor wrote the prescription, she informed him it was purely a _____ and did not expect he would need it.
    a. rationale
    b. compensatory
    c. parameter
    d. precaution

14. Select the meaning of the underlined word in the following sentence:

One of the potential side effects of the medication was <u>constricted</u> blood vessels, resulting in higher blood pressure.

    a. widened
    b. tightened
    c. amplified
    d. impeded

15. What is the best definition for <u>distal</u>?
    a. anatomically decentralized
    b. located away from the heart
    c. related to the liver
    d. related to the spleen

16. What is the best definition for <u>bilateral</u>?
    a. two valves
    b. symmetrical parts
    c. having two sides
    d. involving two parties

17. Though sepsis is still incredibly dangerous, it was once _____ for almost all those who developed the condition.
    a. traumatic
    b. insignificant
    c. fatal
    d. harmless

18. Select the meaning of the underlined word in the following sentence:

In addition to the medications and therapy provided, the doctor recommended other <u>therapeutic</u> modalities to improve recovery time.

    a. detrimental
    b. auxiliary
    c. engaging
    d. healing

19. Select the meaning of the underlined word in the following sentence:

It's important to provide a doctor with all information as a sore throat is a _symptom_ for multiple conditions.

a. pre-existing condition
b. indication
c. placebo
d. contraindication

20. In order to knock out the infection prior to surgery, the doctor prescribed a fairly _____ antibiotic.
a. invasive
b. potent
c. insidious
d. dilute

21. Despite best efforts, it was clear from his inability to get out of bed that Carl's condition was
_____.

a. deteriorating
b. improving
c. insignificant
d. pre-existing

22. What is the best definition for _pathology_?
a. course of action
b. holistic healing
c. medical history
d. study of diseases

23. Select the meaning of the underlined word in the following sentence:

The doctor wrote down his instructions, but then also gave a _verbal_ review to ensure the plan was clear.

a. video
b. performative
c. oral
d. logical

24. What is the best definition for _retain_?
a. to train
b. to put away
c. to test
d. to keep

25. The nurse _____ pressure to the wound to stem the bleeding.
    a. initiated
    b. applied
    c. recurred
    d. suppressed

26. What is the best definition for <u>neurologic</u>?
    a. related to the nervous system
    b. related to the veins, capillaries, arteries
    c. related to the brain
    d. related to the lungs

27. The representative was demonstrating the new dialysis _____ to the team.
    a. bacteria
    b. parameter
    c. device
    d. patent

28. Select the meaning of the underlined word in the following sentence:

    The patient's body was free of lacerations, yet several symptoms suggested <u>internal</u> bleeding.

    a. absent
    b. inside
    c. excessive
    d. minimal

29. Frostbite is the result of _____ to significant cold for prolonged periods.
    a. access
    b. incidence
    c. exposure
    d. transmission

30. Select the meaning of the underlined word in the following sentence:

    Cancer is an <u>insidious</u> disease, and that makes it particularly dangerous.

    a. painful
    b. contagious
    c. fast-moving
    d. slow-moving

31. What is the best definition for <u>dysfunction</u>?
    a. not working as intended
    b. not working at all
    c. making forward progress
    d. a convoluted process

32. Select the meaning of the underlined word in the following sentence:

Sometimes it is medically necessary to <u>suppress</u> labor for the well-being of both mother and child.

   a. force
   b. speed up
   c. hold back
   d. encourage

33. What is the best definition for <u>dilute</u>?
   a. to split apart
   b. to weaken
   c. to repair
   d. to strengthen

34. One of the concerns with football is the potential for head _____, which can cause long-term issues.
   a. lacerations
   b. trauma
   c. bruising
   d. fractures

35. In order to avoid a more _____ procedure, the doctors first tried medications and physical therapy.
   a. invasive
   b. prolonged
   c. costly
   d. ongoing

36. What is the best definition for <u>nutrient</u>?
   a. food choice
   b. dietary restriction
   c. calorie requirement
   d. dietary component

37. Select the meaning of the underlined word in the following sentence:

The doctor conveyed that the condition was chronic and, therefore, likely to <u>recur</u>.

   a. occur over and over
   b. be less severe
   c. not happen again
   d. grow worse

38. The family opted to continue hospice at home, where the environment would be more _____.
   a. insidious
   b. serene
   c. concise
   d. precipitous

39. What is the best definition for <u>posterior</u>?
    a. front
    b. back
    c. delayed
    d. elevated

40. Select the meaning of the underlined word in the following sentence:

    The funds awarded to the family after the malpractice suit were deemed <u>compensatory</u>.

    a. delivered through the court
    b. considered generous
    c. considered frivolous
    d. relief from negative consequence

41. The optometrist warned that, post-exam, the patient's vision would be _____.
    a. inquisitive
    b. serene
    c. impaired
    d. expanded

42. What is the best definition for <u>deficit</u>?
    a. shortage
    b. windfall
    c. plan
    d. unclear

43. _____ is crucial when it comes to wound care.
    a. Parameters
    b. Hygiene
    c. Flexion
    d. Hydration

44. Select the meaning of the underlined word in the following sentence:

    The family called frequently to check on the patient's <u>status</u>.

    a. condition
    b. medication
    c. vital signs
    d. position

45. The hospital was awaiting the _____ of the patient's files from his doctor before admitting him.
    a. patent
    b. extension
    c. chronology
    d. transmission

46. After her heart attack, Rose was transferred to the _____ unit.
   a. renal
   b. etiology
   c. cardiac
   d. hematologic

47. Select the meaning of the underlined word in the following sentence:

   He reported abdominal pain, and testing revealed a gastrointestinal blockage.

   a. related to the central nervous system
   b. related to stomach or intestines
   c. related to the kidney
   d. related to muscles

48. What is the best definition of underline{convulsive}?
   a. creating seizures
   b. with empathy
   c. explosive
   d. extensive

49. The pharmaceutical company filed for a(n) _____ for their new medication.
   a. incidence
   b. patent
   c. parameter
   d. extension

50. Problems with the _____ system tend to occur more frequently with age, causing patients to experience difficulties with pain, stiffness, and movement.
   a. musculoskeletal
   b. cardiovascular
   c. renal
   d. neurologic

51. Select the meaning of the underlined word in the following sentence:

   The nurse noticed that Becky's abdomen had become more distended since her last vitals check.

   a. occluded
   b. suppressed
   c. bloated
   d. impaired

52. Select the meaning of the underlined word in the following sentence:

   Unfortunately, the patient's insurance does not cover preexisting conditions.

   a. during
   b. prior
   c. post
   d. distal

53. What is the best definition for <u>paroxysm</u>?
   a. disease
   b. cough
   c. stroke
   d. attack

54. What is the best definition for <u>cavity</u>?
   a. membrane tissue
   b. tooth decay
   c. hollow space
   d. cardiac chamber

55. Select the meaning of the underlined word in the following sentence:

   The doctor instructed the nurse to <u>elevate</u> Juan's legs to reduce swelling.

   a. raise
   b. move
   c. drain
   d. wrap

Grammar

1. Select the best phrase to complete the sentence.

   By next month, I _____ all my applications.

   a. sent
   b. will send
   c. will send
   d. will have sent

2. Identify the antecedents in the following sentence.

   The lab tech hadn't yet finished the tests, though he said they'd be done by noon.

   a. tech, lab
   b. tech, tests
   c. lab, tests
   d. lab, noon

3. Fill in the blanks with the correct words to complete the sentence.

   I was often reminded to take a deep _____ and remember to _____ deeply.

   a. breath, breathe
   b. breath, breath
   c. breathe, breath
   d. breathe, breathe

4. Which sentence has the correct punctuation?
   a. The new doctor the one who came from New York, is starting today.
   b. The new doctor, the one who came from New York, is starting today.
   c. The new doctor the one who came from New York is starting today.
   d. The new doctor, the one who came from New York is starting today.

5. Select the best word to complete the sentence.

   People complain about hospital food, but our dining center has been named one of the
   _____ in the state.

   a. most fine
   b. most finest
   c. finest
   d. more fine

6. Select the proper noun in the following sentence:

   My friend was lucky enough to get an internship at Weill Cornell Medicine, but she won't start until
   spring.

   a. spring
   b. Weill Cornell
   c. internship
   d. Weill Cornell Medicine

7. Which of the following sentences is correct?
   a. Monica complimented Ruth on how her shoes complemented her rose-colored scrubs.
   b. Monica complemented Ruth on how her shoes complimented her rose-colored scrubs.
   c. Monica complimented Ruth on how her shoes complimented her rose-colored scrubs.
   d. Monica complemented Ruth on how her shoes complemented her rose-colored scrubs.

8. Which pronoun would best replace the words in bold?

   *All staff members were permitted to use the gym on premises, including the **women's** locker room.*

   a. their
   b. hers
   c. our
   d. her

9. Identify the independent clause in the sentence that follows.

   The nursing staff had a meeting on Thursdays, after which they all went to lunch.

   a. the nursing staff
   b. after which they all went to lunch
   c. the nursing staff had a meeting on Thursdays
   d. they all went to lunch

10. Fill in the blank with the word that best completes the sentence.

Radiology is quite busy today _____ maternity is quiet.

a. so
b. because
c. while
d. until

11. Identify the verb in the following sentence:

Cardiology sent the reports to the patient's PCP.

a. reports
b. sent
c. to
d. patient's

12. Select the correct verb to complete the following sentence?

Neither Marco nor Elise _____ able to swap shifts.

a. were
b. been
c. being
d. was

13. Identify the linking verb in the following sentence:

The patient is nervous about her test results, and she won't get them back for at least 48 hours.

a. nervous
b. is
c. get
d. won't

14. Identify the adjective in the following sentence:

All the rooms in the oncology department were outfitted with new furniture.

a. rooms
b. outfitted
c. new
d. department

15. Which of the listed words functions as the subject in the sentence that follows?

Outpatient Services has been moved to the new wing of the hospital as there is more ample parking.

   a. Outpatient Services
   b. wing
   c. hospital
   d. parking

16. Which words in the following sentence are the verbs?

Cardiology needs to recruit more medical students as their numbers are low.

   a. needs, recruit, are
   b. recruit, are
   c. needs, recruit
   d. needs, are

17. Identify the pronoun and antecedent in this sentence:

The critical care team is one of the strongest in the hospital, and they have been recognized for this work.

   a. one, they
   b. hospital, this
   c. team, this
   d. team, they

18. Choose the verb that highlights a past action to complete the following sentence:

Anita _____ to work in urgent care.

   a. choose
   b. chose
   c. choosed
   d. chosed

19. Identify the dependent clause in the following sentence:

Alex was rarely late for his shift, even when he missed the bus.

   a. Alex was rarely late
   b. even when he missed the bus
   c. late for his shift
   d. missed the bus

20. Which of the following word acts as the article in the following sentence?

"Did you request an appointment?" asked Martin.

a. did
b. asked
c. an
d. you

21. In the following sentence, what type of adjective does the word *"which"* function as?

Which cafeteria do you prefer for lunch?

a. Interrogative adjective
b. Demonstrative adjective
c. Possessive adjective
d. Comparative adjective

22. In the following sentence, *"Hey"* is an example of what part of speech?

Hey! Are you heading to the library?

a. a conjunction
b. an article
c. a preposition
d. an interjection

23. Which word in the following sentence is used incorrectly?

Although we graduated as a cohort, its unlikely we'll all work together again.

a. unlikely
b. its
c. cohort
d although

24. Identify the subject pronoun in the following sentence:

We had an hour to complete the charting, but because of computer issues it took a lot longer.

a. but
b. an
c. we
d. a lot

25. Which word in the following sentence is a helping verb?

Learning computerized charting was difficult for many, but they will save time that way.

a. save
b. was
c. will
d. learning

26. Identify the problem with the following sentence:

Maria was running late and nearly missed her bus Joe was the one who told us.

a. run on sentence
b. misplaced modifier
c. sentence fragment
d. dangling modifier

27. Select the best words to fill in the blanks:

Cindy didn't ask for my _____ but I _____ her to apply for the job.

a. advise, advised
b. advice, advised
c. advise, adviced
d. advice, advized

28. Select the best punctuation to complete the sentence:

Though we tried our best___we weren't able to complete a medicine inventory___there just wasn't enough time.

a. , and :
b. ; and ,
c. ; and ;
d. , and ;

29. Which choice is the complete verb in past tense in the following sentence?

The new administrator had done a walking tour before meeting with staff.

a. before meeting
b. had done
c. walking
d. had done walking

30. Select the phrase that best completes the following sentence:

After looking at her picture, Olivia was able to identify the new doctor on _____.

   a. cite
   b. sight
   c. site
   d. cight

31. Identify the adverb in the following sentence:

The doctor advised the patient to walk slowly since she was still recovering.

   a. still
   b. patient
   c. slowly
   d. recovering

32. Select the best phrase to complete the sentence:

Next month, she _____ finally graduate from her nursing program.

   a. will
   b. has
   c. did
   d. was

33. Which of the following words acts as the antecedent in the sentence that follows?

The ambulance driver narrowly avoided an accident on his way back to the hospital.

   a. ambulance
   b. accident
   c. hospital
   d. driver

34. Fill in the blanks with the best-fitting words:

_____ cohort was the first to all score above 85% on the exam. We _____ _____ proud!

   a. Our, were, quite
   b. Are, where, quiet
   c. Our, where, quit
   d. Are, were, quiet

35. Which sentence has the correct punctuation?
   a. The doctor said "Tell the family the patient is out of surgery?"
   b. The doctor said, "Tell the family the patient is out of surgery."
   c. The doctor, said "Tell the family the patient is out of surgery?"
   d. The doctor said Tell the family the patient is out of surgery.

36. Identify the prepositional phrase in the following sentence:

The doctor told the family that the boy would need stitches after attempting to climb over the fence.

    a. would need stitches
    b. attempting to climb
    c. over the fence
    d. told the family

37. Select the sentence with the correct capitalization.
    a. Last Spring, the doctors at St. Joseph's hospital in Houston performed a face transplant.
    b. Last spring, the doctors at St. Joseph's Hospital in Houston performed a face transplant.
    c. Last Spring, the doctors at st. Joseph's Hospital in Houston performed a face transplant.
    d. Last spring, the doctors at St. Joseph's hospital in Houston performed a face transplant.

38. Identify the subject and object in the following sentence:

Gerald was reluctant, but he handed the keys to Orlando.

    a. Gerald, keys
    b. keys, Orlando
    c. Gerald, reluctant
    d. Gerald, Orlando

39. Which pronoun best replaces the word in bold?

*Despite the delays, **Anne's** doctor told her the surgery was scheduled for next week.*

    a. him
    b. her
    c. she
    d. our

40. Identify the collective noun in the following sentence:

A team of nurses was asked to join administrators on a retreat.

    a. nurses
    b. team
    c. administrators
    d. retreat

41. Identify the verbs in the following sentence:

After our shift, we all went to grab a bite to eat.

    a. went, grab
    b. after, went, grab, bite
    c. went, grab, bite
    d. after, went, grab

42. Which of the words functions as a noun in the following sentence?

Exercise is often overlooked as an important part of healthcare.

a. overlooked
b. an
c. important
d. Exercise

43. Identify the adjective in the sentence:

We were counting on the next shift to bring us some relief, as the morning had been long.

a. relief
b. next
c. bring
d. morning

44. Which word best completes the sentence?

The nurse was sure to greet families in the waiting room as _____ as possible.

a. angrily
b. cheery
c. happy
d. cheerfully

45. What is the subject in the sentence that follows?

After the blizzard ended and roads were opened up, the hospital became quite busy.

a. blizzard
b. roads
c. busy
d. hospital

46. Which of the following sentences is correct?
a. The ophthalmologist should of returned to the office by now.
b. The ophthalmologist should have returned to the office bye now.
c. The ophthalmologist should have returned to the office by now.
d. The ophthalmologist should of returned to the office bye now.

47. Fill in the blank to compete the sentence.

Radiology is backed up, _____ there is a long wait for x-rays.

a. for
b. so
c. yet
d. but

48. Which of these is an independent clause?
    a. John ran
    b. another rainy day
    c. never be late again
    d. couldn't ask for more

49. Identify the coordinating conjunction in the following sentence:

    The anesthesiologist and surgeon were nearly ready, but they had to have one more consultation before the surgery.

    a. nearly
    b. more
    c. ready
    d. but

50. Which phrase uses the correct capitalization?
    a. I still need to complete writing, biology, chemistry 101, and Spanish this year.
    b. I still need to complete writing, Biology, chemistry 101, and Spanish this year.
    c. I still need to complete Writing, Biology, Chemistry 101, and Spanish this year.
    d. I still need to complete writing, biology, Chemistry 101, and Spanish this year.

51. Which sentence is grammatically correct?
    a. Dr. Johnson the one who arrived recently from cincinnati is a specialist in rheumatoid arthritis.
    b. Dr. Johnson, the one who arrived recently from Cincinnati is a specialist in rheumatoid arthritis.
    c. Dr. Johnson, the one who arrived recently from Cincinnati, is a specialist in Rheumatoid Arthritis.
    d. Dr. Johnson, the one who arrived recently from Cincinnati, is a specialist in rheumatoid arthritis.

52. In the following sentence, the word *"my"* functions as which of the following?

    I forgot to write my name on the exam.

    a. A noun
    b. An adjective
    c. An adverb
    d. A pronoun

53. Choose the best conjunction for the following sentence:

    We could hear multiple sirens heading towards the hospital, _____ we began to prepare for their arrival.

    a. and
    b. yet
    c. but
    d. for

54. Identify the adverb in the following sentence:

The new RN on the floor worked diligently at learning our routines and schedules.

a. new
b. floor
c. diligently
d. routines

55. Select the best phrases to complete the sentence:

Rose has been a nurse longer _____ Jody or Rob, and both have learned _____ from her.

a. then, a lot
b. than, a lot
c. than, alot
d. then, alot

Biology

1. Consider the following micrographs of several cells. Which figure corresponds to an image taken from a TEM?

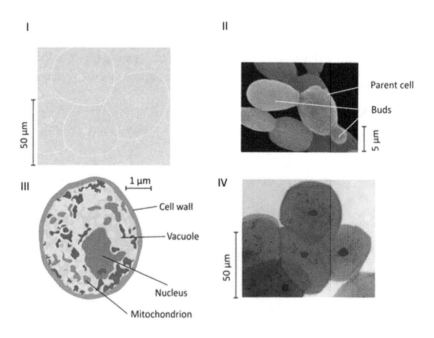

a. I
b. II
c. III
d. IV

2. Which of the following choices are organelles that plants and animals do NOT have in common?
     a. Central vacuole and mitochondria
     b. Mitochondria and chloroplasts
     c. Chloroplasts and central vacuoles
     d. Mitochondria and peroxisomes

3. Integral proteins are found embedded within the plasma membrane of eukaryotes and prokaryotes. Which of the following amino acids, located on the outer surface of the protein, most likely face the inner membrane (tail of the phospholipid)?

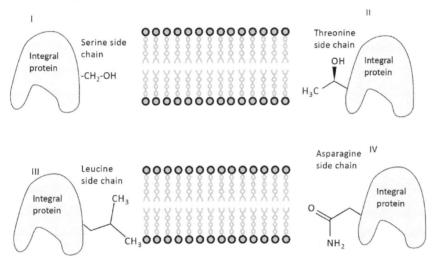

     a. I
     b. II
     c. III
     d. IV

4. The figure below represents the structure of chromosomes and their corresponding components. Which answer choice below is correct regarding the labeling of each chromosome component?

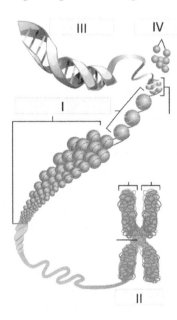

a. I-DNA, II-chromatin, III-protein, IV-chromosome
b. I-chromatin, II-chromosome, III-DNA, IV-protein
c. I-DNA, II-protein, III-chromosome, IV-chromatin
d. I-protein, II-chromatin, III-DNA, IV-chromosome

5. Which of the following statements below is the most accurate regarding the function of the endoplasmic reticulum (ER)?
a. The smooth ER detoxifies drugs by adding hydrocarbon (-CH3) groups to the drug molecules.
b. The rough ER detoxifies drugs by adding hydroxyl groups to the drug molecules.
c. The smooth ER detoxifies drugs by adding hydroxyl groups to the drug molecules.
d. The rough ER detoxifies drugs by adding hydrocarbon (-CH3) groups to the drug molecules.

6. Why are mitochondria and chloroplast believed to have similar evolutionary origins?
a. Both organelles have two membranes and contain DNA.
b. Both organelles have ribosomes and stroma.
c. Both organelles produce ATP and contain a granum.
d. Both organelles contain a single membrane and RNA.

7. In what way are aerobic respiration and gasoline combustion similar to one another?
a. Simple organic compounds are broken down under oxygen to produce complex products such as carbon monoxide, water (H-OH), and heat.
b. Complex organic compounds are broken down under oxygen to produce simple products such as carbon dioxide, water (H-OH), and heat.
c. Simple organic compounds are broken down under oxygen to produce complex products such as carbon dioxide, water (H-OH), and heat.
d. Complex organic compounds are broken down under oxygen to produce simple products such as carbon dioxide, ethanol (CH_3-OH), and heat.

8. Consider the following reaction below. Which compound is reduced?

$$2C_8H_{18} + 25O_2 \rightarrow 16CO_2 + 18H_2O$$

a. O_2
b. H_2O
c. C_8H_{18}
d. CO_2

9. Choose the correct answer below to complete the statement.

During cellular respiration, organic molecules are oxidized, but hydrogen is not attached to oxygen directly. Instead, an electron carrier called _____ traps electrons from glucose which is later transferred to oxygen.

a. $NADH$ (oxidized form)
b. NAD^+ (oxidized form)
c. $NADH^+$ (reduced form)
d. NAD^+ (reduced form)

10. How many electrons and protons does the enzyme dehydrogenase transfer from an organic food molecule to nicotinamide adenine dinucleotide?
a. One electron and two protons
b. Two electrons and two protons
c. One electron and one proton
d. Two electrons and one proton

11. Which choice below corresponds to the correct reduced structure of nicotinamide?

I

II

III

IV

a. I
b. II
c. III
d. IV

12. Which of the following is the correct order of cellular respiration from start to finish?
   a. Pyruvate oxidation, glycolysis, citric acid cycle, oxidative phosphorylation
   b. Glycolysis, citric acid cycle, pyruvate oxidation, oxidative phosphorylation
   c. Glycolysis, pyruvate oxidation, citric acid cycle, oxidative phosphorylation
   d. Oxidative phosphorylation, citric acid cycle, pyruvate oxidation, glycolysis

13. Which of the following statements is accurate regarding the burning of biofuels in cellular respiration?
   a. When biofuels containing many C-H bonds are oxidized to products with many C-O bonds, energy is released as electrons move to a lower energy state.
   b. When biofuels containing many C-O bonds are oxidized to products with many C-H bonds, energy is released as electrons move to a lower energy state.
   c. When biofuels containing many C-H bonds are reduced to products with many C-O bonds, energy is released as electrons move to a lower energy state.
   d. When biofuels containing many C-O bonds are reduced to products with many C-H bonds, energy is absorbed as electrons move to a higher energy state.

14. In eukaryotic cells, which of the following cellular processes occurs outside the mitochondria?
   a. Citric acid cycle
   b. Pyruvate oxidation
   c. Glycolysis
   d. Oxidative phosphorylation

15. Which process occurring in the citric acid cycle results in the production of carbon dioxide?
   a. Citrate to isocitrate
   b. Alpha-ketoglutarate to succinyl CoA
   c. Succinate to fumarate
   d. Malate to oxaloacetate

16. In photosynthesis, light energy (photons) is converted to chemical energy in the form of which two compounds?
   a. ATP and $NADP^+$
   b. ATP and NADPH
   c. ADP and $NADP^+$
   d. ADP and NADPH

17. In photosynthesis, carbon dioxide can reach and enter the chloroplast initially by entering the:
   a. stroma
   b. granum
   c. thylakoid
   d. stomata

18. Photosynthesis consists of two main steps called light and dark reactions. Which of the following statements is correct?
   a. The dark reactions can continually create ADP/$NADP^+$ during the night.
   b. The light reactions can continually create ATP/NADPH during the night.
   c. The light reactions cannot continuously create ATP/NADPH during the night.
   d. The dark reactions cannot continuously create ADP/$NADPH$ during the night.

19. Which pigment absorbs at the longest wavelength of light?
   a. Chlorophyll a
   b. Chlorophyll b
   c. beta-carotene
   d. alpha-carotene

20. Complete the following statement: For every _____ molecule(s) of carbon dioxide that enter(s) the Calvin cycle, _____ net molecule(s) of glyceraldehyde-3-phosphate (G3P) is (are) produced.
   a. two; one
   b. three; one
   c. three; six
   d. one; three

21. Photosystems II and I cooperate in light reactions and contain special chlorophyll a molecules called:
   a. $P500 \ and \ P680$
   b. $P600 \ and \ P700$
   c. $P350 \ and \ P580$
   d. $P680 \ and \ P700$

22. Which of the following choices indicates the correct linear electron flow within PS II and I?

    a. An electron moves from $P680$ to the primary electron acceptor, a photon strikes a pigment, ATP is produced, and a photoexcited electron moves from PS II to PS I.

    b. A photon strikes a pigment, an electron moves from $P680$ to the primary electron acceptor, a photoexcited electron moves from PS II to PS I, and ATP is produced.

    c. A photon strikes a pigment, a photoexcited electron moves from PS II to PS I, an electron moves from $P680$ to the primary electron acceptor, and ATP is produced.

    d. A photon strikes a pigment, an electron moves from $P680$ to the primary electron acceptor, a photoexcited electron moves from PS I to PS II, and ATP is produced.

23. Mitochondria and chloroplasts both generate ATP by what similar mechanism?

    a. Krebs cycle

    b. Citric acid cycle

    c. Calvin cycle

    d. Chemiosmosis

24. What are the phases in order of the Calvin cycle?

    a. Carbon fixation, reduction, and regeneration of the carbon dioxide acceptor called RuBP

    b. Carbon fixation, oxidation, and regeneration of the carbon dioxide donator called G3P

    c. Carbon fixation, oxidation, and regeneration of the carbon dioxide acceptor called RuBP

    d. Carbon fixation, reduction, and regeneration of the carbon dioxide acceptor called G3P

25. What is the initial electron donor in light reactions?

    a. Carbon dioxide

    b. Water

    c. NADPH

    d. Oxygen gas

26. The citric acid and Calvin cycle are similar because both use a starting material that is regenerated. However, there are some metabolic differences. Which set of statements is accurate with respect to the citric acid and Calvin cycle?

    a. The oxidation of acetyl CoA in the citric acid cycle is catabolic since it uses energy to produce ATP. The Calvin cycle is anabolic since it consumes energy to breakdown molecules.

    b. The citric acid cycle is anabolic since it oxidizes acetyl CoA and uses energy to produce ATP. The Calvin cycle is catabolic since it consumes energy to build molecules.

    c. The citric acid cycle is catabolic since it oxidizes acetyl CoA and uses energy to produce ATP. The Calvin cycle is anabolic since it consumes energy to build molecules.

    d. The reduction of acetyl CoA in the citric acid cycle is catabolic since it uses energy to produce ATP. The Calvin cycle is anabolic since it consumes energy to build molecules.

27. The chemical structure of chlorophyll *a* and *b* is shown below. Based on the structure of the porphyrin ring, where might electron loss occur during photoexcitation?

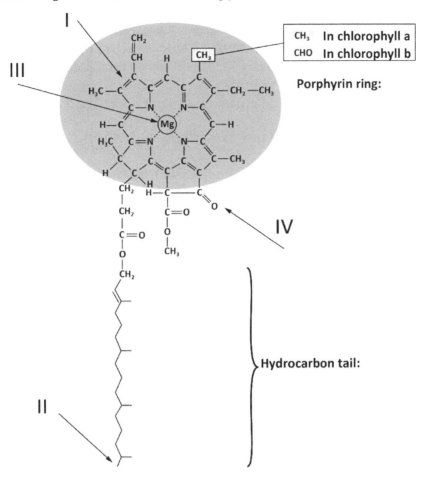

a. I
b. II
c. III
d. IV

28. In cellular respiration, most electrons will do which of the following?
   a. Travel an uphill route from glucose to NADH to ETC to oxygen
   b. Travel a downhill route from glucose to ETC to NADH to oxygen
   c. Travel an uphill route from oxygen to ETC to NADH to oxygen
   d. Travel a downhill route from glucose to NADH to ETC to oxygen

29. In cellular respiration, one glucose molecule produces two ATP molecules in glycolysis and another two ATP molecules in the citric acid cycle. $NADH$ and $FADH_2$ are produced through glycolysis, pyruvate oxidation, and the citric acid cycle. These electron shuttles are eventually oxidized in the ETC. In oxidative phosphorylation, a maximum of twenty-eight ATP and a minimum of twenty-six ATP can be produced. The difference is due to whether $NADH$ or $FADH_2$ is used to shuttle electrons in the cytosol. Which selection below explains how the maximum number of ATP total is initially calculated from all electron shuttles?

   a. Two $NADH$ (glycolysis), two $FADH_2$ (pyruvate oxidation), six $NADH$, and two $FADH_2$ (citric acid cycle)

   b. Two $NADH$ (glycolysis), two $NADH$ (pyruvate oxidation), six $NADH$, and two $FADH_2$ (citric acid cycle)

   c. Four $NADH$ (glycolysis), six $NADH$ (pyruvate oxidation), twelve $NADH$, and six $FADH_2$ (citric acid cycle)

   d. Four $NADH$ (glycolysis), four $FADH_2$ (pyruvate oxidation), twelve $NADH$, and six $FADH_2$ (citric acid cycle)

30. In which of the following ways will electrons travel down the electron transport chain (ETC) in oxidative phosphorylation?

   a. From a less electronegative carrier ($NADH$) to a more electronegative carrier thereby releasing energy

   b. From a more electronegative carrier ($FADH_2$) to a less electronegative carrier thereby releasing energy

   c. From a less electronegative carrier (NAD^+) to a more electronegative carrier thereby releasing energy

   d. From a more electronegative carrier ($NADH$) to a less electronegative carrier thereby releasing energy

Chemistry

1. An element's identity is given by the number of which of the following?

   a. Electrons

   b. Nuclei

   c. Neutrons

   d. Protons

2. Which of the following subatomic particles is negatively charged?

   a. Neutron

   b. Electron

   c. Anion

   d. Proton

3. The total charge on an atom is determined by which of the following?

   a. The number of electrons

   b. The number of neutrons and protons

   c. The number of electrons and neutrons

   d. The number of electrons and protons

4. To find the number of neutrons (N) in an atom, which of the following statements must be true?
    a. The number of neutrons (N) is equal to the mass number minus the number of electrons.
    b. The number of neutrons (N) is equal to the mass number minus the atomic number.
    c. The number of neutrons (N) is equal to the number of electrons minus the number of protons.
    d. The number of neutrons (N) is equal to the atomic number minus the atomic mass.

5. A particular substance has a half-life of 40 days. If the initial sample was 200 g, how many grams will remain after 80 days?
    a. 25 g
    b. 50 g
    c. 75 g
    d. 100 g

6. What is the half-life of an unknown element X if it takes 24 days to decay from 40 g to 10 g?
    a. 4 days
    b. 6 days
    c. 8 days
    d. 12 days

7. How many electrons are found in the p orbitals of oxygen?
    a. 2
    b. 3
    c. 4
    d. 5

8. Within the L shell, how many electrons are found in each orbital for the chlorine element?
    a. 2
    b. 3
    c. 4
    d. 5

9. Which of the following statements is NOT true regarding the modern view of the atomic model?
    a. Protons are positively-charged subatomic particles that are found in the nucleus.
    b. Protons are positively-charged subatomic particles that are dispersed evenly within the atom.
    c. The volume of an atom is mostly unoccupied space.
    d. Electrons are both particles and waves.

10. How many neutrons are present for the nuclide below?
$$^{93}_{36}Kr$$
    a. 129
    b. 93
    c. 36
    d. 57

11. Why were Rutherford and his team surprised when they observed the scattering of some alpha particles?

a. Rutherford believed the alpha particles would easily pass through the nucleus. The protons are found at the center of the atom.

b. Rutherford understood that alpha particles are positively charged; therefore, the deflection should occur because the atom contains protons.

c. Rutherford thought that an alpha particle would pass through the atom unscathed and with minimal deflection because it was initially believed that charges were spread evenly.

d. Rutherford knew that alpha particles are negatively charged particles and should not be deflected because they are attracted to the positively charged particles in a gold atom.

12. What is the classification of the following nuclear reaction if the $_{+1}^{0}e$ particle is detected?

a. Alpha decay

b. Beta decay

c. Electron emission

d. Positron decay

13. Which of the following nuclear reactions involves the conversion of a proton to a neutron?

a. Electron emission

b. Beta decay

c. Electron capture

d. Alpha decay

14. Which of the following is the correct product for the nuclear reaction below?

$$_{24}^{51}Cr + \, _{-1}^{0}e \rightarrow ?$$

a. $_{25}^{51}Mn$

b. $_{23}^{51}V$

c. $_{23}^{50}Mn$

d. $_{22}^{50}Ti$

15. Which of the following is the correct product for the nuclear reaction below?

$$_{15}^{32}P \rightarrow \, _{-1}^{0}e + ?$$

a. $_{14}^{32}Si$

b. $_{16}^{32}S$

c. $_{15}^{32}P$

d. $_{16}^{31}S$

16. One negatively-charged atom and one positively-charged atom form which of the following type of bond?

a. Polar covalent

b. Ionic

c. Coordinate covalent

d. Metallic

17. Electrons that are shared between two atoms form which of the following type of bond?
    a. Ionic
    b. Metallic
    c. Dipole-dipole
    d. Covalent

18. Which of the following types of bonds form due to the free flow of electrons?
    a. Metallic
    b. Hydrogen
    c. Ionic
    d. Covalent

19. Which of the Lewis symbols below is incorrect?

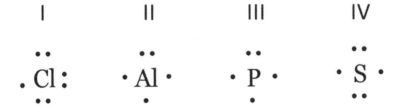

    a. I
    b. II
    c. III
    d. IV

20. Which of the Lewis dot structures below is correct?

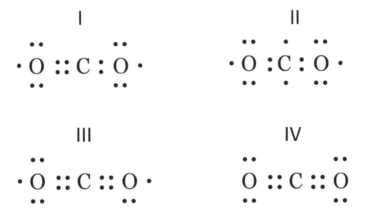

    a. I
    b. II
    c. III
    d. IV

21. Which of the following compounds is nonpolar?
    a. CO
    b. CO_2
    c. CO_3^{2-}
    d. SO_2

22. Which of the following compounds can undergo delocalized bonding?
    a. CH_4
    b. C_2H_6
    c. NO_3^-
    d. NH_3

23. Which of the following compounds does NOT contain a coordinate covalent bond?
    a. NH_4^+
    b. AlH_4^-
    c. $AlCl_3$
    d. H_3O^+

24. Which of the following compounds contains the shortest chemical bond?
    a. C_3H_8
    b. C_2H_6
    c. C_2H_2
    d. C_2H_4

25. Which of the following elements contains eight valence electrons?
    a. Al^{3+}
    b. Cl
    c. Be^{2+}
    d. C

26. Which of the following nuclear reactions does NOT involve the conversion of a proton to a neutron and a neutron to a proton?
    a. Beta decay
    b. Electron capture
    c. Positron emission
    d. Alpha decay

27. A nuclear reaction involves the formation of a daughter nuclide. Which of the following types of nuclear decay involves the formation of a positively-charged particle?
    a. Electron capture
    b. Gamma ray emission
    c. Alpha decay
    d. Beta decay

28. Nuclear fission produces which of the following types of subatomic particles?
    a. Particles of light
    b. Protons
    c. Neutrons
    d. Helium nuclei

29. Exposure to radiation harms DNA and can cause double/single-strand breakages and base damage.

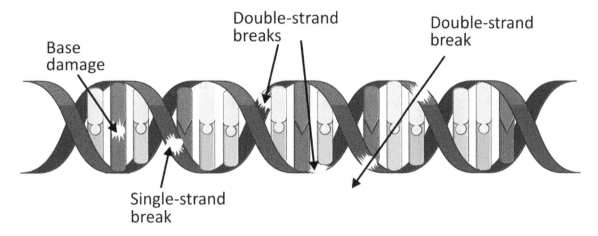

The *rem* is a measurable unit of radiation dosage that helps measure biological damage. It depends on the radiation absorbed dosage (*rads*) and relative biological effectiveness (RBE).

$$rem = rads \times RBE$$

If a person is exposed to 20 rads of alpha, 20 rads of beta, and 250 rads of gamma radiation, which type of radiation causes the greatest biological damage? If 500 rems are considered a lethal dosage, will that exposed person survive? Use the information provided below.

Radiation Type	RBE
α	10
β	1
γ	1
$^{1}_{0}n$	5

    a. Alpha; yes
    b. Beta; no
    c. Gamma; yes
    d. Alpha; no

30. Gold-198 is used to treat ovarian, prostate, and brain cancer and has a half-life of 2.69 days. A hospital needs to have 20 mg of gold-198 for use per day. If it takes 48 hours to deliver gold-198 to the hospital, what amount (milligrams) needs to be ordered?
    a. 24.6 mg
    b. 33.5 mg
    c. 37.2 mg
    d. 40.1 mg

Anatomy and Physiology

1. Which of the following represents the correct order of hormonal gene activation?
    a. The hormone binds to a receptor located on the cell membrane.
    b. The hormone binds to a receptor protein, which then activates an enzyme.
    c. The hormone enters the nucleus to form a hormone-receptor complex, followed by transcription.
    d. The hormone enters the nucleus to form a hormone-receptor complex, followed by translation.

2. What is a hormone that is produced from a polyunsaturated hydrocarbon chain (lipid) called?
    a. Testosterone
    b. Prostaglandin
    c. Peptide
    d. Estrogen

3. Which of the following explains the main reason for the structural differences between the left and right ventricles?
    a. The right ventricle is more powerful and pumps blood over a much longer pathway.
    b. The left ventricle is more powerful and pumps blood over a much shorter pathway.
    c. The right ventricle is less powerful and pumps blood over a much longer pathway.
    d. The left ventricle is more powerful and pumps blood over a much longer pathway.

4. From innermost to outermost, the heart wall is made up of which of the following?
    a. The epicardium, myocardium, and endocardium
    b. The endocardium, myocardium, and epicardium
    c. The fibrous pericardium, pericardial cavity, and epicardium
    d. The epicardium, pericardial cavity, and fibrous pericardium

5. Which of the following is the correct order of blood flow in the circulatory system from the blood capillary beds of the lungs?
    a. The pulmonary arteries, left atrium, systemic circuit, right atrium, and pulmonary veins
    b. The pulmonary arteries, right atrium, systemic circuit, left atrium, and pulmonary veins
    c. The pulmonary arteries, left ventricle, systemic circuit, right ventricle, and pulmonary veins
    d. The pulmonary veins, left atrium, systemic circuit, right atrium, and pulmonary arteries

6. What is the main difference between arteries and veins?
    a. Veins carry oxygen-rich blood away from the heart to the body, and arteries carry oxygen-deficient blood from the body's tissues back to the heart via the venae cavae.
    b. Veins carry oxygen-rich blood away from the heart to the body, and arteries carry oxygen-deficient blood from the body's tissues back to the heart via the aorta.
    c. Arteries carry oxygen-rich blood away from the heart to the body, and veins carry oxygen-deficient blood from the body's tissues back to the heart via the venae cavae.
    d. Arteries carry oxygen-rich blood away from the heart to the body, and veins carry oxygen-deficient blood from the body's tissues back to the heart via the aorta.

7. Which of the following organs of the respiratory system contains the alveoli?
    a. The pharynx
    b. The trachea
    c. The lungs
    d. The larynx

8. Air passes and channels through several organs of the respiratory system. Which of the following organs provides the best initial defense against bacteria or debris found in the air?

a. The respiratory mucosa within the nostrils can moisten the air to trap dust and destroy bacteria.

b. The mucosa in the oral cavity can moisten the air to trap dust and destroy bacteria.

c. The oropharynx can moisten the air and trap foreign debris while destroying bacteria.

d. The ciliated mucosa in the trachea can trap dust and eliminate bacteria with mucus and push it toward the throat where it can be swallowed.

9. What is the correct order of air passage in regard to the respiratory organs?

a. The nasal cavity, pharynx, larynx, trachea, bronchi, bronchioles, and alveoli

b. The nasal cavity, pharynx, larynx, trachea, bronchioles, bronchi, and alveoli

c. The nasal cavity, larynx, pharynx, trachea, bronchi, bronchioles, and alveoli

d. The nasal cavity, larynx, pharynx, trachea, bronchioles, bronchi, and alveoli

10. Alveoli walls contain a single thin layer of tissue that is covered with the capillary walls, together with elastic fibers, to form a fused basement membrane called the respiratory membrane. The membrane allows the gas exchange by simple diffusion. The alveoli walls are most likely what type of epithelial tissue?

a. Simple cuboidal epithelial tissue

b. Simple columnar epithelial tissue

c. Simple squamous epithelial tissue

d. Transitional stratified epithelial tissue

11. The intrinsic nerve plexuses are found in which of the following tissue layers?

a. The serosa

b. The mucosa

c. The visceral peritoneum

d. The submucosa

12. The gastric pits contain specific cells that release chemicals responsible for the stimulation or initiation of the emptying of the stomach. What are these cells called?

a. Enteroendocrine cells

b. Mucous neck cells

c. Parietal cells

d. Chief cells

13. Intrinsic factors are needed for the absorption of vitamin B_{12} in the small intestine. These substances are glycoproteins that are secreted in what part of the alimentary canal?

a. The large intestine

b. The small intestine

c. The stomach

d. The esophagus

14. Most nutrient absorption occurs in which alimentary organ?

a. The small intestine

b. The stomach

c. The large intestine

d. The fundus

15. If the parietal cells were unable to secrete substances into the gastric gland, which of the following scenarios would occur?
    a. Pepsin would not convert to pepsinogen, resulting in the digestion of dietary proteins.
    b. Pepsinogen would not convert to pepsin, resulting in the indigestion of dietary proteins.
    c. Pepsin would convert to pepsinogen, resulting in the indigestion of dietary proteins.
    d. Pepsinogen would convert to pepsin, resulting in the indigestion of dietary proteins.

16. Which muscle component controls the flow of chyme into the small intestine?
    a. The villi
    b. The pylorus
    c. The muscularis externa
    d. The pyloric sphincter

17. The diagram below shows the gross internal anatomy of the stomach. Which of the following labels represents the oblique layer of the stomach?

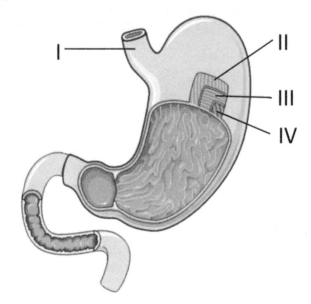

    a. 3
    b. 1
    c. 2
    d. 4

18. Gastric cancer is one of the main causes of cancer-related deaths and the second most deadly cancer throughout the world. Specific cells within the stomach are believed to play a vital role in cancer initiation. These cells have been known to regulate tissue renewal and repair. What are these cells called?
    a. Chief cells
    b. Stem cells
    c. Parietal cells
    d. Enteroendocrine cells

19. What are the three regions of the kidney from the most superficial aspect of the kidneys to the ureter?
    a. The pelvis, medulla, and cortex
    b. The fibrous capsule, perirenal fat capsule, and renal fascia
    c. The cortex, medulla, and pelvis
    d. The renal fascia, perirenal fat capsule, and fibrous capsule

20. A patient visiting a medical clinic tells the doctor that he has been having problems urinating. The doctor notices that the patient had lost a significant amount of weight since he last visited. The doctor most likely suspects that the patient is suffering from hydronephrosis. Which of the following describes this condition?
    a. The fibrous capsule dwindles, causing pressure to build on the kidney tissue.
    b. The fat capsule dwindles, causing the ureters to become kinked.
    c. The renal fascia dwindles, causing pressure to build on the kidney tissue.
    d. The renal pelvis dwindles, causing the ureters to become kinked.

21. The diagram below illustrates several regions of the nephron. Which of the following labels corresponds to a region that protrudes into the renal medulla?

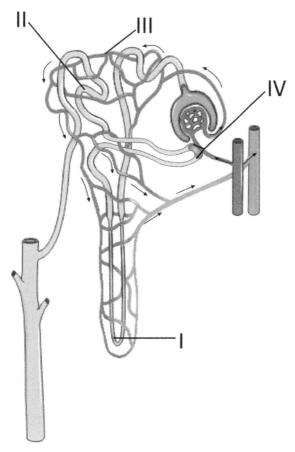

    a. 2
    b. 4
    c. 1
    d. 3

22. Which of the following represents the correct direction of blood flow within the renal blood vessels?
    a. Renal vein, arcuate vein, arcuate artery, renal artery
    b. Interlobar vein, cortical radiate vein, afferent arteriole, cortical radiate artery
    c. Interlobar artery, cortical radiate artery, cortical radiate vein, efferent arteriole
    d. Renal artery, arcuate artery, arcuate vein, renal vein

23. During a vasectomy, a surgeon makes a small incision in the scrotum and ties which of the following accessory organs?
    a. The ejaculatory duct
    b. The ductus deferens
    c. The ampulla of ductus deferens
    d. The prostatic urethra

24. In the female duct system, there is no contact between the ovaries and the uterine tubes. What specific part of the uterine tube helps carry the oocyte toward the uterus?
    a. The fimbriae
    b. The infundibulum
    c. The cilia
    d. The broad ligaments

25. The appearance of the follicular antrum signals which of the following developmental stages?
    a. Formation of the primary follicle called the vesicular follicle
    b. Formation of the ruptured follicle called the corpus luteum
    c. Formation of the corpus luteum following ovulation
    d. Formation of the secondary follicle called the vesicular follicle

26. Considering the structure of sperm, where are the mitochondria and DNA located, respectively?
    a. The head; the midpiece
    b. The head, the tail
    c. The midpiece; the head
    d. The tail; the head

27. Which of the following labels corresponds to the peritoneal cavity?

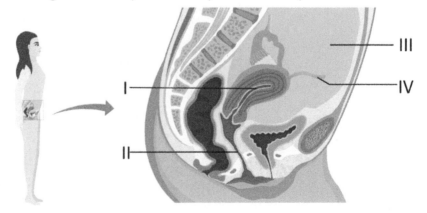

    a. 3
    b. 4
    c. 1
    d. 2

28. A woman's anatomy is more vulnerable to infection for several reasons. For example, a woman's vagina is covered by a thin and more delicate mucous membrane that allows bacteria and viruses to pass through more readily. Which of the following is another reason why women are at higher risk for infections spreading within the reproductive tract?

    a. Contact between the uterine tube and ovaries causes infections to spread more readily into the peritoneal cavity.

    b. Contact between the uterine tube and ovaries is minimal, causing infections to spread more easily into the peritoneal cavity.

    c. Contact between the fimbriae and ovaries is minimal, causing infections to spread more readily into the peritoneal cavity.

    d. Contact between the infundibulum and ovaries causes infections to spread more readily into the peritoneal cavity.

29. The diagram below illustrates the frontal view of the male reproductive organs and accessory glands. The following choices represent several accessory glands and organs. Which choice does not contribute to the composition of semen?

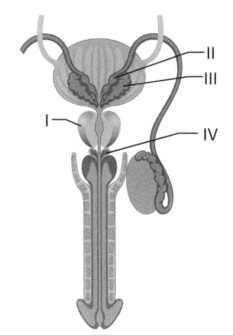

    a. 1
    b. 2
    c. 3
    d. 4

30. For the most part, the glands, ducts, and organs found within the male and female systems have similar functions. Which of the following does NOT have a reproductive role?

    a. The testes and ovaries
    b. The bulbourethral and greater vestibular glands
    c. The gonads in men and women
    d. The male and female urethra

Answer Explanations #2

Mathematics

1. B: There are three decimal places in 0.081. Therefore, write 81 over a denominator of 1 with three zeros, or 1,000.

2. C: There are two decimal places in 33.75. Therefore, write 3375 over a denominator of 1 with two zeros, or 100. $\frac{3375}{100}$ reduces to $\frac{135}{4}$ in lowest terms.

3. A: The denominator is a power of ten, and it has three zeros. Therefore, move the decimal in the numerator to the left three places, resulting in 0.567.

4. C: The denominator is a power of ten, and it has two zeros. Therefore, move the decimal in the numerator to the left two places, resulting in 567.9.

5. C: When comparing two negative decimals, compare digits from left to right. The number with the smaller first digit is larger. Therefore, -5.677 is the largest because it has the smallest value in the hundredths place.

6. B: The thousandth place is three digits to the right from the decimal, so its value is 7. The number to the right of it is 8, so 7 rounds up to 8 and everything to its right becomes a zero. The answer is 8.568.

7. D: When comparing two positive decimals, compare digits from left to right. The number with the first different digit that is larger is the greater value. Therefore, 1.2192 is the largest because it has the largest value in the ten thousandths place.

8. B: The hundredths place is two digits to the right from the decimal, so its value is 9. The value to the right of it is 9, so it rounds up. 9 rounds up to 10, so a 1 is added to the tenth place, resulting in -6.9.

9. D: The ones place is one digit to the left of the decimal, so its value is 5. The value to its right is a 7, so 5 rounds up to 6, and everything else becomes a zero. The answer is 16.

10. B: To write a fraction as a decimal, divide. $17 \div 25 = 0.68$.

11. D: To write a fraction as a decimal, divide. $2 \div 9 = 0.22222 \ldots$ This is a repeating decimal, and it is written with a bar over the part that repeats. Therefore, the answer is $0.\overline{2}$.

12. B: To write a fraction as a decimal, divide. $7 \div 24 = 0.2916666$, which is a repeating decimal. Rounded to the nearest hundredths place, it is equal to 0.29.

13. C: The ratio 18 to 40 can be written as a fraction as $\frac{18}{40}$; however, it must be simplified into lowest terms. Therefore, the correct ratio is $\frac{9}{20}$.

14. C: To find his speed in miles per hour, divide the total distance traveled by the time. $565 \div 9.5 = 59.47368 \ldots$ Rounded to the nearest tenth, the speed is equal to 59.5 mph.

15. B: To find the best buy, find the unit cost of each option. Divide the cost by the ounces. The corresponding unit costs are $0.56/ounce, $0.50/ounce, $0.53/ounce, and $0.52/ounce. The lowest unit cost is $0.50/ounce, which corresponds to the 24-ounce option.

16. A: To solve the proportion, first, cross-multiply. This step results in $54x = 35$. Then, divide both sides by 54, resulting in $x = \frac{35}{54}$.

17. B: To solve the proportion, first, cross-multiply. This step results in $3y = 19.11$. Dividing both sides by 3 gives the solution $y = 6.37$.

18. D: This problem can be solved using the following proportion:

$$\frac{12}{15} = \frac{x}{60}$$

Cross-multiplication results in $15x = 720$. Dividing each side by 15 results in $x = 48$. Therefore, 48 pounds of ham are needed.

19. A: This problem can be solved using the following proportion:

$$\frac{0.5}{75} = \frac{x}{90}$$

Cross-multiplication results in $45 = 75x$. Dividing each side by 75 results in $x = 0.6$. Therefore, the distance is equivalent to 0.6 in. on the map.

20. A: This problem can be solved using the following proportion:

$$\frac{214}{x} = \frac{18}{92}$$

Cross-multiplication results in $19{,}688 = 18x$. Dividing each side by 18 results in $x = 1093.777\ldots$ This amount rounded to the nearest whole number is 1,094.

21. C: This problem can be solved using the following proportion:

$$\frac{4}{12} = \frac{14}{x}$$

Cross-multiplication results in $4x = 168x$. Dividing each side by 4 results in $x = 42$. Therefore, the building is 42 ft tall.

22. B: Similar triangles have corresponding sides lengths with the same ratio. For this triangle, a proportion of side lengths is $\frac{4}{10} = \frac{a}{15}$. Cross-multiplying results in $60 = 10a$. Dividing each side by 10 results in $a = 6$.

23. A: Because there are 12 inches in a foot, multiply 9.5 times 12, resulting in 114 inches.

24. A: Because there are 5,280 feet in one mile, there are $6(5{,}280) = 31{,}680$ feet in 6 miles. There are 3 feet in 1 yard, so there are $31680 \div 3 = 10{,}560$ yd is 6 mi.

25. B: To convert kilometers to meters, move the decimal point three places to the left, adding zeros if necessary. Therefore, 1 m = 1,000 km.

26. C: To convert cm to mm, move the decimal point one place to the right. Therefore, 56.78 cm = 567.8 mm.

27. B: To convert cm to km, move the decimal point five places to the left. Therefore, 34,598 cm = 0.34598 km.

28. C: There are 2.54 cm in 1 inch and 12 inches in 1 ft. Therefore, there are $12(2.54) = 30.48$ cm in 1 ft. Multiplying this amount by 3 shows that there are $3(30.48) = 91.44$ cm in 3 feet, which is rounded to 91.4.

29. C: There are 4 qt in 1 gal, so there are $18(4) = 72$ qt in 18 gal. There are 2 pt in 1 qt, so there are $72(2) = 144$ pt in 18 gal. There are 2 cups in 1 pt, so there are $144(2) = 288$ cups in 18 gal. Finally, there are 8 oz in 1 cup, so there are $288(8) = 2,304$ oz in 18 gal.

30. A: There are 2 cups in a pint and 2 pints in a quart, so there are 4 cups in a quart. Dividing 8,490 by 4 results in 2,122.5 qt.

31. D: Because 1 cc = 1 mL, there are 750 cc in 750 mL of the medicine.

32. A: To convert milliliters to liters, move the decimal point three places to the left. Therefore, 7,500 mL is equal to 7.5 L.

33. C: Because there are 2,000 pounds in 1 ton, there are $2000(4) = 8,000$ pounds in 4 tons.

34. D: Because there are 16 ounces in 1 pound, there are $16(8) = 128$ ounces in 8 pounds.

35. B: To convert g to kg, move the decimal 3 places to the left. Therefore, there are 89.452 kg in 89,452 g.

36. D: To convert g to mg, move the decimal 3 places to the right, adding zeros if necessary. Therefore:

$$675.2 \text{ g} = 675,200 \text{ mg}$$

37. B: The freezing point of water is 0°C or 32°F.

38. B: The formula to convert Fahrenheit to Celsius is $C = \frac{5}{9}(F - 32)$. Therefore:

$$C = \frac{5}{9}(214 - 32) = \frac{5}{9}(182) = 101.1 \text{ rounded to the nearest tenth}$$

39. D: The formula to convert Celsius to Fahrenheit is $F = \frac{9}{5}C + 32$. Therefore,

$$F = \frac{9}{5}C + 32 = \frac{9}{5}(45) + 32 = 113$$

40. A: Large numbers can be converted to Roman numerals by breaking the number up into thousands, hundreds, tens, and ones and writing each number in its equivalent form using the Roman numeral system. 3,786 is equal to 3,000 + 700 + 80 + 6. 3,000 in Roman numerals is MMM. 700 in Roman

Numerals is DCC. 80 in Roman numerals is LXXX. Finally, 6 in Roman numerals is VI. Combining them in order results in 3,786 = MMMDCCLXXXVI.

41. C: Large numbers can be converted to Roman numerals by breaking the number up into thousands, hundreds, tens, and ones and writing each number in its equivalent form using the Roman numeral system. 2,765 is equal to 2,000 + 700 + 60 + 5. 2,000 in Roman numerals is MM. 700 in Roman Numerals is DCC. 60 in Roman numerals is LX. Finally, 5 in Roman numerals is V. Combining them in order results in 2,765=MMDCCLXV.

42: D: To convert a time after noon to military time, add 12 to the hour and drop the p.m. Thus, 8 +12 = 20, so 8:45 p.m. is equal to 20:45 or 2045.

43: B: Because the military time is greater than 12, subtract 12 from the time, resulting in 3:30. Also, attach p.m. because the time is after noon.

44: C: To find out how many tablets this patient needs daily, use cross-products. Let x be the number of tablets. Therefore:

$$150 \text{ mg} \times x = 375 \text{ mg}$$

Dividing by 150 results in:

$$x = \frac{375}{150} = 2.5$$

Therefore, 2.5 tablets need to be given to this patient daily.

45. D: To determine how many ml she receives each day, cross-products can be used. Let x be the unknown quantity of cough syrup. Therefore,

$$25 \frac{\text{mg}}{\text{ml}} \times x = 125 \text{ mg}$$

Dividing both sides by $25 \frac{\text{mg}}{\text{ml}}$ results in $x = 6$ ml. Therefore, 6 ml of the cough syrup need to be administered once daily orally to this patient.

46. A: To convert 0.00005 to a percent, move the decimal point two places to the right and attach the % symbol. Therefore, 0.00005 = 0.005%.

47. D: To convert 0.04% to a decimal, move the decimal point two places to the left and drop the % symbol. Therefore, 0.04% = 0.0004.

48. B: To find 95% of 1,895, multiply the decimal form of 95% times 1,895. Therefore,

$$0.95 \times 1895 = 1800.25$$

49. C: To find the answer, divide 38 by the decimal form of 45%, which is 0.45. Therefore, $\frac{38}{0.45} = 84.4444 \ldots = 84.\overline{4}$.

50. C: To find the percentage, divide 65 by 140 and convert the decimal to a percentage. Therefore,
$$\frac{65}{140} = 0.464 = 46.4\%$$

51. A: Plugging 5 in for x and 7 in for y, we have:

$$5 \times 5^3 - 4 \times 7^2$$

$$5 \times 125 - 4 \times 49$$

$$625 - 196 = 429$$

52. D: First, subtract 5 from both sides, resulting in $8x = 64$. Then, divide both sides by 8 to obtain the solution $x = 8$.

53. D: First, distribute the 12 throughout the parentheses to obtain $12x - 108 = 120$. Add 108 to both sides to obtain $12x = 228$. Then, divide both sides by 12 to obtain the solution $x = 19$.

54. B: First, subtract 7.2 from both sides, resulting in $1.1y = 11$. Then, divide both sides by 1.1, resulting in the solution $y = 10$.

55. C: Substituting 2 in for x and 4 in for y, we have:

$$2(2)^2 + 8(4)^3$$

$$2 \times 4 + 8 \times 64$$

$$8 + 512 = 520$$

Reading Comprehension

1. C: According to the text, "public health groups have suggested [...] the Motion Picture Association of America assigning an R rating to any movie with tobacco imagery, unless it portrays an actual historical figure who used tobacco or depicts the negative effects of tobacco use." Based on that information, there are only two occasions under which those groups would find the inclusion of tobacco use acceptable. Whether the character is the bad guy (Choice A), unlikeable (Choice B), or over the age of 21 (Choice D) is not a factor.

2. D: The main point of the passage is that the increase in depictions of tobacco usage in youth-targeted films is concerning and should be addressed so as not to further degrade the progress made in decreasing tobacco use in media watched by American youths. While multiple suggestions are made to address the issues, banning tobacco usage is not among them, so Choice A is incorrect. Choice B and Choice C are supporting details and so are both incorrect.

3. A: According to the passage, "During 2010–2018, the number of PG-13 biographical dramas with tobacco incidents approximately tripled." Therefore, none of the other choices is correct.

4. C: The concern is that it will normalize tobacco usage, potentially raising rates of teen smoking. While Choices A and C are possibilities, they are not mentioned in this passage. Because there is a clear concern noted in the passage, Choice B is incorrect.

5. B: According to the passage, "All major motion picture companies have policies to reduce tobacco depictions in youth-rated movies; however, Disney and Viacom were the only companies with no tobacco use in youth-rated movies in 2018." This quote renders choices A, C, and D incorrect.

6. B: The text reports, "Even many cancer survivors with private insurance coverage reported borrowing money, being unable to cover their share of medical care costs, going into debt, or filing for bankruptcy." As noted in the passage, cancer patients and survivors have considerable out-of-pocket expenses, so choice *A* is incorrect. Choice *C* and choice *D* are not discussed in this passage and so are therefore incorrect as well.

7. C: According to the text, the findings in this report might lead to increased awareness in all sectors of the public health and medical community that the rising cost of cancer care is a major barrier to survivors' well-being. Choice *A* is not discussed. Choice *B* is mentioned, but as a fact, not as an outcome of the report. Choice *D* is mentioned, and may be an outcome of raised awareness, but it is not an outcome of the report.

8. D: Choice D is correct. According to the first paragraph, "Further, approximately one-fourth of cancer survivors reported having material financial hardship."

9. C: The final paragraph discusses what interventions would be useful, including screening for financial hardship. It is likely that in some cancer diagnoses, a genetic or family history screening may occur (Choice *A*), but it's not the focus of this passage and is, therefore, incorrect. Choices *B* and *D* would also be helpful, but both have likely already occurred.

10. A: Based on the tone and subject of the passage, *adverse*, in relation to the financial consequences of cancer treatment, means harmful. Choices *B* and *C* are both the opposite of what is discussed and, therefore, incorrect. While *immense* makes sense, Choice *D* is incorrect as it doesn't necessarily convey the damage done by the consequences.

11. C: According to the text, "only about half of adolescents are up-to-date on [their HPV] vaccine."

12. B: According to the text, "no state met the Healthy People 2020 objective for HPV vaccination."

13. B: According to the text, "Cervical cancer is the only HPV-associated cancer for which screening is routinely recommended." While the other cancers are mentioned as associated with HPV, they are not routinely screened for.

14. D: The research shows that "Catch-up vaccination is not recommended for all adults aged older than twenty-six years because the benefit of HPV vaccination decreases in older age groups." As they have this data, choice *A* is incorrect because it appears to have been studied. Neither choice *C* nor *D* are explicitly stated as the cause for the reduced efficacy, so one cannot draw either of those as a conclusion without textual support.

15. A: The topic of this passage is HPV. While choices *B*, *C*, and *D* are discussed in the passage, they are done so in relation to the topic of HPV and the cited data and research.

16. A: According to the text, "A more recent study among young children enrolled in WIC reported that the overall obesity prevalence decreased from 15.9% in 2010 to 13.9% in 2016 and statistically significant decreases were observed in all age, sex, and racial/ethnic subgroups." While data was difficult to track at the state level, suggested in choice *D*, it was trackable as a whole. Therefore, the other choices are incorrect.

17. B: As noted in the text, "Comprehensive approaches that create positive changes to promote healthy eating and physical activity for young children from all income levels, strengthen nutrition education and breastfeeding support among young children enrolled in WIC [...] could help maintain or accelerate these declining trends." There is no mention of choice A or choice C in the passage, so they are both incorrect. Choice D is not mentioned either, though could be a positive change.

18. D: The main idea of this passage is that WIC has successfully decreased obesity levels in children and could do more. While choices A and B are both established in the passage, they are not the main idea. Choice C is not a conclusion established by the data in the passage or the writers/researchers.

19. A: WIC is a program of the USDA, as noted midway through first paragraph. While it could easily be a program of the CDC to prevent obesity and the issues that stem from that (Choice B) or a program of HHS (Choice D), those are both incorrect. It is also not its own entity (Choice C).

20. C: According to the first sentence of the passage, "Obesity negatively affects children's health because of its associations with cardiovascular disease risk factors, type 2 diabetes, asthma, fatty liver disease, victimization stemming from social stigma and bullying, and poor mental health (e.g., anxiety and depression)." There is no mention to cancer risk (Choice A) in this passage nor Osgood-Schlatter (Choice D). While diabetes is mentioned, type 1 is not associated with obesity (Choice B).

21. D: According to the text, "opportunities for risk factor prevention and management among younger adults are of particular importance given the increase in heart disease mortality observed from 2010 to 2015 among adults aged thirty-five to sixty-four years in approximately half of U.S. counties." For this reason, this subset of high-risk individuals was identified as a population to focus on. While seniors (Choice A) and sedentary adults of all ages (Choice B) are of concern, they are not the groups discussed specifically in this passage. Similarly, individuals aged twenty-one to thirty-three (Choice C) are not mentioned.

22. B: Million Hearts 2022 has set "at the community level, a 20% reduction in the prevalence of combustible tobacco product use and of physical inactivity, and a 20% reduction in mean daily sodium intake are targeted." Choice A and choice C are noted but the targets are incorrect. Similarly, choice D is an overall goal, though not named, and not at that target level.

23. C: The research notes several disparities among racial groups in particular. "Compared with whites, Hispanics were less likely to use aspirin for secondary prevention or take a statin when indicated, Blacks were less likely to have their blood pressure under control, and persons of other racial/ethnic groups, including American Indians and Alaska Natives, were more likely to use combustible tobacco products. Other studies confirm the existence of these disparities." Choices A, B, and D are not noted in this research.

24. B: The clinical strategies noted are "self-measured blood pressure monitoring with clinical support, standardized treatment protocols, reduced out-of-pocket costs and adherence approaches for medications, clinician-driven tobacco assessment and treatment increasing awareness of the effect of particle pollution (including tobacco smoke, automobile or diesel exhaust, and wood smoke) on persons with known heart disease, and using clinical data to identify persons with undiagnosed conditions." Choice A, though unsupervised, is noted in community strategies. While choices C and D may be beneficial, they are not suggested here.

25. A: The final paragraph reiterates the main idea when it states, "Heart disease and stroke are leading causes of death in the United States; their risk factors are prevalent in the general population and are particularly high among certain subgroups. Evidence-based strategies for preventing acute cardiovascular events exist, with 213 million opportunities for better risk factor prevention and management." While choice *D* is discussed in this passage, the main focus is not whether this two-pronged strategy is best. Choices *B* and *D* are both supporting details.

26. D: According to the first two sentences of the passage, "E-cigarettes were introduced to the U.S. market in 2007. In 2018, 20.8% of high school students reported current e-cigarette use." 2007 to 2018 is approximately eleven years.

27. C: According to the text, "Given the vast number of chemicals used in e-cigarette, or vaping, products, it is important to link epidemiologic data with findings from laboratory analyses of products and clinical specimens from patients." While the other choices are likely important to the research, particularly choice *B*, they are not the focus. Choice *A* is information likely already available for the product to be on the market at all. Choice *D* is similarly regulated by law in states where marijuana is available for sale.

28. D: The study notes the following reasons for inability to conduct interviews as "patient refusal, loss to follow-up, persons who were too ill or died before they could be interviewed." Choices *A* and *C* would be addressed prior to the study. Choice *B* is not noted as an obstacle or issue in this passage.

29. A: According to the data, E-cigarette use is markedly lower among U.S. adults than among youths;" and "current e-cigarette use is slightly higher among males than females for both adults and youths." Thus, Choice *A* is the best answer.

30. B: In reference to the products and effort to link to patient data, "Federal, state, and private laboratories are working to collect and analyze products obtained from patients with lung injury associated with e-cigarette use, or vaping." While data for choice *A* and choice *C* is noted here, it is important as part of the overall research, but is not the focus. Choice *D* is not mentioned.

31. B: According to the second paragraph, medications for joint pain are accompanied by adverse side effects. Choices *A*, *C*, and *D* are not mentioned as issues related to this treatment.

32. C: According to the passage, "Adults who are unable to meet the aerobic guideline because of their condition (e.g., those with severe joint pain) should engage in regular physical activity according to their abilities and avoid physical inactivity." This advice contradicts Choice *A*. Choice *B* is not mentioned (and most recommend against it), and there is no data here to suggest that medicating prior to exercise (Choice *D*) helps.

33. A: The main idea of this passage is that physical exercise can and should be a strategy to manage and mitigate pain associated with arthritis. While choices *B*, *C*, and *D* are discussed in this passage, they are all supporting ideas.

34. A: According to the passage, "Arthritis-appropriate, evidence-based, self-management programs and low-impact, group aerobic, or multicomponent physical activity programs are designed to safely increase physical activity in persons with arthritis." Choices *B* and *C* are contradicted by this advice. While choice *D* may be beneficial, it's not specified here.

35. D: According to the passage, "These [exercise] programs are available nationwide and are especially important for those populations that might have limited access to health care, medications, and surgical interventions (e.g., those in rural areas, those with lower income, and racial/ethnic minorities)." There is no mention of the other choices having been identified as specifically needing targeted exercise programs.

36. C: The passage focuses fairly heavily on the need for research to determine occupational hazards as they relate to COPD in adult nonsmokers. While Choice *A* is the discussed in relation to which occupations have higher risk, there is no recommendation to avoid those careers. Choice *B* is not supported in the passage. That is, it may be true, but there is no data to support that. Choice *D* is not the subject of the passage. While it is discussed, the prevalence of those two conditions as they relate to COPD is not fully clear.

37. B: According to the study, "office and administrative support workers (including secretaries, administrative and dental assistants, and clerks), protective service workers, and information industry workers (including publishing, telecommunications, broadcasting, and data processing workers) had the highest COPD prevalence."

38. C: Among both smokers and nonsmokers, "among those who ever smoked and those who never smoked was similar (e.g., highest proportions with COPD were among those who were diagnosed with chronic bronchitis)." Though emphysema (Choice *A*) was reported among the two groups, chronic bronchitis was reported nearly twenty times more frequently. While choice *B* may result in COPD, it was not noted as a common complaint of the two groups, nor was choice *D* discussed.

39. D: According to the passage, "known respiratory irritants...have been associated with bronchitis, emphysema, and COPD." There is no mention in this passage of choices *A*, *B*, or *C*, though certainly one can't rule out that those may also be issues related to respiratory irritants; there is just no evidence or data to draw such conclusions here.

40. B: The evidence of nonsmokers developing COPD after exposure to air contaminants and pollutants supports the claim that the poor air quality can cause COPD, so *confirms* is the best synonym for *corroborates*. Choice *A* and choice *C* would both mean the opposite, meaning the evidence didn't support the claim; therefore, they are both incorrect. To *underscore* (Choice *D*) is to emphasize; therefore, this choice is incorrect.

41. A: As outlined in the concluding paragraph, and noted throughout, educational efforts regarding heart attacks and the appropriate responses to symptoms all need to be improved. Choices *B*, *C*, and *D* are all supporting details rather than main ideas.

42. D: According to the study, "approximately half of respondents (50.2%) knew all five common heart attack signs and symptoms," making Choices *A*, *B*, and *C* incorrect.

43. B: According to the passage, "Consistent messaging campaigns should be complemented with regular contact with a health care provider because screening and evaluation might lead to early intervention." While choices *A*, *C*, and *D* may impact the retention of information regarding the signs and symptoms, none are mentioned in the passage.

44. C: In regard to the goals for awareness, "estimates for certain subpopulations remained below the HP2020 target, including racial/ethnic minorities and adults with less than a high school education." Choices *A* and *B* were not mentioned. Choice *D* is the opposite of one of those sub-populations (those with high risk).

45. A: According to the text, "Clinical, community, and public health efforts are needed to continue to systematically improve the awareness of heart attack symptoms throughout the United States." While individuals (Choice *B*) and institutions (Choice *C*) may play a role, that is not outlined or specified here.

Choice *D* is incorrect as it is not a group or an organization, but rather the focus of the groups/organizations.

46. B: The primary focus of this passage is second-hand smoke in the workplace. While smoke-free policies (Choice *A*), deaths (Choice *C*), and nonsmoking workers (Choice *D*) are mentioned, they are all discussed as supporting details or in relation to second-hand smoke in the workplace.

47. C: According to previous studies, "the absence of a policy restricting or prohibiting smoking at the worksite put workers at higher risk for workplace SHS exposure." While Choice *A* is discussed (construction, transportation, and mining), the data covers more industries than the two mentioned. Choice *B* is not mentioned. Choice *D* is mentioned in relation to the impact on the construction industry, but not workers overall.

48. C: According to the research, "Based on NHIS data for 2014–2016, 34.3% of workers in the construction, 30.4% of workers in the mining, and 30.2% of workers in the transportation industries used some form of tobacco." Therefore, Choices *A*, *B*, and *D* are incorrect.

49. A: According to the passage, "A recent study determined that indoor workers who reported working at a worksite having a 100% smoke-free policy had significantly lower odds of smoking combustible tobacco than did those reporting a partial or no smoke-free policy."

50. B: According to the passage, "Furthermore, workplace SHS exposure has been recognized as one of the top occupational hazards that contributes substantially to the prevalence of occupational cancer among nonsmokers." While it may be a workplace complaint (Choice *A*), contribute to difficulty quitting smoking (Choice *C*), or a be a reason to leave a workplace (Choice *D*), none of those are mentioned in this passage.

51. D: According to the passage, "For children aged two to six, AAPD recommends that dental health care personnel provide sealants for caries-susceptible primary molars and permanent molars, premolars, and anterior teeth." Canines (Choice *A*) and incisors (Choice *B*) are not mentioned. However, sealant is clearly recommended for some teeth, so choice *C* (none) is also incorrect.

52. A: The passage notes "A major barrier to successful implementation of these programs is low consent rates." The passage does not mention that access to schools is the issue (Choice *B*) or a lack of dentists (Choice *C*). Further, it notes that these programs would be cost-effective; therefore, choice *D* is also incorrect.

53. B: According to the text, "because dental care is reduced among low-income and racial/ethnic minority families and among parents with only very young children, relying on dental professionals to provide sealant information is problematic." Choice *A* is not discussed and is, therefore, incorrect. There is no data or information in this passage to support choice *C*. While it is true that the sealants are underutilized, the cause of this is outlined in the passage itself (educational and access issues) and is not tied to dentist refusal. There is no information to support that claim, so choice *D* is incorrect.

54. B: Education should be targeted at the communities that most need the information including "low-income and racial/ethnic minority parents and parents with only young children could reduce disparities in sealant knowledge and untreated dental caries." Choice *A* is incorrect because parents of children under age six are targeted. There is no mention of choice *C*, parents who may have their own dental issues. Finally, school nurses are mentioned as part of the potential solution; thus, choice *D* is incorrect.

55. C: The primary focus of the passage goes beyond the usefulness of sealants (Choice *D*) and really focuses in on the need for education among specific communities regarding the benefits. Thus, choice *C* is the best answer. While choice *A* is mentioned, it is a supporting detail. The text suggests that dentists are not the best people to provide the information/education, as many of the groups that need the education do not see the dentist as often as they should. Therefore, choice *B* is incorrect.

Vocabulary

1. D

2. A

3. A

4. B

5. C

6. C

7. D

8. A

9. C

10. C

11. B

12. A

13. D

14. B

15. A

16. C

17. C

18. D

19. B

20. B

21. A

22. D

23. C

24. D

25. B

26. A

27. C

28. B

29. C

30. D

31. A

32. C

33. B

34. B

35. A

36. D

37. A

38. B

39. B

40. D

41. C

42. A

43. B

44. A

45. D

46. C

47. B

48. A

49. B

50. A

51. C

52. B

53. D

54. C

55. A

Grammar

1. D: Choice *D* is correct as it is the correct conjugation of the verb tense to suggest that an event will happen in the future. Choices *A, B*, and *C* all offer the wrong verb tenses.

2. B: There are two pronouns in the sentence, *he* and *they*, and two nouns in the sentence, *tech* and *tests*. *Tech* is the antecedent of *he,* and *tests* is the antecedent of the word *they*. Choice *B* is the correct answer.

3. A: *Breath* is the air taken in <u>or</u> out. *Breathing* is the act of taking air in <u>and</u> out. So, to *take a deep breath* means to only take air in, but to *remember to breathe* is to do both. Therefore, Choice *A* is correct.

4. B: As a non-essential element and dependent clause, *the one who came from New York*, should contain a comma before and after, so Choice *B* is correct.

5. C: Choice *C* is correct as *finest* is the correct superlative adverb. Superlative adverbs often end in *-est* and they compare 3 or more items.

6. D: Proper nouns name specific people, places, or things. So, in this sentence *Weill Cornell Medicine* is the proper noun, so Choice *D* is the correct answer.

7. A: *To compliment* means to express praise. On the other hand, *to complement* means to pair well with and to complete to perfection. Choice *A* demonstrates correct usage of both of these words; therefore, it is the correct choice.

8. A: Because the word *women's* is a third-person plural noun, the correct answer must be a third person plural pronoun; therefore, Choice *A* is correct.

9. C: Independent clauses are clauses that can stand alone because they include a subject, a verb (predicate), and a complete idea. Of all the options presented, only Choice *C* is an independent clause.

10. C: The word *while* can mean "although" or "even though," so Choice *C* is the best word to contrast the two departments. Choice *A* and Choice *B* are both conjunctions that show causation, but it is unlikely that there would be a cause-and-effect relationship between these two unrelated departments. Similarly, the word *until* suggests that radiology is busy right up to the point when maternity got quiet, but the two are not related in this way, so Choice *D* is not correct.

11. B: Choice *B*, *sent*, is the verb. *Reports*, Choice *A*, is a noun. *To*, Choice *C*, is a preposition. *Patient's*, Choice *D*, is a possessive noun.

12. D: Marco and Elise are treated as singular, as they function independently and not as a group. This means that the sentence requires a singular past tense verb—*was*. Choice *D* is correct.

13. B: Choice *B* is correct. In this case, the subject is *the patient,* which is linked to *nervous.* This suggests how the patient feels. *Nervous,* Choice *A*, is an adjective. While *get*, Choice *C*, and *won't*, Choice *D*, are verbs, they are not linking verbs. Linking verbs connect a subject to more information about the subject.

14. C: The word *new*, Choice *C*, modifies the noun *furniture,* and is, therefore, an adjective. *Rooms,* Choice *A*, is a noun. *Outfitted*, Choice *B*, is a verb and *department*, Choice *D*, is a noun.

15. A: The subject of the sentence states who or what the sentence is about. *Wing* (Choice *B*)*, hospital* (Choice *C*), and *parking* (Choice *D*) are only important as they relate to the subject.

16. A: While Choices *B, C,* and *D* include at least one verb (*are, needs*), the only choice that includes ALL of the verbs is Choice *A.*

17. C: Choice *A* includes two pronouns. Choice *B* includes a noun and an adjective. Choice *C* includes a noun and an adjective. Choice *D*, however, includes the pronoun *they* and its antecedent *team.*

18. B: Because the choice happened in the past, the sentence requires the singular past tense of the verb, which is *chose.* To *choose,* is present tense, *choosed* (Choice *C*) and *chosed* (Choice *D*) are both incorrect conjugations.

19. C: *Alex was rarely late for his shift* is the independent clause. There is no need for any additional information because it can stand on its own. *Even when he missed the bus* is a clause that requires more information to be complete. It is dependent on the rest of the sentence; therefore, Choice *C* is correct.

20. C: Choice *C* is the only answer option that offers an article— *an.* The rest of the options are verbs and a pronoun.

21. A: Interrogative adjectives include *which* and *what,* and they typically begin question statements; therefore, Choice *A* is the correct answer. Choice *B*, demonstrative adjectives, include *this*, *that*, *these*, and *those*. Choice *C*, possessive adjectives, are possessive pronouns that modify nouns. Choice *D*, comparative adjectives, compare two items and include words like *better*, *larger*, etc.

22. D: Interjections are often found at the start of a sentence and are followed by an exclamation point. Therefore, choice *D, interjection*, is correct.

23. B: Choice *B* is the correct choice, as the sentence requires the contraction of the words *it* and *is* (which is *it's*) and not the pronoun *its.*

24. C: The subject of a sentence states who or what a sentence is about. In this case, the subject is a pronoun; therefore, Choice *C* is correct.

25. C: Helping verbs are paired with main/action verbs to provide more information about the verb tense of the time the action occurred. Choice *C* is correct as the verb phrase *will save* includes the helping verb. While Choice *B, was*, is a verb, it is not a helping verb.

26. A: The sentence in this question is a run on, Choice *A*, as it is two independent clauses fused together. One would need to add punctuation or a coordinating conjunction to join the two clauses appropriately and fix the problem.

27. B: Choice *B* is correct as *advice* is a noun that means guidance and *advise* is a verb that pertains to the act of giving guidance. In the example, the pronoun *my* acts as an adjective to modify the noun and provides a clue that the next word in the sentence is not a verb. Therefore, Choice *A* is incorrect. Choices *C* and *D* both contain spelling errors.

28. D: Choice *D* is correct as *Though we tried our best* is an introductory clause that requires a comma. The absence of a semicolon right before the word *there* would make it a run-on sentence.

29. B: Choice *B* is correct. *Before meeting*, Choice *A*, is an adverb phrase. Choice *C* and Choice *D* both includes an adjective.

30. B: Choice *B* is correct because *sight* means one's ability to see. This gives a clue to the correct word with the clause *After looking at her picture*, which implies sight or visual recognition.

31. C: Choice *C* is the correct answer. *Slowly* describes how the patient was told to *walk*; therefore, *slowly* is an adverb.

32. A: *Will* is the most appropriate word to complete the sentence. It denotes future tense, suitably matching the tense of the introductory element *next month*.

33. D: In this sentence, the pronoun is *his,* which refers to the driver as the antecedent. Therefore, the correct answer is Choice *D*.

34. A: *Our* is the first person collective personal pronoun whereas *are* is a form of the verb *to be*, so the first blank should be filled in with the word *Our*. *Were* is the correct verb and *quite* is an adverb that means acute or to a specific degree. Therefore, Choice *A* is correct. The other answers include incorrectly used words.

35. B: The speech tag, *The doctor said*, requires a comma. Quotation marks must be opened and closed as they should always be used as a set, and the punctuation is placed before the closing quotation mark. In this case, the direct quote is a statement; thus, it requires a period. Therefore, Choice *B* is correct.

36. C: Prepositional phrases provide more information about where or when something happens, and more information about its object. In this case, the object is the fence thus the prepositional phrase is *over the fence*. Choice *C* is the correct answer.

37. B: Proper nouns in this sentence include: *St. Joseph's Hospital* and *Houston. Spring*, as a season, does not get capitalized. Therefore, Choice *B* is correct.

38. D: The subject of a sentence talks about whomever or whatever the sentence is about, which, in this case, is *Gerald*. The object of the sentence talks about whomever or whatever the subject interacts with, which, in this case, is *Orlando*. Therefore, Choice *D* is correct.

39. C: Because *Anne's doctor* is the subject of the sentence, the pronoun that replaces it needs to be a subject pronoun; therefore, Choice *C* is the correct answer.

40. B: Collective nouns are nouns that name a group of individuals. Of all the options listed, *team*, Choice *B,* is the collective noun.

41. A: In this sentence, *after* is an adverb, and *bite* is a noun. Therefore, Choice *A*, which lists *went* and *grab* as the verbs, is correct.

42. D: Nouns name people, places, and things thus *exercise* is the noun in this sentence, and Choice *D* is correct. Choice *A*, *overlooked*, is a verb. Choice *B*, *an*, is an article. Choice *C*, *important,* is an adjective.

43. B: Adjectives modify or describe nouns; therefore, Choice *B*, *next*, which modifies the word *shift* and states which one, is the correct answer. Choice *A*, *relief*, is a noun. Choice *C*, *bring*, is a verb. Choice *D*, *morning*, is also a noun.

44. D: This is a question of both meaning and grammar. In other words, the word in the blank should modify *greet* and describe how the *nurse greeted families*. However, the adverb should also be appropriate for the situation based on meaning; therefore, Choice *D* is correct.

45. D: The subject of a sentence answers the question who or what, and though several nouns come before the subject in this example, the sentence is about the hospital. Choice *D* is correct.

46. C: Choice *C* is the correct answer. The contraction *should've* is often confused for *should of*, but the contraction involves the words *should* and *have*. *By* is a preposition that attributes action or time as in *by now*. Choices *A*, *B*, and *D*, all include misused words.

47. B: The most appropriate conjunction is *so*, Choice *B*, as it establishes cause—*radiology is backed up*—and effect—*there is a long wait for x-rays.*

48. A: Independent clauses should be able to stand alone, so they should include a subject, a verb, and a complete idea. Only Choice *A* includes all three of these requirements. Choices *B*, *C*, and *D* are all incomplete fragments.

49. D: Coordinating conjunctions are words that connect phrases and clauses within a sentence. Choice *D* is correct as it is the coordinating conjunction.

50. D: Choice *D* is correct because named courses like *Chemistry 101* need capitalization.

51. C: Non-essential elements like *the one who arrived recently from Cincinnati* require commas, and proper nouns like *Dr. Johnson, Cincinnati*, and *Rheumatoid Arthritis* all require capitalization. Therefore, Choice *C* is correct.

52. B: Choice *B* is correct because the word *my* in this sentence modifies *name*, which is a noun. Therefore, *my* acts as an adjective.

53. A: Choice *A* is correct, as the relationship between both independent clauses references two events that happen jointly. Choice *B* and Choice *C* both suggest contrast, while Choice *D* suggests cause and effect. These relationships are not how the two clauses are connected and, therefore, these answers are not the best fit.

54. C: The main verb in the sentence is *worked,* while *diligently* describes how the new RN worked. Because adverbs modify verbs, Choice *C* is the correct answer.

55. B: The word *than* sets up contrast (i.e., *Rose has been a nurse longer than Jody and Rob)*; therefore, it belongs in the first blank. *A lot* is always two words. Based on these grammar rules, Choice *B* is the correct answer.

Biology

1. C: Figure III presents a cross-sectional view of a cell and is characteristic of a TEM. In addition, the organelles of the cell are clearly seen at a resolution of one micrometer. Light microscopes don't generally have the resolution needed to visualize each organelle with distinguishing details, although super-resolution microscopy (using fluorescent labeling) makes it possible. Choice *A* represents an image taken from a light microscope using a brightfield setting. However, the image has little contrast since the cells are not stained. Choice *B* represents an image taken from a scanning electron microscope, which can reveal the topography and 3-D shape of the cell. No other image shows a 3-D image. Choice *D* represents an image taken from a light microscope using a brightfield setting where the specimen is stained with a dye. Staining improves the contrast of a cell but also kills cells in the process.

2. C: Only plants contain organelles such as chloroplasts and central vacuoles, and both are not seen in animals. Choice *A* is incorrect because plants and animals have mitochondria, but central vacuoles are only seen in plants. Choice *B* is incorrect because plants both have mitochondria and chloroplasts, but animals only contain mitochondria. Choice *D* is incorrect because both plants and animals contain mitochondria and peroxisomes.

3. C: Leucine represents a hydrophobic chain and is relatively nonpolar since it contains hydrocarbons similar to the tails of the phospholipids. Because the amino acid chain is structurally similar to the nonpolar phospholipid tail, leucine will be oriented towards the lipid membrane's hydrophobic region. As a general rule regarding the mixing of substances, remember that "like dissolves like," which means that structurally similar compounds/molecules will be attracted to each other. The remaining choices represent polar amino acids.

4. B: Selection I points to chromatin, a segment of the chromosomes that coils into several bundles (nucleosomes) to create a fiber. The chromosomes are characterized by an X shape, as indicated by selection II. DNA, selection III, is characterized by a double-strand that has the shape of a double helix. Selection IV corresponds to proteins called histones, which are wrapped together by DNA to form a nucleosome. Choices *A*, *B*, and *D* misidentify two or more of chromosome components.

5. C: Enzymes within the smooth ER act to detoxify drugs by adding hydroxyl groups to the drug molecules. These toxic substances become more soluble within the cell and can be flushed out of the body. Choice *A* is incorrect because the smooth ER enzymes don't add hydrocarbon groups; the drug would become even more insoluble if these groups were combined. Drugs such as phenobarbital initially contain hydrophobic groups, but by adding a hydroxyl group, they become more soluble. Choices *B* and *D* are incorrect since the function of the rough ER is not to detoxify drugs.

6. A: Mitochondria and chloroplasts were believed to evolve from a type of prokaryote engulfed by an ancestor of a eukaryotic cell. The reasons were attributed to the double membranes that both organelles had, in addition to the existence of genetic material (DNA, RNA). Mitochondria and chloroplasts both contain ribosomes, which are used to produce proteins/compounds. Therefore, both organelles are somewhat autonomous since they grow and reproduce inside the cell. Choices *B* and *C* are incorrect since stroma and granum are specific to the chloroplasts. Choice *D* is incorrect because both organelles contain a double membrane.

7. B: Both aerobic respiration and gasoline involve the breakdown of complex molecules such as glucose (respiration) and the hydrocarbon octane (combustion). The net reaction produces carbon dioxide, water, and energy (ATP + heat). Complex molecules are typically carbohydrates that

346

include monosaccharides such as glucose, sucrose, and fructose. These sugar molecules act as cellular fuel. In respiration and combustion, the reactants are generally complex molecules since they have more atoms compared to the products (water, carbon dioxide), which have fewer atoms. Therefore, Choices A and C are incorrect because the initial compounds are not "simple" but relatively complex. Choice D is incorrect because ethanol is not a typical byproduct that is expelled. Under anaerobic conditions, the muscle will produce lactic acid, while yeast will produce ethanol.

8. A: In this reaction, oxygen gas is reduced. When a substance is reduced, it gains electrons from another substance. When a substance is oxidized, it loses electrons to another substance. Oxygen gas (O_2) is reduced because it gains electrons from octane (C_8H_{18}). Oxygen gains electrons or has electrons closer to it through the addition of hydrogen. When oxygen is reduced to water to form an O-H bond, the electrons move closer to the oxygen atom since it's more electronegative than hydrogen. In general, the addition of hydrogen to a substance results in the reduction of that substance. The addition of oxygen to a substance results in oxidation of that substance. Octane is oxidized to carbon dioxide because the C-H bond is replaced with a C-O bond. The electrons are distributed closer to the oxygen atom in the C-O bond since oxygen is more electronegative. Octane is the reducing agent since it's oxidized to CO_2; it loses electrons to oxygen (loses H). Oxygen gas is the oxidizing agent since it's reduced to water; it gains electrons from octane (accepts H).

9. B: The oxidized form of nicotinamide adenine dinucleotide acts as an electron shuttle by accepting two electrons and one proton. Dehydrogenase reduces NAD^+ to $NADH^+$. Specifically, two electrons and a proton are transferred to nicotinamide. Choice A is incorrect since $NADH$ contains "H" and makes it the reduced form that already contains the added electrons. Choice C is incorrect since the reduced form of $NADH^+$ should not be positively charged at the nitrogen atom in nicotinamide and will, therefore, not take up electrons. Choice D is incorrect since NAD^+ is an oxidized form of the electron carrier.

10. D: The oxidized form of nicotinamide (NAD^+) accepts two electrons and one proton to form the reduced form of nicotinamide ($NADH$). Although the enzyme removes two protons and two electrons (a pair of hydrogen atoms), only one proton is transferred to nicotinamide. The remaining proton goes into the surrounding aqueous solution.

11. B: The reduced form of nicotinamide contains one ring structure without the positive charge on the nitrogen atom. A proton is added para to the nitrogen atom or on the opposite side of the ring. Choices A and D do not correspond to the structure of nicotinamide but to the nucleobase called adenine.

Choice *C* is incorrect because the proton is added ortho to the nitrogen (carbon next to nitrogen). The correct reduction mechanism is shown below.

12: C: Cellular respiration begins with glycolysis whereby a glucose molecule is broken down into two pyruvate molecules. As pyruvate enters the mitochondria, it is oxidized to acetyl-CoA. In the citric acid cycle, acetyl-CoA is transformed into carbon dioxide. Oxidative phosphorylation is the last stage whereby the electron transport chains transform chemical energy needed for the production of ATP. Choice *A* is incorrect because pyruvate is formed from glucose in glycolysis. Choice *B* is incorrect since acetyl CoA must be created first via pyruvate oxidation. Choice *D* is incorrect and is the reverse process of cellular respiration.

13: A: Biofuels such as carbohydrates (glucose, $C_6H_{12}O_6$), lipids, and proteins contain several C-H bonds. These molecules are generally oxidized to products such as carbon dioxide, which contain C-O bonds. Biofuel is oxidized, while the oxidizing agent (oxygen) is reduced to water. Biofuels contain "hilltop" electrons since they contain C-H bonds. As the reaction occurs, energy is released to the surroundings since electrons lose their potential energy when shared unequally. For example, the electrons in the C-O bond spend more time near the electronegative oxygen atom. Choice *B* is incorrect since electrons transferred from a reactant with several C-O bonds to a product with C-H bonds would be reduction. Choice *C* is incorrect because the word "reduced" should be "oxidized." Choice *D* is incorrect because it's the reverse process of cellular respiration.

14: C: Glycolysis, the first metabolic stage, takes place inside the cytosol. After glucose is broken down into two pyruvate molecules, each pyruvate molecule moves into the mitochondria and is oxidized to acetyl-CoA. Choices *B, C,* and *D* are not accurate since they occur within the mitochondria.

15: B: Two redox reaction steps in the citric acid cycle involve the formation of carbon dioxide. The first redox reaction is the oxidation of isocitrate to α- ketoglutarate and the reduction of NAD^+ to $NADH$, which creates a molecule of carbon dioxide. The second redox reaction, which generates carbon dioxide, is the oxidation of α- ketoglutarate to succinyl-CoA and reduction of NAD^+ to $NADH$.

16. B: Using light energy, $NADP^+$ is reduced to $NADPH$, where two electrons and one proton are added. Since electrons are added (reduction), $NADPH$ can store potential energy in the form of chemical energy. ADP contains two phosphate groups, while ATP contains three phosphate groups. Through phosphorylation, ADP combines with one phosphate group to form ATP. The addition of a negative phosphate group to ADP increases the molecule's negative charge (more electrons).

17. D: Carbon dioxide is nonpolar, so it can first enter the leaf cell membrane via the stomata. The stomata are microscopic pores found in the epidermis of leaves and stems. The stomata's main function is to allow for gas exchange by permitting carbon dioxide (CO_2) to enter and oxygen gas (O_2) to exit. Stomata can open and close with the help of guard cells. These cells can control their solute concentrations by taking up or losing water. Stomata tend to stay open during the day and close at night. Eventually, carbon dioxide will enter the chloroplast membrane to reach the stroma.

18. C: Both the light and dark cycles are interdependent and cannot occur without one another. Even though the dark reactions (Calvin cycle) don't require direct light, the dark cycle typically occurs in the daylight because light reactions can continuously supply $ATP/NADP$. For example, during the daytime, the light cycle will use light energy to create ATP and $NADPH$. The dark cycle uses both molecules ATP and $NADPH$ to convert carbon dioxide into sugar. However, the dark cycle produces ADP and $NADP^+$, which are both needed by the light cycle. In other words, the light cycle cannot continuously create ATP and $NADPH$ without the dark cycle. Choice A is incorrect since ADP and $NADP^+$ cannot be generated if $ATP/NADPH$ is not created from the light cycle at night. Choice B is incorrect since light reactions need light from the sun (daytime) to produce $ATP/NADPH$. Choice D is incorrect since dark reactions don't create $NADPH$.

19. A: The longest wavelength of light in the visible spectrum corresponds to the red region of the spectrum (~700 nm). The absorption intensity of chlorophyll *a* peaks near 425 and 675 nm. Choice B is incorrect since chlorophyll *b* absorbs light near 460 nm and 640 nm. Choices C and D, collectively called the carotenoids, are incorrect since most of the absorbed light occurs near 460 and 480 nm.

20. B: For every three molecules of carbon dioxide that enter the Calvin cycle, one net molecule of $G3P$ is produced. In particular, Choice C is incorrect since the remaining five molecules of $G3P$ are used to complete the Calvin cycle. The five molecules are used to regenerate three molecules of Ribulose bisphosphate ($RuBP$).

21. D: In photosystem II, the reaction center of chlorophyll a is P60 since that pigment can absorb light at 680 nm (red light). In photosystem I, the reaction center containing chlorophyll *a* is known as $P700$ since it absorbs light at 700 nm (far-red spectrum). Both chlorophyll *a* molecules are similar and absorb in the red region. The number following "P" corresponds to the wavelength of absorbed light. Chlorophyll *a* also absorbs near 450 nm. Therefore, Choices A, B, and C are incorrect since they contain wavelength numbers that don't match the absorption spectrum of chlorophyll *a*.

22. B: The correct order of linear electron flow is: a proton strikes a pigment, an electron moves from $P680$ to the primary electron acceptor, an enzyme catalyzes the splitting of water (not shown), a photoexcited electron moves from PS II to PS I, and then ATP is produced. Remaining steps include the transfer of light energy to the PS I reaction center containing $P700$. The photoexcited electron is passed in a series of redox reactions down a second ETC through a ferredoxin protein. Lastly, an enzyme $NADP^+$ reductase catalyzes the transfer of electrons from ferredoxin to $NADP^+$.

23. D: Chemiosmosis is a process seen in both the mitochondria and chloroplasts. Electron transport chains pump hydrogen ions (protons) across a membrane with low proton concentration to one where there is a high concentration. As protons diffuse back through the ATP synthases, within the membrane, it results in ATP production. Choices A and B are incorrect since these processes occur only in the mitochondria. The citric acid cycle is also called the Krebs cycle. Choice C is incorrect since the Calvin cycle is specific to chloroplasts.

24. A: The correct order of phases is carbon fixation, reduction, and regeneration of the carbon dioxide acceptor called $RuBP$ (carboxylase-oxygenase called rubisco). Choice B is incorrect since the electrons are reduced to 1,3-bisphosphoglycerate to form $G3P$. Choice C is incorrect because the reduction is occurring in the second phase. Choice D, like Choice B, is incorrect because rubisco, not $G3P$, is the carbon dioxide acceptor (not donator).

25. B: In step 3 of the linear electron flow process, an enzyme catalyzes water into two protons and an oxygen atom. Two electrons are transferred to P680 of PS II. Choice A is incorrect because carbon dioxide enters the Calvin cycle. Choice C is incorrect since $NADPH$ is formed through a reduction process within the light cycle. Choice D is incorrect since oxygen gas is a byproduct of the light cycle.

26. C: The citric acid cycle is catabolic because it breaks down glucose to form acetyl CoA. As acetyl CoA moves along the citric acid cycle, it is oxidized, and energy is used to create ATP. Carbon dioxide is produced. In contrast, the Calvin cycle is catabolic since it takes carbon dioxide and uses energy to build a three-carbon sugar called $G3P$. Therefore, Choice A is incorrect because the Calvin cycle does not breakdown molecules; it builds molecules. Choice B is incorrect since the citric acid cycle is a catabolic process, breaking down sugar. Choice D is incorrect because acetyl CoA is oxidized and not reduced.

27. C: Electron loss will occur at magnesium since metals tend to lose electrons (less electronegative) compared to nonmetals. The porphyrin ring contains several carbon double bonds. Therefore, the electron density within the ring is much greater than the hydrocarbon tail. Electrons will tend to flow within the ring to the metal, which oxidizes during photoexcitation. During linear electron flow (Stage 3 and 6), an electron in chlorophyll a ($P680$ and $P700$) is photoexcited and transferred to a primary electron acceptor. The oxidation of magnesium creates an electron-hole. Consequently, the movement of electrons to that hole is facilitated in both photosystems. Chlorophylls ($P680^+$ or $P700^+$) will act as electron acceptors.

28. D: Cellular respiration occurs in various stages and not in one exergonic step. An exergonic reaction indicates that energy will be released in cellular respiration. Therefore, electrons are traveling down the potential energy well. Glucose contains stored chemical energy, which is released when broken down. NAD^+ accepts two electrons and a proton and is reduced to $NADH$. The electron transport chain (ETC) breaks the fall of electrons into smaller steps. Some of the released energy is stored to make ATP. Two electrons, two protons, and oxygen combine to form water. In the ETC, oxygen gas (O_2) is reduced to water.

29. B: $NADH$ pumps a specific number of protons that results in the production of 2.5 ATP, and $FADH_2$ will result in the formation of 1.5 ATP. In the ETC, the reduction of each molecule drives the pumping of protons from the mitochondrial matrix into the intermembrane space. Ubiquinone and cytochrome C ferry electrons (from $NADH$ and $FADH_2$) between complexes. During chemiosmosis, the concentration of protons increases in the intermembrane space, and protons flow back down a gradient into the matrix via ATP synthases. The synthases will harness the proton motive force to create ATP.

Therefore, we can calculate the number of ATP molecules produced as follows:

Two *NADH* (glycolysis), two *NADH* (pyruvate oxidation), six *NADH*, and two $FADH_2$ (citric acid cycle)

$$2\ NADH \times 2.5\frac{ATP}{NADH} + 2\ NADH \times 2.5\frac{ATP}{NADH} + 6\ NADH \times 2.5\frac{ATP}{NADH} + 2FADH_2 \times 1.5\frac{ATP}{FADH_2} = 28\ ATP$$

Choice *A* is incorrect because the maximum number of *ATP* produced occurs with two *NADH* from pyruvate oxidation, not $FADH_2$. Choices *C* and *D* are incorrect since they don't show the correct number of electron shuttles.

30. A: Electrons move from a less electronegative carrier (*NADH*) to a more electronegative carrier. *NADH* is oxidized to NAD^+ and electrons travel along the chain with cytochrome a3 as the last carrier. Choices *B* and *D* are incorrect since the electrons will flow towards the most electronegative electron carrier. Choice *C* is incorrect since NAD^+ is not an electron carrier for the ETC.

Chemistry

1. D: Each element on the periodic table has an assigned atomic number. The atomic number (Z) gives the number of protons, which is specific to that element. An element can still retain its identity even if the number of electrons (e.g., cation or anion) or the number of neutrons changes. For example, carbon-12 and carbon-13 have the same number of protons but a different number of neutrons. A sodium cation and a neutrally-charged sodium atom have the same number of protons but a different number of electrons.

2. B: Electrons are the lightest particle and are negatively charged. Protons and neutrons have approximately the same mass, but protons are positively charged, and neutrons are neutrally charged.

3. D: The number of electrons and protons determines the atom's charge. A proton is a nuclear particle that carries a positive charge. An electron is a negatively-charged particle that is much lighter than a proton. Both an electron and a proton have a charge that is equal in magnitude but opposite in sign. Therefore, the atomic charge on an atom will depend on the number of electrons and protons.

4. B: The number of neutrons must be equal to the mass number (A) minus the atomic number (Z):

$$N = A - Z$$

Choice *A* would give a similar answer because the number of protons is typically equal to the number of electrons. However, if the atom has a charge (e.g., Na^+), Choice *A* would not be correct. For example, let's consider the nuclide $^{23}_{11}Na^+$. Choice *A* would give N = A – (number of electrons) = 23 – 10 = 13. However, the actual number of neutrons is given by Choice *B*: N = A – Z = 23 – 11 = 12.

5. B: The final amount of the substance can be calculated in two steps:

First, find the rate constant using the following formula:

$$k = \frac{0.693}{t_{1/2}} = \frac{0.693}{40\ days} = 0.017325\ days^{-1}$$

Next, calculate the final amount using the following equation (note that $[B]_0$ = 200 g):

$$[B]_t = [B]_0 e^{-kt} = 200\ g \times e^{-(0.017325\ days^{-1} \times 80\ days)} = 50\ g$$

After 40 days, the initial amount will reduce by half, from 200 to 100 g, (e.g., the half-life is 40 days). After another 40 days, the previous amount of 100 g will reduce by half, from 100 to 50 g.

6. D: The half-life can be determined in two different ways. The first method involves the use of a table.

Time (Days)	Amount (Grams)
0	40
x = 12	20
24	10

After 24 days, the amount of the unknown element is equal to 10 g. Half of 40 g is 20 g. So, half of 24 days is 12 days. Therefore, the half-life (12 days) is the amount of time that it takes for half the amount of the element to decay (20 g). The second method requires using the following two formulas:

$$k = -ln\left(\frac{[B]_t}{[B]_0}\right)\frac{1}{t} , t_{1/2} = \frac{0.693}{k}$$

The term $[B]_t = 10$ g and $[B]_0 = 40$ g. The value of t is 24. The rate constant is:

$$k = -ln\left(\frac{10.0}{40.0}\right)\frac{1}{24\ days} = 0.05776\ days^{-1}$$

The half-life can now be calculated using the following formula:

$$t_{1/2} = \frac{0.693}{0.05776\ days^{-1}} = 12\ days$$

7. C: The atomic number of oxygen is 8 (Z = 8). For a neutrally-charged oxygen atom, there are eight electrons. Within the K shell, two electrons are found in the s orbital. The total number of valence electrons is equal to the group number (six valence electrons). For example, oxygen belongs to group VIA and will have six electrons in the L shell. The L shell contains one 2s orbital and three 2p orbitals. Two electrons will occupy the s orbital, and the remaining four electrons will occupy the p orbitals.

8. A: According to the Pauli exclusion principle, only two electrons can occupy a single orbital with the restriction that each electron has an opposite spin. Regardless of the shell and the number of orbitals per shell, only two electrons, with opposite spin, can occupy a single orbital.

9. B: The atom contains electrons, protons, and neutrons. Rutherford's alpha-scattering experiments indicated that a majority of the mass was centered in a small space called the nucleus. The protons (positively charged) and neutrons (neutrally charged) are found within the nucleus, whereas electrons are dispersed around the nucleus. Electrons move inside a space that is devoid of mass. Choice B is incorrect because Rutherford's scattering experiments were not in agreement with the plum-pudding model.

10. D: The atomic number of krypton is Z = 36, and the mass number is A = 93. Therefore, the number of neutrons is A − Z = N, or 93 − 36 = 57.

11. C: Based on the plum-pudding model, Rutherford initially believed the charge within the atom was evenly spread throughout. Choice C is correct because if the atom contained electrons that were evenly spread with a positively-charged sphere, the bombardment of alpha particles should pass through the atom with a small deflection. Large deflections are observed in Rutherford's gold foil experiment because the alpha particles bombard the protons at the center of the nucleus. Choice A is incorrect because if all the alpha particles managed to hit the nucleus, all the particles should be deflected. Most of the alpha particles passed through the atom because the atom is mostly empty space. A few were deflected because they managed to hit the nucleus. Choice B is incorrect because most alpha particles pass through the nucleus; deflection does not always occur. Choice D is incorrect because alpha particles are positively charged (helium without two electrons.)

12. D: Positron decay or positron emission is a type of radioactive decay that produces beta (β^+) particles ($_{+1}^{0}e$). The particle has an identical mass to an electron except that it has a positive charge. Positron emissions result in the conversion of a proton to a neutron.

13. C: An electron capture nuclear reaction means that a nuclide will collide with an electron to form a daughter nuclide that has the same mass number as the parent nuclide. However, the chemical identity of the daughter nuclide is different (e.g., the atomic number decreases by 1). Like positron emission, electron capture involves the conversion of a proton to a neutron. The daughter nuclide has the same mass number as the parent nuclide but with one less proton.

14. B: The correct balanced nuclear equation is:

$$_{24}^{51}Cr + _{-1}^{0}e \rightarrow _{23}^{51}V$$

The nuclear reaction describes electron capture whereby a proton is converted to a neutron. Chromium is bombarded with an electron, and one proton is converted to a neutron to form vanadium.

15. B: The emission of an electron indicates that the nuclear reaction is an example of beta decay whereby a neutron is converted to a proton. The mass number of the daughter nuclide will remain the same, but the atomic number will increase by one. The balanced nuclear equation is:

$$_{15}^{32}P \rightarrow _{-1}^{0}e + _{16}^{32}S$$

16. B: Ionic bonds contain an atom that has lost electrons to the other. Because the electron is not shared, there is a positive charge on one atom and a negative charge on the other. Metals tend to lose electrons. Electron loss for metals results in an octet or electron configuration that is similar to a noble gas. For example, the loss of one electron from rubidium produces a cation that has an electron configuration similar to krypton. Nonmetals such as chlorine will gain an electron to obtain an electron configuration similar to argon. Rubidium chloride ($RbCl$) is an example of an ionic compound.

17. D: If electrons are shared between two atoms, the bond is covalent. Nonpolar, polar, and coordinate covalent bonds are examples of bonds that contain electron pairs that are shared. Choice C is not a bond but a dipole-dipole force. Dipole forces are relatively weaker than covalent bonds and are intermolecular forces that exist between two or more atoms (e.g., hydrogen bonding).

18. A: Metallic bonds generally contain elements that belong to the main metals (groups I and IIA) and transition metals (groups IIIB-VIIIB). These elements are electron-deficient or positively charged. The delocalization or free flow of electrons across the metal cluster creates an attractive electrostatic force between each metal. For example, at a specific point in time, an atom from a metal may be electron-deficient and another atom may be electron-rich due to the localization of the electron cloud. Even though there is a small difference in electronegativity between each metal atom, the sea of electrons moves easily within the cluster because the valence electrons in the metal (*s* and *p* electrons) are easily removed.

19. B: The chlorine atom belongs to group VIIA (7A) and should have seven dots or electrons. Phosphorous is a group VA (5A) element and contains five valence electrons. Sulfur is a group VIA (6A) element and will have six valence electrons. Choice *B* is the correct answer because aluminum belongs to group IIA (3A) and can only have three valence electrons or dots. The Lewis dot symbol that is shown indicates five dots; therefore, it is incorrect.

20. D: Oxygen and carbon will follow the octet rule and must contain eight valence electrons. Choices *A* and *B* are incorrect because carbon needs to be surrounded by eight electrons, not six. Choices *C* and *D* indicate the correct number of valence electrons for carbon (e.g., carbon has an octet). However, Choice *C* indicates that both oxygen atoms don't have an octet of electrons. Choice *D* is correct because oxygen and carbon contain an octet. In addition, for a neutral compound, the total number of electrons must equal the sum of all valence electrons. For example, there are two oxygen atoms (12 electrons total) and one carbon atom (4 electrons), so the total number of electrons or dots is equal to 16.

21 B: A nonpolar compound does not necessarily mean that all bonds are nonpolar. Carbon monoxide, Choice *A*, is an example of a polar compound because the oxygen atom is more electronegative than carbon. Carbonate ion, Choice *C*, contains two negatively-charged oxygen atoms and one neutrally-charged oxygen atom with carbon located at the center. The compound is polar because one side of the structure is electron-rich and the other side electron-deficient. Sulfur dioxide is a polar compound because the overall dipole moment points toward the oxygen atoms. Carbon dioxide contains two bond dipoles that cancel each other, thereby making the compound nonpolar because the overall dipole is 0.

22. C: Charged polyatomic anions such as nitrate can undergo electron delocalization. The lone electron pairs on the oxygen atoms can be shared with the nitrogen atom. As an N-O bond forms, another shared electron pair between nitrogen and oxygen will delocalize to an oxygen atom and form a nonbonding electron pair. Several resonance structures exist for the nitrate ion, but the true structure is a hybrid structure that incorporates all three resonance structures.

23. C: Coordinate covalent bonds are generally present in electrically-charged compounds that contain atoms that donated or accepted an electron pair. Choices *A*, *B*, and *D* contain a coordinate covalent bond or a bond that results when one atom donates an electron pair to share with another atom. For Choice *A*, the nitrogen atom in ammonia donates its lone pair to a hydrogen proton to form ammonium. For Choice *B*, a hydride ion (H^-) donates its lone pair to a vacant *p* orbital on aluminum hydride to form aluminum hydride ion. For Choice *D*, the nonbonding pair from the oxygen atom within the water molecule is donated to a free proton, thereby producing a hydronium ion. Aluminum chloride, Choice *B*, does not contain a coordinate covalent bond. Aluminum belongs to group IIIA, and like boron, it will generally follow the sextet rule unless a lone pair is donated.

24. C: The structural formulas of each answer choice are shown below.

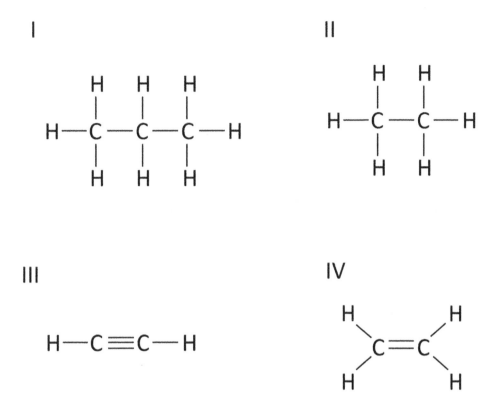

I

II

III

IV

Choice C contains the shortest bond because the carbon-carbon bond is a triple bond. Choice D contains a carbon-carbon double bond. Choices A and B contain the longest chemical bonds because each bond is a single bond.

25. A: A neutral aluminum atom contains 13 electrons. An aluminum cation with a charge of 3+ contains 10 electrons and has the same number of electrons as neon (Ne, Z = 10). There are eight valence electrons in Al^{3+} that are located in the L shell. Two valence electrons are found in the 2s orbital, and six valence electrons spread through the three 2p orbitals.

26. D: Positron emission involves the conversion of a proton to a neutron, and beta decay involves the conversion of a neutron to a proton. Electron capture, like positron emission, converts a proton to a neutron. Alpha decay, unlike the other radioactive decays, produces a daughter nuclide and an alpha particle. The parent nuclide breaks into smaller components, and the mass number changes. Beta decay, electron capture, and positron emission produce a nuclide that does not change its mass number.

27. C: Electron capture results in the formation of x-rays. Gamma ray emission involves the formation of gamma rays or high-energy photons. Beta decay involves the formation of negatively charged beta particles (e.g., electrons). Alpha decay, Choice C, is the correct answer because alpha particles are helium nuclei without any electrons. The helium nuclei are positively charged and have a 2+ charge. Positron emission also produces positively charged particles called positrons or antielectrons.

28. C: In nuclear fission, heavy nuclides such as uranium-235 are bombarded with neutrons. The nuclear reaction results in the formation of a lighter daughter nuclide (e.g., krypton-94 and barium-139) and three neutrons. The produced neutrons then bombard another uranium-235 nuclide, thereby creating a chain reaction.

29. C: The amount of radiation can be determined by using the provided equation and information from the table:

$$Alpha: rem = 20 \times 10 = 200 \; rems$$

$$Beta: rem = 20 \times 1 = 20 \; rems$$

$$Gamma: rem = 250 \times 1 = 250 \; rems$$

Gamma radiation causes a greater amount of damage, primarily because the RBE value is the greatest. The total amount of rems is equal to 200 + 20 + 250 = 470 rems and slightly below the lethal dosage. The person would barely survive radiation exposure.

30. B: The amount of gold-198, 20 mg, is the minimum amount that is needed. During transport, the amount of gold-198 will reduce over time, so 20 mg can be considered the final or minimum amount needed. Given the final amount and the half-life, the initial amount that needs to be ordered can be found using the following equations:

$$t_{1/2} = \frac{0.693}{k}$$

$$[B]_t = [B]_0 e^{-kt}$$

First, solve for k.

$$k = \frac{0.693}{t_{1/2}} = \frac{0.693}{2.69 \; days} = 0.25762 \; days^{-1}$$

Next, calculate the initial amount $[B]_0$ that needs to be ordered using the following equation. The value of t is equal to the transport time (48 hours = 2 days).

$$[B]_0 = \frac{[B]_t}{e^{-kt}} = \frac{20.0 \; mg}{e^{-(0.25762 \; days^{-1} * 2 \; days)}} = 33.5 \; mg$$

Choice B is the correct answer. The initial amount of 33.5 mg of gold-198 needs to be delivered to have a final amount of 20 mg for usage in a day.

Anatomy and Physiology

1. C: After the hormone-receptor complex is formed, it binds to DNA with the cell. Transcription of mRNA in the nucleus will take place, followed by translation of mRNA in the cytoplasm. Choice A is incorrect because it refers to the first step of the second-messenger system in which the steroid hormone attaches to a receptor located on the cell membrane. Choice B is incorrect because it refers to the second and third steps of the second-messenger process. In this process, the receptor becomes activated and sets off a series of reactions that activate an enzyme. Choice D is incorrect because transcription of mRNA precedes mRNA translation.

2. B: Prostaglandins are lipid compounds called eicosanoids. These types of hormones are derived from lipids, enzymatically, from the fatty acid called arachidonic acid. A prostaglandin contains twenty carbon atoms and a five-carbon ring. Fatty acids typically contain long hydrocarbon chains that are polyunsaturated. Choice *A* is incorrect. Testosterone is a male sex hormone and steroid; it is derived from the cholesterol molecule. Testosterone molecules don't contain long, polyunsaturated chains but are composed of several six-membered and five-membered rings. Choice *C* is incorrect because peptides are composed of amino acid chains. A peptide chain contains many peptide bonds that consist of an amide functional group. These groups contain a nitrogen atom bonded to a carbonyl group (-NH-(CO)-). Choice *D* is incorrect. Estrogen is a female sex steroid hormone that is derived from and similar in structure to cholesterol.

3. D: The systemic circulation is a second circuit that supplies oxygen- and nutrient-rich blood. Oxygen-rich blood from the capillary beds moves into the pulmonary veins, left atrium, and left ventricle of the heart. Because the left ventricle wall is thicker than the right ventricle, it is a more powerful pump, which allows it to pump over longer distances or over a longer pathway throughout the body. Choice *A* is incorrect because the right ventricle wall is thinner, thereby making it a weaker pump. Choice *B* is incorrect because the left ventricle pumps over a longer pathway, from the left ventricle to the body tissues and then back to the atrium. The pathway is the second circuit called the systemic circulation pathway. Choice *C* is incorrect. Although the statement indicates that the right ventricle is a less powerful pump, it does not pump over a longer pathway. Blood is pumped a shorter distance and moves from the right ventricle to the pulmonary arteries and then to the capillary beds and back to the left atrium.

4. B: The heart wall is made up of, from inner to outer, the endocardium, myocardium, and epicardium. Note that the prefix -endo means "internal" or "within," and the prefix -epi means "over." Therefore, the term *epicardium* should be the innermost layer and the term *endocardium* the outermost layer. Choice *A* is incorrect because the epicardium is not the innermost layer. Choice *A* shows the arrangement of terms in the reverse order. Choices *C* and *D* are incorrect because they are not technically part of the heart wall. The pericardium is a sac that is made up of three layers. Note that the pericardial layer is more of a cavity than a layer.

5. D: Gas exchange occurs at the capillary beds of the lungs. The oxygen-rich blood flows into the pulmonary veins, left atrium/ventricle, aorta/branches, and systemic circuit. After gas exchange at the capillary beds of the body tissue, the oxygen-poor/carbon dioxide–rich blood flows out of the systemic circuit to the venae cavae, right atrium, right ventricle, and pulmonary arteries and back into the capillary beds of the lungs. Choice *A* is incorrect because the pulmonary arteries are not directly connected to the left atrium. Choice *B* is incorrect because the flow of blood is the reverse of Choice *D*. Choice *C* is incorrect because, like Choice *A,* the pulmonary arteries are not directly connected to the left or right ventricles.

6. C: To summarize, arteries carry blood out of the heart, and veins carry blood into the heart. The *aorta* leads to other arteries, and the *venae cavae* returns blood from the veins. The pulmonary vessels are arteries that carry oxygen-poor blood from the right ventricle to the lungs. The pulmonary veins carry oxygen-rich blood back to the left atrium. The systemic vessels are arteries that transport oxygen-rich blood from the left ventricle to the body's tissues. The oxygen-poor blood then moves through the veins back to the right atrium. Choice *A* is incorrect because veins don't carry oxygen-rich blood away from the heart; veins carry oxygen-rich blood into the heart (pulmonary) or oxygen-deficient blood from the body into the heart (*venae cavae*). Choice *B* is incorrect because arteries (not veins) carry oxygen-rich blood away from the heart (aorta). Choice *D* is incorrect because oxygen-deficient blood flows from the body back to the heart via the veins or *venae cavae* (not the aorta).

7. C: The lungs contain the terminal air sacs called alveoli. Oxygen and carbon dioxide gas exchange within the blood takes place only in the alveoli. Choices *A*, *B*, and *D* are incorrect because these structures are merely conducting passageways and do not contain alveoli. Choice *A*, the pharynx, commonly known as the *throat,* is the common passageway for air and food. Choice *B*, the trachea, is known as the *windpipe* and extends four inches below the larynx. It is a wall that is composed of C-shaped rings that expand when food is swallowed. Choice *D*, the larynx, is the voice box that plays a role in speech and routes air and food toward the proper channels.

8. A: The respiratory mucosa sits on thin-walled veins that warm up the air that is breathed in through the nose. Within the nasal cavity, the mucus that is produced by the goblet cells and mucous glands can moisten the air, causing bacteria and dust to be trapped. Choice *B* is incorrect because the oral mucosa cannot perform the same functions as the respiratory mucosa. Choice *C* is incorrect because the pharynx's main function serves as a passageway for food and air. Lysozymes in the mucus of the nasal cavity will destroy the bacteria, and the ciliated cells of the nasal mucosa create a current that moves the contaminated mucus toward the pharynx. Choice *D*, although true, is not the best answer because, unlike the mucosa lining in the nasal cavity, it does not have the enzymes needed to break down bacteria.

9. A: The correct order of air passage from the nostrils to the lungs is the nasal cavity, pharynx, larynx, trachea, bronchi, bronchioles, and alveoli. All the answer choices have the first (nasal cavity) and last organs (alveoli). Between Choice *A* and *B*, the difference lies with the ordering of the bronchi and bronchioles. The primary bronchi are divided into a right and left bronchus and are the result of the division of the trachea. The left and right bronchus run obliquely and then dive into the medial depression, called the hilum, of the left or right lung. The main bronchi divide into smaller, tree-like branches and then reach the bronchioles, the smallest air-conducting passageways. Therefore, Choice *B* cannot be correct because bronchioles should not be placed before bronchi. Choices *C* and *D* are incorrect because air flows through the pharynx before the larynx.

10. C: Simple squamous epithelial tissue rests on a basement membrane and contains extremely thin walls that allow for gas exchange and filtration. The tissue is found in both the alveoli and the walls of the capillaries. Choice *A* is incorrect because cuboidal epithelial tissue is found mostly in the salivary glands or pancreas, the surface of the ovaries, and the tubules of the kidneys. Choice *B* is incorrect because columnar epithelial tissue is found on the walls of the stomach or digestive tract. Choice *D* is incorrect because it is found in the urinary bladder and parts of the urethra. Although the transitional stratified epithelial tissue can undergo considerable stretching and become squamous-like, this type of tissue contains two or more layers of skin instead of a single layer.

11. D: The submucosa contains the nerve endings, blood vessels, lymphatic vessels, and lymphoid tissue. Specifically, the submucosal nerve plexus is one of two nerve fibers within alimentary canal walls. The myenteric nerve plexus is the other nerve type that is found on or within the muscularis external. Specifically, the nerves can be found within the longitudinal and inner circular muscle. Choice *A*, the serosa, is incorrect because it is the outermost layer of the wall. Choice *B*, the mucosa, is incorrect because it is the innermost layer and mucous membrane that lines the lumen of an organ. Choice *C*, the visceral peritoneum, is incorrect. It is part of the serosa and is made of a single layer of flat cells that produce a serous fluid.

12. A: The enteroendocrine cells produce gastrin, a local hormone that is vital for regulating digestive activities in the stomach. Once food is in the stomach, gastrin is released and stimulates the release of gastric juice and stomach emptying. Choice *B*, the mucous neck cells, is incorrect. These cells produce a thin acidic (low pH) mucus that contains mucin proteins. The mucus has an unknown function that is different from the secretions of the mucous cells from the mucosa. Choice *C*, the parietal cells, is incorrect because these cells produce a corrosive acid called hydrochloric acid (HCl). The acid creates an acidic environment in the stomach and activates enzymes. For example, pepsinogen is converted to pepsin. Choice *D*, the chief cells, is incorrect because these are responsible for producing inactive protein-digesting enzymes called pepsinogens.

13. C: Within the gastric mucosa, specific stomach cells called parietal cells produce an intrinsic factor. The intrinsic factor is a glycoprotein that is important for the absorption of cobalamin (B_{12}) in the intestine. Without the production of the glycoprotein, red blood cell count will decrease, a condition known as pernicious anemia, causing a weakened stomach lining, fatigue, and even heart and nerve damage. Choices *A*, *B*, and *D* are incorrect because these organs don't contain parietal cells. They are found in the gastric glands within the lining of the fundus and the stomach's cardia.

14. A: The small intestine is the longest portion of the alimentary tube (7–13 feet). Because of its length and availability of enzymes (from the pancreas) and emulsifiers (bile from the liver), chemical breakdown of food is facilitated and allows most nutrient absorption to occur within the small intestine. Choices *B* and *D* are incorrect. The stomach, Choice *B*, holds food and breaks it down while moving food along the tract. Specifically, the stomach will churn, mix, and pummel food into small fragments. The fundus of the stomach, Choice *D*, refers to the upper region of the stomach that is the farthest from the stomach openings (esophagus and pyloric region). The function of the fundus is to store gases and undigested food that are formed when chemical digestion occurs. Choice *C*, the large intestine, is incorrect. Its function is to dry out indigestible food through the absorption of water. The large intestine eliminates residues from the body in the form of feces.

15. B: If the parietal cells were unable to secrete corrosive hydrochloric acid, pepsinogen could not be converted to pepsin. Consequently, pepsin would not form, and dietary proteins would remain undigested. Choice *A* is incorrect because indigestion can still occur if pepsin is not produced. Choice *C* is incorrect because pepsin does not convert to pepsinogen readily. Pepsin is a lower molecular weight enzyme compared to pepsinogen. The conversion of pepsin to pepsinogen would require a new enzyme. Choice *D* is not correct because pepsin would result in the digestion, not indigestion, of dietary proteins.

16. D: The pyloric sphincter controls the flow of chyme into the small intestine. Chyme is a semi-fluid mass of processed food that is thick like heavy cream and enters the small intestine via the pyloric sphincter. Choice *A* is incorrect because the villi are extensions of the mucosa within the small intestine. The villi contain rich capillary beds that make it well suited for nutrient absorption. Choice *B* is incorrect because the pylorus refers to the terminal funnel-shaped opening of the stomach that connects to the small intestine. Choice *C* is incorrect because it refers to the three types of muscle layers found in the stomach—the longitudinal, circular, and obliquely arranged muscles—that function in the movement and pummeling of food.

17. D: Label 4 represents the oblique layer of the stomach. The walls of the alimentary canal organs generally have a muscularis externa that is composed of a longitudinal and circular layer. However, the stomach contains an oblique layer that helps the stomach physically break down food. Therefore, the longitudinal layer is the outermost muscle layer, the circular muscle layer is in the middle, and the oblique layer is the innermost muscle layer. Choice *A* is incorrect because the circular muscle keeps food from moving backward. Choice *B* is incorrect because the cardia is the initial part of the stomach right below the esophagus. The cardia contains the cardia sphincter, a thin ring of muscle that keeps contents from leaving the stomach into the esophagus. Choice *C* is incorrect because the longitudinal muscle layer shortens the gastrointestinal tract.

18. B: Stem cells can regenerate resident cells that secrete substances within the gastric glands. Stem cells are important for replenishing the surface epithelium. Choice *A*, chief cells, is incorrect. These cells are responsible for producing inactive protein-digesting enzymes called pepsinogens. However, researchers have discovered that chief cells can transform into stem cells in response to an injury along the stomach wall. Chief cells are located at the base of the gastric gland. During the transformation of chief cells to stem cells, a mutation may occur. The mutation of these stem cells is a major source of tumors located at the base of these glands. With that said, Choice *B*, *stem cells,* is the better choice. Choice *C* is incorrect because parietal cells are responsible for the secretion of hydrochloric acid. Choice *D* is incorrect because enteroendocrine cells are responsible for the production of local hormones.

19. C: The cortex, medulla, and pelvis represent three main aspects of the kidney. Choice *A* is incorrect because the ordering of each aspect is in reverse, from deep to superficial. Choices *B* and *D* are incorrect because they refer to protective layers of the kidney. If the question asked for the correct order of the protective layers from superficial to deep, Choice *D* would be correct.

20. B: The fat capsule is a fatty mass or tissue that surrounds each kidney. Hydronephrosis is a condition in which fatty tissue dwindles when rapid weight loss occurs. Consequently, the kidneys shift to a lower position, a condition known as ptosis. Due to the shift, urine is unable to exit the kidneys because the ureters are kinked. Pressure on the kidney tissue builds because urine gets backed up, thereby causing urination problems and kidney damage. Choices *A*, *C*, and *D* are incorrect because the fibrous capsule, renal fascia, and renal pelvis are not fatty masses.

21. C: Label 1 corresponds to the loop of Henle, also called the nephron loop. Specifically, the descending component of the loop (left side) has low permeability to urea and ions but is permeable to water. The ascending loop (right side) is permeable to ions but impermeable to water. The loop of Henle protrudes into the renal medulla and makes a sharp bend. Choice *A* is incorrect because it refers to the distal convoluted tubule (DCT) that is located within the renal cortex and is connected to the ascending portion of the loop of Henle. Choice *B* is incorrect because it refers to a segment called the juxtaglomerular apparatus, an area between the loop of Henle and the DCT that meets the cortical radiate artery. Choice *D* is incorrect because it points to the proximal convoluted tubule (PCT), which is surrounded by peritubular capillaries. The PCT lies between Bowman's capsule and the loop of Henle and is found within the renal cortex.

22. D: The order of blood flow, as shown in the diagram below, is renal artery, arcuate artery, arcuate vein, and renal vein. An important note is that the arteries carry the oxygenated blood, and the veins carry the deoxygenated blood (venous blood). Choice *A* is incorrect because the order is reversed and indicates that oxygenated blood would flow through the renal vein. Similarly, Choice *B* is incorrect because the interlobar vein does not carry oxygenated blood, and the pathway is given in reverse with respect to blood flow. Choice *C* is incorrect because blood flows into the afferent arteriole before it reaches the cortical radiate vein.

23. B: A portion of the vas deferens lies within the scrotum. *Vasectomy* means "cutting the vas." In a vasectomy procedure, the surgeon makes a small incision at the scrotum to cut the vas deferens. At least one end of the vas deferens is sealed off by a cauterizing, suturing, or clamping technique. Choices

A and D, the ejaculatory duct and prostatic urethra, are incorrect and close to one another. Surgery at these sites would be invasive and most likely lead to urination complications because the bladder is connected indirectly. Choice C, the ampulla of ductus deferens, is incorrect because surgery would be too invasive, leading to other complications. For example, the diameter of the ampulla is much greater than the vas deferens. Because the organ is larger, it may present more of a challenge to seal or close off.

24. A: The fimbriae are finger-like projections that partly surround the ovary. During ovulation, the oocyte leaves the ovary, and the fimbriae move in a wave-like manner to create fluid currents that propel the oocyte into the uterine tube. Choice B is incorrect because, although part of the uterine tube, the infundibulum is a funnel-shaped cavity where the oocyte will pass to move toward the uterus. Choices C and D are incorrect because they are not part of the uterine tube. Choice C, the cilia, is generally found in the oviduct or fallopian tube. The cilia protect and cover the egg as it moves through the fallopian tube, from the ovary to the uterus. Choice D, the broad ligaments, is peritoneum that connects the sides of the uterus to the walls of the pelvis. It provides structural support for the female reproductive organs.

25. D: The antrum is the part of the ovarian follicle that contains follicular fluid. When the antrum appears, it signals the next stage of maturation and formation of the secondary follicle called the mature vesicular (Graafian) follicle. Choice A is incorrect because the primary follicle does not have an antrum. Choice B is incorrect because, once the follicle ruptures, the antrum is no longer present. Choice C is incorrect because the corpus luteum does not contain an antrum.

26. C: Mitochondria are located in the midpiece, and DNA is located in the nucleus of the head. Choice A is incorrect because it's in the reverse order. Choice B is incorrect because mitochondria are not stored in the head, and DNA is not found in the tail. Choice D is incorrect. It would seem to be a likely choice because the mitochondria produce ATP to power the movement of the tail. However, because the tail undergoes rapid whip-like movements, the tail would not be a suitable place to hold the mitochondria, which has a wrapped nonlinear structure. In contrast, the midpiece filament remains rigid compared to the axial filament of the tail.

27. A: Label 3 points to the peritoneal cavity. In females, the peritoneal cavity is not completely closed. The uterine tubes are open to this cavity. Consequently, bacterial infections traveling up the vagina, uterine cavity, and uterine tubes can move into the peritoneal cavity and cause diseases such as pelvic inflammatory disease. Choice B is incorrect because it points to the round ligament. Choice C is incorrect because it points to the uterus cavity. Choice D is incorrect because it points to the vagina.

28. C: The fimbriae are found at the end of the fallopian tube and are the closest to the ovary. However, there is minimal contact between the ovaries and the fimbriae. Consequently, the ovary is also open to the peritoneal cavity, which can result in the lost eggs within the cavity. Infections can spread from the reproductive tract into the peritoneal cavity. Infections in the cavity can cause severe inflammation and lead to a type of pelvic inflammatory disease in which the uterine tubes close, thereby resulting in female infertility. Both Choices A and B are incorrect because the uterine tubes do not connect directly to the ovaries. Choice D is incorrect because the infundibulum and ovaries are not directly connected.

29. B: Label 2 represents the ampulla of ductus deferens. The ampulla is an enlarged and terminal section of the ductus deferens that acts as a reservoir for sperm. Choice A is incorrect because it represents the prostate. The prostate contributes to approximately 25 to 30 percent of the semen. Choice C is incorrect because it corresponds to the seminal vesical, an accessory gland that produces approximately 65 to 75 percent of the semen. Choice *D* is incorrect because it corresponds to the bulbourethral glands. These glands secrete a mucous fluid that makes up approximately 1 percent of the semen.

30. D: Unlike the male urethra, the female urethra is separated from the main reproductive tract. For example, in males, the male urethra carries both the sperm and urine toward the exterior of the body. The male urethra serves both the reproductive and urinary systems, and the female urethra serves only the urinary system. Choice *A* is incorrect because the testes and ovaries produce sex cells. Choice *B* is incorrect because both glands produce mucus that functions in lubrication. Choice *A* and Choice *C* are incorrect because the gonads are the sex organs and refer to the testes in males and ovaries in females.

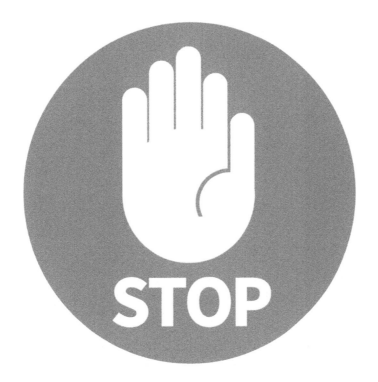

Free Exam Tips Videos/DVD

We have created a set of videos to better prepare you for your exam. We would like to give you access to these **videos** to show you our appreciation for choosing Exampedia. **They cover proven strategies that will teach you how to prepare for your exam and feel confident on test day.**

To receive your free videos, email us your thoughts, good or bad, about this book. Your feedback will help us improve our guides and better serve customers in the future.

Here are the steps:

   1. Email **freevideos@exampedia.org**

   2. Put **"Exam Tips"** in the subject line

Add the following information in the body of the email:

   3. **Book Title:** The title of this book.

   4. **Rating on a Scale of 1–5:** With 5 being the best, tell us what you would rate this book.

   5. **Feedback:** Give us some details about what you liked or didn't like.

Thanks again!

Made in the USA
Coppell, TX
16 March 2022